MCAT Chemistry and Organic Chemistry

Content Review

blueprint

2nd Edition Acknowledgments
Reviewers: Elizabeth Flagge and Mackenzie Perkins
Editors: Allison Chae, Patricia Eldredge PhD, Paul Forn, Michael Leung, Brian McGrew, Yizhu Sun, Michael Yao, and Maureen Yargeau PhD
Copywriters: Aislinn McCormack, Zoe Mikel-Stites, and Emily Soto
Cover Design: Becca Roth and Lona Ryan

Special thanks to all of the writers, editors, and reviewers involved in prior editions

Printed in the United States of America

First Printing, 2022

ISBN 978-1-944935-37-5

Blueprint Education Subsidiary Holdings LLC
6080 Center Drive
Suite 520
Los Angeles, CA 90045

Second Edition

This page left intentionally blank.

Group→1
↓Period

Period	1	2	3	4	5	6	7	8	9	10	11	12	13	14	15	16	17	18
1	1 H																	2 He
2	3 Li	4 Be											5 B	6 C	7 N	8 O	9 F	10 Ne
3	11 Na	12 Mg											13 Al	14 Si	15 P	16 S	17 Cl	18 Ar
4	19 K	20 Ca	21 Sc	22 Ti	23 V	24 Cr	25 Mn	26 Fe	27 Co	28 Ni	29 Cu	30 Zn	31 Ga	32 Ge	33 As	34 Se	35 Br	36 Kr
5	37 Rb	38 Sr	39 Y	40 Zr	41 Nb	42 Mo	43 Tc	44 Ru	45 Rh	46 Pd	47 Ag	48 Cd	49 In	50 Sn	51 Sb	52 Te	53 I	54 Xe
6	55 Cs	56 Ba	57 La *	72 Hf	73 Ta	74 W	75 Re	76 Os	77 Ir	78 Pt	79 Au	80 Hg	81 Tl	82 Pb	83 Bi	84 Po	85 At	86 Rn
7	87 Fr	88 Ra	89 Ac **	104 Rf	105 Db	106 Sg	107 Bh	108 Hs	109 Mt	110 Ds	111 Rg	112 Cn	113 Nh	114 Fl	115 Mc	116 Lv	117 Ts	118 Og

*	58 Ce	59 Pr	60 Nd	61 Pm	62 Sm	63 Eu	64 Gd	65 Tb	66 Dy	67 Ho	68 Er	69 Tm	70 Yb	71 Lu
**	90 Th	91 Pa	92 U	93 Np	94 Pu	95 Am	96 Cm	97 Bk	98 Cf	99 Es	100 Fm	101 Md	102 No	103 Lr

STOP! READ THIS FIRST!

Welcome and congratulations on taking this important step in your MCAT prep process!

The book you're holding is one of Blueprint's six MCAT review books, and contains concise content review with a specific focus on the science that you need for MCAT success. To get the most out of this book, we'd like to draw your attention to some distinctive aspects of our book set and their role in MCAT prep.

First and foremost, **books are not enough** for MCAT prep. Realistic practice is absolutely essential, and should include both MCAT-targeted practice questions and an ample number of full-length practice exams that simulate the MCAT itself.

Second, **our books reflect our experience**. Our book editing team is made up of a combination of people: they represent people who have been in your shoes and have excelled on the MCAT, people who are truly experts in the field of Chemistry, and people who are experienced tutors and instructors with a focus on MCAT prep (not to mention a few skilled copywriters and communicators to keep us on our toes!). Our books recognize that the MCAT is **primarily a test of thinking**—and more specifically, a test that reflects how the American Association of Medical Colleges encourages future physicians to think. The "MCAT Strategy" sidebars throughout the book call out specific points to be aware of as you study, and in general, our approach to presenting science is informed by how science is tested on the MCAT—that is, in a way that draws upon passages, builds connections across subject areas, and prioritizes an understanding of fundamental principles. In a nutshell, it's our hope that by studying with these books, you can benefit from our team's unparalleled MCAT expertise.

Third, after completing a chapter, we urge you to test your knowledge with all of the online practice materials that were included with your Blueprint course: our Learning Modules, Qbank, End of Chapter Quizzes, and of course our Practice Tests.

Best,

The Blueprint MCAT Team

This page left intentionally blank.

TABLE OF CONTENTS

This page left intentionally blank.

Atomic Structure and Periodic Trends

CHAPTER 1

0. Introduction

The study of matter is the foundation of all chemistry. Matter is any substance that occupies space and has mass. Atoms, for example, have matter and interact with other atoms in generally predictable, but still fascinating ways. In this chapter, we will discuss how atoms are characterized and the trends we can use to predict their behavior. These may seem like easy concepts you almost certainly learned in your college or even high school chemistry courses. For this reason, you might be tempted to rush through this chapter to save time to focus on more challenging concepts, such as electrochemistry or kinetics. However, MCAT chemistry—like the exam in general—requires a knowledge of basic concepts, and a thorough understanding of the material in this chapter will help you draw connections to later topics or even separate subjects.

1. Atomic Structure and Identity

Atoms are the building blocks of molecules. An element is a pure substance composed of like atoms, such as gold or helium. Molecules are made up of a group of one or more atoms; examples include O_2 and S_8. If molecules include atoms of different elements they form a **compound**, such as ammonia (NH_3) or carbon dioxide (CO_2). Atoms are composed of subatomic particles, which constitute a large and complex field of study in advanced physics. Have you ever heard of quarks? How about bosons or leptons? However, the MCAT, however, only focuses on three types of subatomic particles: protons, neutrons, and electrons.

Protons carry a positive charge and have a mass of 1 atomic mass unit (amu) or 1 dalton (Da), which is based on the mass of a particular form of carbon. The actual charge on a single proton is approximately 1.6×10^{-19} coulombs (C), a magnitude that is termed the elementary charge (e). However, while this value is used in some calculations, the designated charge of a proton is + 1. Protons reside in the nucleus, or central core of the atom. All atoms must contain at least one proton.

Neutrons derive their name from their neutral charge. The mass of one neutron is similar to that of one proton, so they, too, have a mass of 1 amu. Neutrons also reside in the atomic nucleus. As such, both neutrons and protons are called "nucleons."

MCAT STRATEGY >>>

As you build your chemistry foundation, you will become familiar with the fact that 1 amu corresponds to a mass of 1 g/mol. In this way, the number of protons and neutrons in an atom can be used to determine its molar mass. Don't worry, however; you are given a periodic table on the exam, where the mass of each element in amu is given.

Finally, **electrons** carry a negative charge and have a mass so small as to be considered insignificant in their contribution to the mass of an atom. The approximate charge on an electron is -1.6×10^{-19} C, which is the same magnitude but opposite in sign of the charge on a proton. An electron's charge is typically simplified as -1. Because the charge of a proton and an electron are opposite in sign, they are electrostatically attracted to one another. Electrons reside in an **electron cloud** around the nucleus (Figure 1). You may have seen descriptions of electrons as existing in regularly-spaced spherical orbits, or shells, surrounding the center of the atom. While this model is useful to conceptualize the atom, it is now outdated. The electron cloud model, proposed by Erwin Schrödinger, is more modern. This model states that we cannot know *exactly* where an electron is located at any given time, but it is more probable that it exists in certain regions of space, or clouds, rather than in others. The farther away an electron is from the nucleus, the higher its potential energy due to its electrostatic attraction to the nucleus. The electrons in the farthest from the nucleus are called valence electrons and play a vital role in chemical bonding, as you will see in Chapter 2. As shown below in Figure 1, atoms are mostly empty space, with the nucleus occupying a small area at the center. The diameter of a helium nucleus with 2 protons and 2 neutrons is about 1 femtometer (1 x 10^{-15} m) while the diameter of the full atom, including the electron cloud, is 100,000 fm.

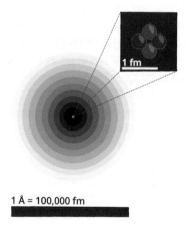

1 fm

1 Å = 100,000 fm

Figure 1. Atomic structure of helium

MCAT STRATEGY >>>

Don't get too caught up in high-level chemical theories, as fascinating as they are. The MCAT is not designed to quiz you on the history of chemistry, and it similarly is usually not trying to trick you on the minute points of theoretical chemistry. Instead, focus on the basics: what are protons and electrons, and how do they affect how an atom behaves?

Now that we are familiar with subatomic particles, let's think about how this information can be used to determine the unique identity of any given atom. The atoms of each element are associated with a certain number of protons, termed the **atomic number** (Z). The atomic number gives each element its unique identity. For example, every nitrogen atom (Z = 7) contains 7 protons. If an atom contains more or fewer than 7 protons, it cannot possibly be a nitrogen atom.

In contrast, the **mass number** (A) of an atom is the total number of neutrons and protons in the nucleus. Recall that the mass contributed by electrons is negligible, so they are excluded in this calculation. Atomic number and mass number are usually represented as shown in Figure 2.

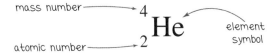

Figure 2. The mass and atomic number of helium (He)

While no two atoms of the same element can have different numbers of protons, they certainly can vary in their number of neutrons. Atoms of the same element that have different numbers of neutrons are called **isotopes**. For example, carbon-12 and carbon-13 are isotopes: these possess 6 protons plus 6 and 7 neutrons, respectively. In fact, an amu is defined as 1/12 the mass of an atom of carbon-12 (1 amu = 1.7 x 10^{-24} g). Even hydrogen has several isotopes. As you may know, hydrogen is the lightest element; it contains only a single proton. The form of hydrogen with which we are most familiar is protium (^{1}H), which contains no neutrons and thus has a mass number of 1. Deuterium (^{2}H, or D) is a hydrogen isotope with one proton and one neutron, and tritium (^{3}H) contains one proton and two neutrons. Deuterium in particular may appear on the MCAT for the purpose of labeling hydrogens and tracking their movement through the course of an organic reaction; it will behave similarly to a regular protium atom.

Two concepts related to mass number are atomic mass, often referred to as atomic weight, and molar mass, or molecular weight. The mass of an individual atom of an element is an extremely small number, so it is measured in amu. For a specific isotope of an element, the mass of a single atom is equal to its mass number. For example, the mass of a carbon-12 atom is 12 amu. Most elements exist naturally as a mixture of different isotopes. The periodic table shows the mass of each element given as the weighted average of all its naturally occurring isotopes. For example, carbon exists naturally as carbon-12 (99% abundant), carbon-13 (1% abundant), and carbon 14 (~10^{-10}% abundant), so the atomic mass of carbon is 12.01 amu, which is closest to the mass of the more abundant isotope, carbon-12.

> **>> CONNECTIONS <<**
>
> Chapter 10 of Physics

Because most measurements are not practical on the scale of individual atoms, the mole is a common unit used by chemists. One mole is defined as the number of atoms contained in 12 grams of carbon-12, and has the value of a mole 6.022 x 10^{23}, called Avogadro's number. The mass in grams of one mole of atoms of any element is equal in number to the mass of one atom of that element in amu. For example, one mole of carbon atoms would have a molar mass equal to 12.01 g, since one carbon atom has a mass of 12.01 amu.

Neutral atoms have an equal number of protons and electrons, but they can gain or lose electrons to become **ions**, which carry a net charge. The two main types of ions are **cations**, which carry a net positive charge, and **anions**, which carry a net negative charge. For example, a calcium (Ca) atom that contains 20 protons and 20 electrons is considered neutral. By losing two electrons, calcium will become a cation with a charge of + 2, which is expressed as Ca^{2+}.

We can determine a charge by comparing the numbers of protons and electrons. If an atom contains nine protons, it must be fluorine (F), the element with atomic number 9 in the periodic table. A neutral fluorine atom also has 9 electrons, but what if it has 10 electrons? In this case, the overall charge on the atom is (+ 9) + (−10) = −1, which corresponds to a fluoride ion. In general, when you see negative species (anions), you should think "electron-rich," and when you see positive species (cations), you should think "electron-deficient" or "proton-rich."

Monoatomic ions follow a few simple nomenclature rules. Cations are called by the name of their original atom. For instance, a sodium ion is Na⁺. If there is more than one ionic form of an element, the positive charge can be represented by Roman numerals. This is common for metals such as iron, which can form both +2 and +3 ions.

Simple anions take the root name of the parent element with the suffix *-ide*.

Fe^{2+}	Iron (II)	Ferrous ion
Fe^{3+}	Iron (III)	Ferric ion
H^-	Hydride	O^{2-} Oxide

Polyatomic ions are ions that contain multiple atoms that are connected by bonds. We'll focus here on oxyanions, polyatomic anions that contain oxygen and that are common in biological systems. Oxyanions use the suffix *-ite* and *-ate* for compounds with fewer and greater numbers of oxygen atoms, respectively. The prefix *hypo-* is added for oxyanions with one fewer oxygen than *-ite* ions, and *per-* is added for ions with one more oxygen than *-ate* ions.

		ClO^-	Hypochlorite
NO_2^-	Nitrite	ClO_2^-	Chlorite
NO_3^-	Nitrate	ClO_3^-	Chlorate
		ClO_4^-	Perchlorate

If the polyatomic anion includes a hydrogen (H^+) ion, *hydrogen* or *dihydrogen* is added to the name of the parent anion.

CO_3^{2-}	Carbonate	HCO_3^-	Hydrogen carbonate
PO_4^{3-}	Phosphate	$H_2PO_4^-$	Dihydrogen phosphate

2. The Bohr Model

In 1913 Niels Bohr and Ernest Rutherford introduced their revolutionary model of the atom, building on Rutherford's earlier work. The **Bohr model** described the electronic structure of the hydrogen atom; this is a useful, albeit simplified, model, of the structure of the atom.

In the Bohr model, electrons orbit the nucleus in spherical shells that vary in their distance from the nucleus. Positively-charged protons in the nucleus exert an attractive force on electrons in constant motion within their orbit. As you can imagine, the electrons closest to the nucleus experience the greatest attractive force, and thus the closer an electron is to the nucleus (and the smaller the shell's radius), the greater its stability and the lower its energy. However, an electron located farther from the nucleus will have a higher potential energy and will be less stable.

Each shell is numbered by its proximity to the nucleus (n = 1, 2, 3...) and is associated with a unique energy level. An electron in its lowest energy level is closest to the nucleus and is said to be in its **ground state**. For hydrogen (with only a single electron) this is n = 1, but for larger atoms with multiple electrons, the ground state is not necessarily n = 1.

If a ground-state electron absorbs energy equal to the difference in energy between a higher energy level and the energy of the ground state, it can be promoted to the higher-energy orbit. The electron is no longer in the ground state, but rather is now in an excited state. An electron in an excited state can move to a lower energy level by emitting a photon of energy that corresponds exactly to the difference in energy between the two orbits. A photon is a subatomic particle that makes up light. Since the energy gaps between orbits have specific energy values, the energy of the emitted photons are "quantized," meaning that they can only contain certain discrete amounts of energy. In the reverse process, an electron is said to relax, or decay, if it is in an excited state and moves to a lower energy level. A photon is emitted with exactly the same energy required for promotion of the electron between the two orbits.

Energy is emitted and absorbed in the form of **electromagnetic radiation**, which is radiation that includes both electric and magnetic fields. The electromagnetic spectrum includes a continuum of electromagnetic radiation, which includes visible light, radio waves, gamma rays, X-rays, and more.

> > **CONNECTIONS** < <

Chapter 9 of Physics

The many forms of electromagnetic radiation differ in their energies, frequencies, and wavelengths. The energy of electromagnetic radiation is given by Equation 1, which was proposed by the physicist Max Planck.

Equation 1.
$$E = hf$$

Here, h is **Planck's constant** (approximately 6.63×10^{-34} J·s) and f is the frequency of the light. Since the frequency of a wave (f) is equal to the speed of light (c, or 3.00×10^8 m/s in a vacuum) divided by its wavelength (λ), the energy of a photon can also be expressed as the following (Equation 2).

Equation 2.
$$E = hf = \frac{hc}{\lambda}$$

Because energy is absorbed or released in quanta, the absorption or emission of electromagnetic radiation results in a characteristic atomic **absorption spectrum** and atomic **emission spectrum** that are unique for each element. Every element has both an absorption spectrum and an emission spectrum.

Figure 3. The atomic emission spectrum of iron (Fe)

These spectra contain distinct lines that represent quantized energy levels. Absorption lines are dark because they correspond to the absorption of energy, and emission lines are bright because photons of energy is emitted. Equations 3 and 4 below show how the energy levels of an electron can be related to the energy absorbed or emitted during an electron transition from one energy level to another. Equation 3 is the Rydberg formula, in which R_H is the Rydberg constant, n_i is the initial electron energy level, and n_f is the final electron energy level. Substituting the Rydberg formula into Equation 2, the energy of the electron, gives Equation 4, where ΔE is the energy change in Joules (kg m^2/s^2). ΔE will be negative for electron transitions from higher to lower energy levels, where energy is emitted, and positive for electron transitions from lower to higher energy levels, where energy is absorbed.

Equation 3.

$$\frac{1}{\lambda} = R_H \left(\frac{1}{n_i^2} - \frac{1}{n_f^2} \right)$$

Equation 4.

$$\Delta E = 2.18 \times 10^{-18}\,\text{J} \left(\frac{1}{n_i^2} - \frac{1}{n_f^2} \right)$$

MCAT STRATEGY >>>

The MCAT test-makers will generally provide you with the values of constants in chemistry and physics formulas. However, be certain to memorize the value of the speed of light in a vacuum (3.00×10^8 m/s), as this is one they expect you to know.

Let's try an example: say you are asked to calculate the energy of the emitted photon when an electron is promoted from the $n = 2$ to the $n = 4$ energy level. A photon of energy is absorbed as the electron moves from a lower energy orbit to a higher one. Substituting into our equation with $n_i = 2$ and $n_f = 4$, we obtain the energy of the photon:

$$\Delta E = 2.18 \times 10^{-18}\,\text{J} \left(\frac{1}{n_i^2} - \frac{1}{n_f^2} \right)$$

$$= 2.18 \times 10^{-18}\,\text{J} \left(\frac{1}{2^2} - \frac{1}{4^2} \right)$$

$$= 4.09 \times 10^{-19}\,\text{J}$$

Notice that a $+\Delta E$ means that energy is absorbed, and a $-\Delta E$ means energy is released.

3. Quantum Numbers and Electron Configuration

While the Bohr model of the atom provided us with an enormously useful foundation to build upon, a later description of atomic structure determined that we cannot be fully certain where an electron is and how it is behaving at a certain point in time. Specifically, the **Heisenberg uncertainty principle** posits that it is impossible to accurately know *both* the exact position and the momentum of a given electron at the same time.

The quantum model describes electrons as existing in **orbitals**, or regions of space in which an electron is likely to be located. Each electron in an atom is associated with four quantum numbers that describe its position, the shape of its orbital, its orientation, and its angular momentum, and can be thought of as an electron's address in space. In fact, the Pauli exclusion principle states that no two electrons in a given atom can have the exact same values for all four quantum numbers.

The first quantum number is the **principal quantum number**, or n and corresponds to the Bohr radii. This denotes the energy level of the electron. The higher the principal quantum number (e.g., $n = 2$ rather than $n = 1$) the greater the energy, and the greater the distance from the nucleus. The periodic table is arranged in rows corresponding to increasing values of n. Sodium (Na), for example, is in the third period, or row. This element has a principal quantum number of $n = 3$.

The **azimuthal**, or **angular momentum**, **quantum number** (l) describes the shape of an orbital's subshell. Each type of subshell has its own characteristic orbital shape(s); s orbitals are spherical, p orbitals are dumbbell-shaped, and d and f orbitals have shapes that are more complex. Notice that there is one s orbital, there are 3 p orbitals, 5 d orbitals, and 7 f orbitals.

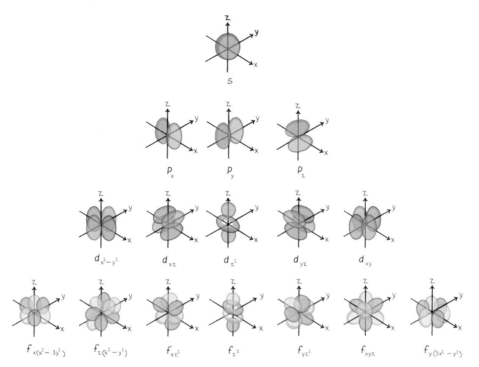

Figure 4. Shapes of the orbitals of different subshells. From top to bottom: *s, p, d, f.* Note that the *p, d,* and *f* subshells have multiple possible shapes

Next, the **magnetic quantum number** (m_l) describes the spatial orientation of the orbital region of space with respect to an applied magnetic field.

Finally, the **spin quantum number** (m_s) describes the spin orientation of the electron in an external magnetic field. The two possible spin orientations are $m_s = +\frac{1}{2}$ (up) and $m_s = -\frac{1}{2}$ (down), so each orbital can contain a maximum of two electrons (one spin up and one spin down). Two electrons in the same orbital are said to be spin paired and must have opposite spins. Because of the spin orientations, notice that an s orbital can contain a maximum of two electrons, *p* orbitals a maximum of 6 electrons, *d* orbitals 10 electrons, and *f* orbitals 14 electrons.

The **electron configuration** of an atom describes the arrangement of electrons about the nucleus. The notation consists of a series of symbols containing a number, a letter, and a superscript. For example, the lowest-energy subshell is 1*s*; if this subshell were filled with two electrons, its corresponding term in the electron configuration would be $1s^2$, with the superscript denoting the number of electrons in that subshell. A 3*d* subshell that contains eight electrons would be denoted as $3d^8$, and so on. According to the Aufbau principle, electrons fill lower-energy orbitals first to create the most stable electron configuration. Electrons fill orbitals in order of increasing energy level, as depicted in Figure 6.

MCAT STRATEGY >>>

We're seeing quite a few similar terms here: shell, subshell, orbital, etc. While the MCAT is generally not designed to trick you, reading questions very carefully is absolutely essential.

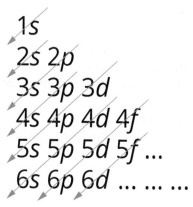

Figure 6. Order of orbital filling. Begin with 1s and follow each consecutive arrow from tail to tip (1*s*, then 2*s*, 2*p*, 3*s*, 3*p*, etc.)

To describe the electron configuration of a neutral chlorine (Cl) atom, we begin by finding the total number of electrons. A neutral Cl atom has 17 protons, and thus the neutral atom must have 17 electrons (its atomic number is 17). We know that each s subshell can hold 2 electrons, and each p subshell can hold 6 electrons. Electrons will fill orbitals from lower to higher energy levels, filling low-energy orbitals first. The first two electrons will fill the 1s subshell, the next two will fill the 2s subshell, and so forth, until all 17 electrons have been accounted for. This gives us an electron configuration of $1s^2 2s^2 2p^6 3s^2 3p^5$, which is shown in Figure 7 using a common form of arrow notation for spin up and spin down.

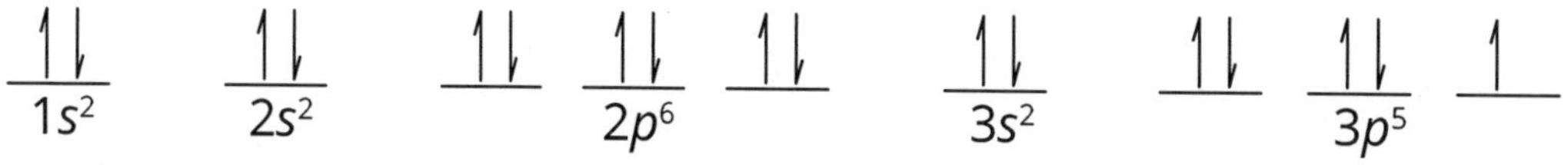

$$\underset{1s^2}{\uparrow\downarrow} \qquad \underset{2s^2}{\uparrow\downarrow} \qquad \underset{2p^6}{\uparrow\downarrow \quad \uparrow\downarrow \quad \uparrow\downarrow} \qquad \underset{3s^2}{\uparrow\downarrow} \qquad \underset{3p^5}{\uparrow\downarrow \quad \uparrow\downarrow \quad \uparrow}$$

Figure 7. The electron configuration of a neutral chlorine atom

Another important principle to remember when dealing with electron configuration is **Hund's rule**. Recall that each orbital can hold up to two paired electrons with opposite spin. Like charges repel, so electrons will occupy orbitals with the lowest energy configuration first. That is, they will align with the magnetic field, occupying orbitals in a spin up configuration, before they are forced to spin pair with one aligned against the magnetic field.

We can easily illustrate Hund's rule with an example. A neutral nitrogen atom has seven electrons. The first four of these electrons fill the 1*s* and 2*s* orbitals. For the next three, note the diagram below; the electrons occupy the orbitals spin up. We should never see two paired electrons in the same orbital until all orbitals are half-filled.

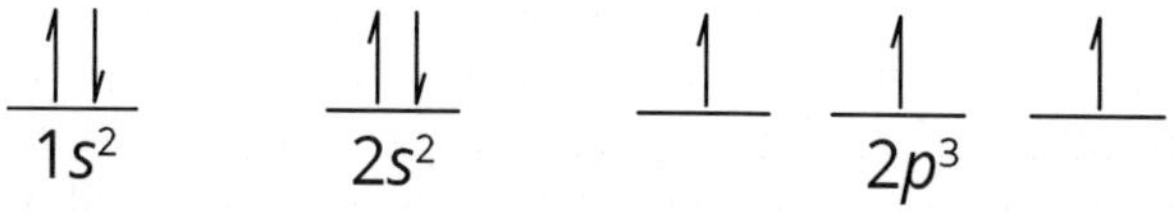

$$\underset{1s^2}{\uparrow\downarrow} \qquad \underset{2s^2}{\uparrow\downarrow} \qquad \underset{2p^3}{\uparrow \quad \uparrow \quad \uparrow}$$

Figure 8. The electron configuration of neutral nitrogen

A direct method for determining the electron configuration of an atom is to divide the periodic table into blocks (Figure 9). The **s-block** consists of the first two columns (or groups) on the left (along with helium), while the **p-block** includes the last six groups on the right. The **d-block** contains transition metals, and the **f-block** contains the lanthanide and actinide series, which are usually shown below the s, p, and d blocks of a periodic table. Columns on the periodic table are called Groups and rows across are called periods. Lithium is in Group 1 (it has a single s electron), period 2 of the periodic table. Therefore, its valence shell is n = 2, and its valence electron configuration is $2s^1$. Lithium has three electrons in its neutral state, so its complete electron configuration is $1s^2 2s^1$. Nitrogen is also in period 2, but in group 15, placing it in the p block. Therefore its valence shell is n = 2; it has a full s subshell, $2s^2$, and 3 p electrons, $2p^3$. This is confirmed by the full electron configuration for nitrogen shown in Figure 8.

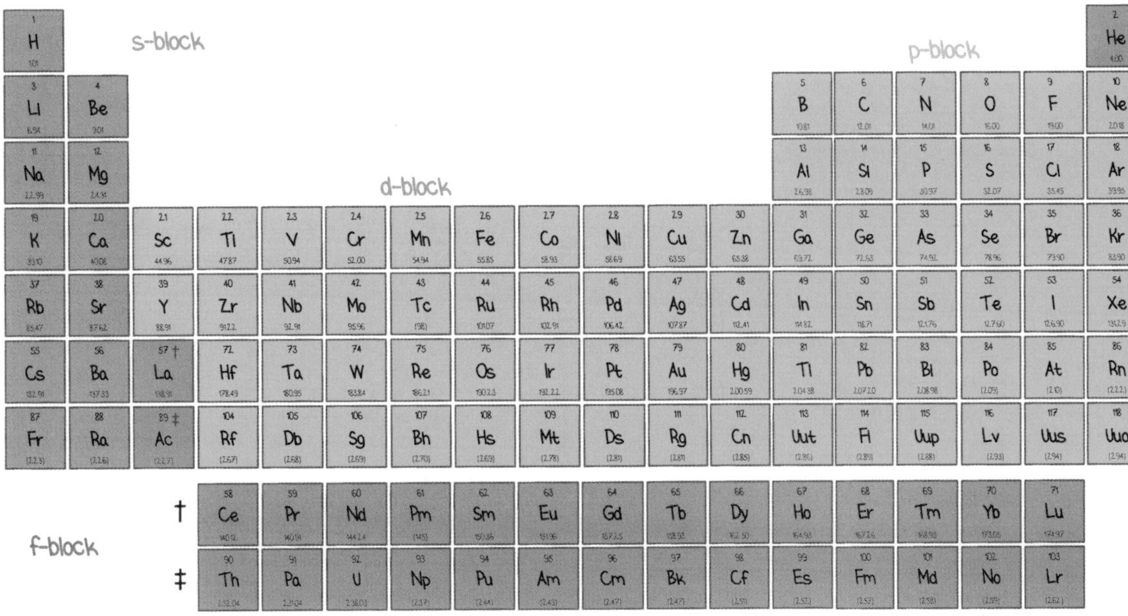

Figure 9. Element blocks of the periodic table

Electrons fill the valence shell from left to right in the periodic table. The elements of groups 18, the noble gases, have filled valence shells. For a given atom, the electron configuration can be abbreviated by placing the noble gas from the prior row in brackets to represent the electron configuration of its inner shell electrons. The abbreviated electron configuration of potassium, then, is [Ar] $4s^1$. Oxygen is found in the p-block of the second period of the periodic table, so its abbreviated electron configuration is [He] $2s^2 2p^4$.

> **MCAT STRATEGY >>>**
>
> Valence electrons play a key role in chemical bonding. This will be discussed in much more depth in Chapter 2 of this book; for now, just know that they are particularly important.

From the Aufbau principle (Figure 6), the d block fills as *n*-1 and the f block as *n*-2. Thus, for example, Fe has a valence electron configuration of [Ar]$4s^2 3d^6$ and Cd of [Kr]$4d^{10} 5s^2$.

What if we want to determine the electron configuration of an ion? Remember, negative ions (anions) have an excess of electrons, while positive ions, or cations, are electron-deficient. For the Ca^{2+} ion, first write out the configuration of neutral Ca: $1s^2 2s^2 2p^6 3s^2 3p^6 4s^2$. Now, since Ca^{2+} has a +2 charge, we must remove two electrons. We remove them from the highest-energy subshell, which is 4s, as it has the highest principal quantum number. This leaves us with $1s^2 2s^2 2p^6 3s^2 3p^6$, which, in its abbreviated form, is [Ar].

We have already seen from the Aufbau principle that orbitals are filled from lowest energy to highest energy, so the $4s$ subshell fills before the $3d$ subshell. Once the d orbitals begin to fill, though, the $4s$ subshell is higher in energy than the $3d$. This means that when forming cations, the $4s$ electrons are lost first. This is important to remember for the MCAT: Electrons populate the valence s orbital before the d orbital, but electrons are *removed* from the valence s orbital first. Thus, while Fe has an electron configuration of $[Ar]4s^2\,3d^6$, Fe^2+ is $[Ar]3d^6$.

Finally, it can be very helpful to ask yourself one question whenever you learn a new chemistry concept: *do any exceptions exist*? When describing electron configurations the answer is "yes." Half-filled subshells, which minimize electron-electron repulsions, and fully-filled subshells, with all electrons spin paired, are more stable than subshells filled with some other number of electrons. For a p subshell, then, it is energetically favorable to contain either three or six electrons; similarly, a d subshell will be especially stable if it contains either five or ten electrons.

The exceptions to understand for the MCAT are the transition metals in the same groups as chromium (Cr) and copper (Cu). Specifically, these constitute exceptions to the Aufbau principle. We would expect the electron configuration of chromium to be $[Ar]\,4s^2 3d^4$. However, a more energetically stable configuration is obtained if an s electron is promoted to the d orbital. This gives two half-filled orbitals and is a more stable arrangement. The electron configuration of chromium is thus $[Ar]\,4s^1 3d^5$. Similarly, we might use the Aufbau principle to predict the electron configuration of copper as $[Ar]\,4s^2 3d^9$. In reality, however, it is $[Ar]\,4s^1 3d^{10}$ to achieve a half filled and filled subshell. Remember these exceptions on Test Day!

4. Structure of the Periodic Table

The **periodic table**, the initial version of which was proposed by Dmitri Mendeleev in 1869, is an elegant system for organizing an enormous amount of information. The modern periodic table arranges the known chemical elements by atomic number, although Mendeleev sorted his table according to atomic weight. Mendeleev's table positioned elements with similar properties in the same column, leaving some gaps where no known elements yet existed. Interestingly, Mendeleev was able to use his table to predict information about these then-unknown elements, and when they were subsequently discovered, his predictions largely held true. This is but one example of the tremendous utility of the periodic table.

The rows of the periodic table are called periods, while the columns are called groups or families. Across a period, the number of valence electrons increases until the valence shell is full. For example, in the second period, lithium has one valence electron, beryllium has two, boron has three, carbon has four, and so on until neon, which has a full valence shell of 8 electrons. Since elements belonging to the same group (or column) have the same number of valence electrons, they tend to share physical and chemical properties. Atoms may donate or gain electrons to obtain a full valence shell, which confers stability.

Groups are numbered from 1 to 18, without distinguishing the transition metals separately, as indicated in older versions of the periodic table.

The elements B, Si, Ge, As, Sb, Te, and At lie along a diagonal line and are known as semimetals, also called metalloids. They separate metals from nonmetals and have many of the characteristics of both. Metals lie to the left of the metals and nonmetals lie to the right. Group 1 elements are commonly referred to as **alkali metals**. Metals are good electrical conductors and are typically solid under standard conditions, although exceptions such as mercury exist. They are shiny, or lustrous, and they exhibit ductility, or the property of being easily stretched into wires. They are opaque, rather than transparent, and they can be made to form other shapes or sheets, a property termed malleability. Some—but not all—metals have multiple oxidation states, which will be discussed further in Chapter 8 of this book. All alkali metals share these metallic properties with the exception of hydrogen (H), which is not an alkali metal at all but a nonmetal and a gas at room temperature. The lone valence electron (ns^1) makes alkali metals highly reactive, as they will readily donate their valence electron to other atoms to form cations with a + 1 charge, giving them the valence electron configuration of a noble gas. In fact, some alkali metals, in particular sodium and potassium, are so reactive that they explode in water if exposed to it in their solid metal forms.

Group 2 elements, or **alkaline earth metals**, have a metallic character. Alkaline earth metals have two valence electrons (ns^2), which they will donate to form +2 cations. Again, this gives them the valence electron configuration of a noble gas. In their solid states they are reactive, a property they share with alkali metals.

The elements in groups 3-12 are the **transition metals**. Transition metals include some of our most precious elements, such as gold (Au) and platinum (Pt), which are valued for their luster and other unique properties. Transition elements are hard, durable metals that readily conduct electricity, and they often take on vivid colors due to electronic transitions between d orbitals. The number of electrons a transition metal can lose varies, so most have multiple oxidation states. For example, iron (Fe) is most commonly found with oxidation numbers of +2 or +3.

Now that we have discussed the alkali metals, alkaline earth metals, and transition metals, we will begin to describe elements that are *not* metallic in nature. In particular, the nonmetals have many traits that are opposite those of metals. **Nonmetals** are not lustrous (shiny); as examples, consider oxygen gas or solid carbon. Nonmetals are also poor electrical conductors. The **semimetals**, or **metalloids**, share traits of both metals and nonmetals. The metalloids you are most likely to see on the MCAT are boron and silicon, a major component of Earth's crust. Metalloids vary in their characteristics, but in general, they are brittle, are poor to decent electrical conductors, and tend to act like nonmetals in chemical reactions, although even this can vary.

Group 13 elements include boron (B) and aluminum (Al). Boron is a semimetal, while the rest of the elements in this group are categorized as metals. Some form + 3 cations, as they have three valence electrons. By losing them they achieve a noble gas configuration.

Group 14 elements belong to the **carbon family**. These elements also have properties of both metals and nonmetals and are capable of forming oxides (CO_2, SiO_2, etc.). The study of organic chemistry can be thought of as the study of carbon-containing compounds, so pay close attention whenever you see carbon in your MCAT prep! Group 14 elements have four valence electrons. Carbon can take many forms, including that of diamond (a very hard solid), although carbon in its standard state exists as a gray mineral termed graphite. Next, Group 15 elements belong to the

MCAT STRATEGY >>>

The individual characteristics of each element can get overwhelming, so note that you do *not* need to memorize most of them. Instead, pay special attention to those elements that play a biologically relevant role.

>>CONNECTIONS<<

Chapter 7 of Chemistry

nitrogen family. These elements have five valence electrons and display properties of both metals and nonmetals.

Group 16 elements are the **chalcogens**, which include oxygen (O) and sulfur (S). Chalcogens have mostly non-metallic characteristics. Their nearly filled valence shell (ns^2np^4) causes them to react with other atoms to gain two electrons, forming −2 anions and achieving a noble gas configuration. These elements, especially oxygen, are enormously important components of organic molecules, so you will encounter them regularly in biochemistry, biology, and of course chemistry.

Group 17 elements are called **halogens**, which are reactive species with a nearly-filled valence shell (ns^2np^5). A halogen atom contains seven valence electrons, so it will readily accept one electron from an alkali metal or other species to form an anion with a -1 charge and a noble gas configuration. The halogens include fluorine (F) and chlorine (Cl), which exist as diatomic gases (F_2, and Cl_2), bromine (Br), which exists as a diatomic liquid (Br_2), and iodine (I), which exists as a diatomic solid (I_2), at room temperature. Note that the halogens are nonmetals.

Finally, Group 18 elements are the inert or **noble gases**. Noble gases have a non-metallic character and are very unreactive due to their filled valence shell. As you may have guessed from the term "gas," these elements have low boiling points, causing them to exist in the gaseous state under standard conditions (Contrast this with most metals and even nonmetals, such as carbon, which exist in the solid form at room temperature).

5. Periodic Trends

We've now discussed the organization of the periodic table, but this is only a small amount of the information the table gives us. Let's say we want to compare an alkali metal (located on the far left of the table) with a chalcogen (found in the same group as oxygen). Can we predict at least some relationships between the two, even without having memorized the specific parameters of these groups? Of course we can! This is where **periodic trends** come into play.

The periodic trends you should be familiar with for the MCAT are atomic/ionic radius, electronegativity, electron affinity, and ionization energy. Luckily, these four trends follow an overarching pattern. Ask yourself this: why do chemists spend so much time dwelling on the positioning of electrons? Electrons determine the nature of the atom's behavior. While each atom has a nuclear charge denoted as Z, the actual attractive force of the positively-charged nucleus on the atom's valence electrons is termed the **effective nuclear charge (Z_{eff})**. Because inner electrons shield outer electrons from the nucleus, the electrostatic attraction between the nucleus and the outer electrons decreases. This is known as the shielding effect. Valence electrons shield each other poorly, so the shielding effect is lower across a row. Down a group, however, the shielding effect is significant. Consider, for example, what it's like to sit in the back row of theater. Your experience with the performers on stage will be significantly diminished compared to those in the front row. Only hydrogen experiences no shielding effect, so $Z = Z_{eff}$. For all other elements, $Z_{eff} < Z$. As the number of protons in the nucleus and the number of electrons increases from left to right across a period, the electrostatic force increases, so Z_{eff} also increases. However, moving down a group, as the principal quantum number increases, more layers of core electrons shield the valence electrons from the positive nuclear charge. Thus, Z_{eff} decreases as one moves down a group.

Periodic trends in Z_{eff} help explain other trends on the periodic table. **Atomic size**, or **radius**, decreases from left to right across a period as more protons and electrons are added (Recall that valence electrons shield each other poorly).

In contrast, atomic radius increases down a column as *n* increases and shielding effects increase. Thus, atoms with the largest radii are found nearest the bottom left of the periodic table.

A concept that relates closely to atomic radius is ***ionic* radius**, or the radius of a charged species (for example, F^-). Because electron-electron repulsions are reduced when an electron is removed from a valence shell, and the remaining valence electrons experience a greater average positive charge, *cations* (positive ions) tend to have smaller ionic radii than the atomic radii of the corresponding neutral atom. On the other hand, for *anions* (negative ions), the ionic radius is typically larger than the corresponding atomic radius. Additional valence electrons increase electrostatic repulsions, and the average nuclear attractive force decreases, so the radius of an anion is larger than that of the neutral atom. Thus, in order of increasing radius, $Na^+ < Na < Na^-$.

Ionization energy (IE) is the energy required to remove one valence electron from a neutral atom in the gaseous state. Ionization energy is positive, since it requires an input of energy to remove an electron from the nucleus. As you might imagine, the first ionization energy (the energy required to remove one electron from a neutral species) is always smaller than the second ionization energy (the energy required to remove a second electron), and so on, because additional electrons are being removed from increasingly positively charged species. Ionization energy is directly related to Z_{eff}, as atoms with a greater Z_{eff} require more energy to remove electrons that are more tightly held. Thus, in general, IE increases as one moves up and to the right along the periodic table. One important point, however, is that this trend does not hold true perfectly. For example, one might assume that oxygen would have a higher first IE than nitrogen, as oxygen is found to the right of nitrogen in the second period. In reality, nitrogen has the higher first IE of the two. Remember what you have learned about electron configuration; nitrogen has a half-filled $2p$ subshell, which is particularly stable because it has no paired electrons. It is thus more difficult to remove a valence electron from nitrogen than from oxygen, which has an additional $2p$ electron. In fact, there is a significant increase in IE when removing an electron from a half-filled or filled subshell. Thinking about relationships between seemingly-distinct general chemistry concepts will be immensely helpful on the MCAT!

> **MCAT STRATEGY >>>**
>
> It can be easier to retain information about chemistry concepts if you pair each concept with an example. Here, we could say that Mg^{2+} has a smaller radius than Mg (s), while Cl^- has a larger radius than uncharged Cl.

Our next periodic trend is **electron affinity** (EA). This quantity denotes the amount of energy released when an electron is *added* to an atom. Atoms that can more readily accept an electron, such as halogens, have higher electron affinities. For most species, the addition of an electron is an exothermic process, meaning that energy is released (-EA). However, if energy must be added to the system to produce an anion, the electron affinity is positive (+EA). For example, the halogens have very negative electron affinities (they readily accept an electron), whereas Be has a positive EA (gaining an electron is destabilizing). Like ionization energy, electron affinity is directly related to Z_{eff}, because atoms with a more positive nuclear charge have a greater affinity for electrons. This causes atoms closer to the top right of the periodic table to have higher electron affinity values. A key exception to this trend is the noble gases, which, in spite of their position on the far right of the table, have near-zero electron affinities as they already possess full valence shells.

> **>>CONNECTIONS<<**
>
> Chapter 4 of Chemistry

Finally, **electronegativity** refers to the tendency of an atom to attract electrons that are shared in a chemical bond. Since atoms with high electron affinities will naturally attract electrons more strongly, electronegativity is also directly related to Z_{eff} (In fact, students often confuse electronegativity with electron affinity, but the only difference to know for the MCAT is that electronegativity directly relates to behavior *within a chemical bond*). Electronegativity increases from left to right along a period as radii decrease, and decreases as one moves down a group from an increase in *n* and shielding effects, which cause electrons to have a lower electrostatic attraction to the nucleus. An easy way to remember this trend is to commit to memory that fluorine, near the top right of the table, is the most electronegative element. Figure 10 summarizes these trends; be sure to understand them as well as memorize them if you want to ensure that your chemistry foundation is strong for the coming chapters!

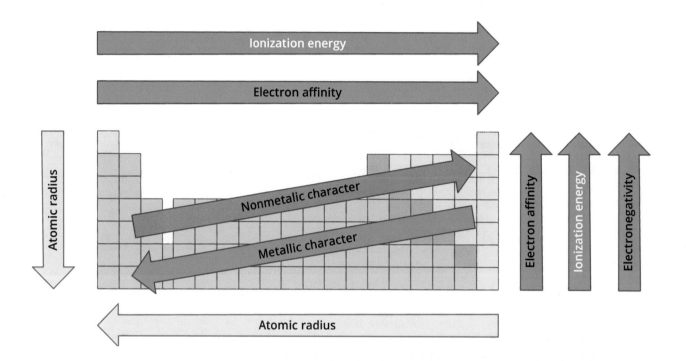

Figure 10. Periodic trends

6. Must-Knows

> All matter is composed of atoms, which in turn are composed of subatomic particles.
>   — Protons have a designated charge of +1 and a mass of 1 amu.
>   — Neutrons are uncharged and have a mass of approximately 1 amu. Both protons and neutrons are found in the nucleus. Together they are called nucleons.
>   — Electrons are nearly massless and have a designated charge of −1.
> Atomic number (Z): number of protons in an atom, determines chemical identity.
> Mass number (A): total number of protons and neutrons in the nucleus.
> Isotope: same number of protons, different number of neutrons (different mass number).
> Cations are positively charged ions, while anions are negatively charged ions.
> Bohr model of the hydrogen atom: electrons orbit the nucleus in spherical shells.
>   — When energy is absorbed, electrons are promoted to higher energy levels, farther from the nucleus.
>   — When energy is released/emitted, electrons decay from higher to lower energy levels, closer to the nucleus.
> Four quantum numbers describe the region of space occupied by each electron in an atom.
>   — n = principal quantum number; corresponds to the orbital radius.
>   — l = azimuthal quantum number; denotes shape and subshell identity (s, p, d, or f).
>   — m_l = magnetic quantum number; denotes the orientation of an orbital within a subshell.
>   — m_s = describes electron spin (+½ or −½).
> Pauli exclusion principle: no two electrons in the same atom can have the same set of four quantum numbers.
> Aufbau principle: lower energy orbitals fill first.
>   — Watch out for exceptions: Cr, Cu, and other elements in their groups.
> Hund's rule: within a subshell, each orbital will fill with one electron before they spin pair.
> Periodic table: periods = rows, groups = columns (elements in same group often share properties).
> Periodic trends:
>   — Atomic radius increases moving down and to the left along the table.
>   — Ionization energy, electron affinity, and electronegativity increase moving up and to the right.

End of Chapter Practice

The best MCAT practice is realistic, with a focus on identifying steps for further improvement. For those reasons, we recommend completing practice questions in an online setting that simulates the real MCAT interface, and taking advantage of advanced analytic features to help you determine how best to move forward in your MCAT study journey.

With that in mind, online end-of-chapter questions for Biology, Biochemistry, Chemistry + Organic Chemistry, Physics, and Psychology/Sociology are available through your Blueprint MCAT account.

As a further supplement, given the importance of active learning for effective studying, we also suggest that you consult the Must-Knows as a basis for creating a study sheet, in which you list out key terms and test your ability to briefly summarize them.

This page left intentionally blank.

This page left intentionally blank.

Bonding, Molecules, and Intermolecular Forces

0. Introduction

If atoms are the building blocks of molecules, chemical bonds are the glue that holds molecules together. The molecules in your own body contain countless types of bonds, which are broken and re-formed in very specific ways to keep your physiological functions intact. Moreover, many more interactions take place other than those involving chemical bonds, such as the interactions between distinct molecules in close physical proximity. In this chapter, we will discuss molecules in general, then cover intra- and intermolecular attractions. This portion of the book also includes some topics that you may remember from your early undergraduate years, such as formal charge, VSEPR theory, and molecular geometry.

1. Molecules

As mentioned in Chapter 1, a **molecule** consists of multiple atoms that are either like or unlike and are bonded together. When atoms combine to form a molecule, the masses of the individual atoms combine to form the molecular weight of the overall species. For example, the molecular weight of water (H_2O) is the sum of the masses of two moles of hydrogen atoms and one mole of oxygen atoms: 1 g/mol + 1 g/mol + 16 g/mol = 18 g/mol.

A molecule is held together by chemical bonds, but what, exactly, *is* a bond? Before we can answer this question, we must outline some fundamental concepts that were alluded to in Chapter 1. First, the electrons in an element's outermost shell are termed **valence electrons**, and it is

> **MCAT STRATEGY >>>**
>
> You may see periodic tables give more numerically exact values for atomic weight, such as 15.999 amu for oxygen. On the MCAT, it is virtually always acceptable to round values to make math faster and easier. Of course, be sure to check to ensure that the available answer choices are sufficiently far apart before rounding.

these electrons that are involved in the formation of chemical bonds (Inner electrons are called core electrons, and these play no direct role in bonding). A simple bonding model devised by G.N. Lewis, known as the **octet rule**, is based on *s* and *p* orbitals and posits that each atom will act in such a way as to obtain eight electrons to fill its valence shell—a highly stable state. When using the octet rule, each lone pair of electrons surrounding an atom counts as two electrons, and each single bond to that atom also counts as two electrons. Double bonds count as four, while triple bonds count as six. Structures drawn using the octet rule are known as Lewis electron structures.

As an example, consider the diatomic oxygen (O_2) molecule in Figure 1. On its own, an oxygen atom possesses six valence electrons (it is in Group 16). However, if it forms a chemical bond as pictured here, each oxygen atom will have four electrons from its lone pairs and four from the double bond, for a total of eight. As such, the formation of O_2 is predicted to be favorable, as it leads to a stable state.

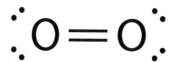

Figure 1. A molecule of O_2, in which each oxygen atom possesses a full octet

For such a simple model however, the octet rule is not without exceptions. Consider hydrogen (H), for example. One neutral hydrogen atom has a single electron in its $1s$ orbital, meaning that a molecule of H_2 will contain a total of only two. In fact, two valence electrons is the *maximum* number that an s orbital can have. As such, a H atom will be stable with a single bond and no lone pairs. This ability to exist in a stable bonded state with fewer than eight valence electrons is termed an incomplete octet. Other atoms that form incomplete octets are helium (which also has only a $1s$ orbital and has a maximum of two valence electrons), lithium (with 3 electrons), beryllium (with 4 electrons), and boron (with 6 electrons).

Lewis did not describe his structures based on anything other than s and p orbitals, but can structures form that have more than eight valence electrons? This, too, is possible. For example, consider the compound phosphorus pentafluoride (PF_5). A central phosphorus atom has a single bond to each fluorine. Since each single bond constitutes two electrons, this central P atom has a total of $2 \times 5 = 10$ valence electrons. This is termed an expanded octet. Phosphorus is not the only atom that can accomplish this; in fact, atoms in the third period ($n = 3$) and higher tend to form expanded octets readily because they are not limited to having just s and p subshells

The octet rule also doesn't hold if there is an odd number of electrons. Radicals, for example, have an unpaired, or "free", electron. As a classic example, nitric oxide (NO) possesses five valence electrons from nitrogen (Group 15) and six from oxygen (Group 16). With a total of eleven valence electrons, a distribution of eight around each component atom is impossible.

2. Bond Types

Two forms of bonding you are likely to see on the MCAT that involve *intramolecular forces*—that is, bonds that hold together atoms in a compound or atoms in a single molecule—are **ionic bonds** and **covalent bonds**. Recognize that purely ionic and purely covalent bonding represent extremes. A vast number of intramolecular bonding interactions lie between the two extremes.

Ionic bonds are strong chemical bonds that hold together ions of opposite charge. These interactions are between positively charged cations and negatively-charged anions. In an ionic bond, electrons are completely transferred from one species to another, forming the cation and anion. This electron transfer occurs when the two species have a large difference in electronegativity such that one will readily accept electrons from the other. The Pauling scale, assigns the most electronegative element, fluorine, an electronegativity value of 4.0. In contrast, the alkali metals on the other side of the periodic table have Pauling electronegativity values close to 1.0. An oft-cited rule is that ionic bonds only form when the difference between the Pauling electronegativities of the two species is 1.7 or greater. However, you are not given an electronegativity table for the MCAT, so recognize that metals (especially alkali and alkaline earth metals, Groups 1 and 2) tend to form ionic bonds with nonmetals (especially halogens, Group 17). For example, table salt used to season food is made of sodium chloride (NaCl), which is an ionic salt formed by Na^+ cations and Cl^- anions. Ionic compounds tend to have a highly-ordered crystal lattice structure, high melting points due to the strong electrostatic forces holding them together, and are brittle. When an ionic compound dissociates in aqueous solution, the resulting solution conducts electricity, which explains why they are often termed "electrolytes."

In contrast to ionic bonding, **covalent bonding** involves the sharing of an electron pair between two atoms. The electrons within a covalent bond are attracted to the positive nuclei of both atoms. Compared to ionic compounds, the electronegativity difference between covalently bonded atoms is small. Bond strengths and melting and boiling points of covalent compounds are generally lower than those of ionic compounds. Diamond, for example, contains only carbon-carbon covalent bonds, yet its boiling point is substantially higher than that of NaCl, an ionic compound (4027 °C vs 801 °C).

Nonpolar covalent bonds form between atoms that have very similar or identical electronegativity values when the electrons are shared equally. For example, the two chlorine atoms in a molecule of Cl_2 have equal electronegativity values, so the Cl_2 bond is nonpolar covalent. Generally speaking, electronegativity differences of less than 0.5 correspond to nonpolar covalent bonds. In contrast, atoms with a moderate electronegativity difference—greater than nonpolar covalent but less than ionic, or an electronegativity difference between 0.5 and 1.7—form **polar covalent bonds**. The more electronegative atom will attract the shared electrons more strongly, gaining a partial negative charge (δ−), while the less electronegative atom will gain a partial positive charge (δ+). An example of this sign convention is shown in Figure 2.

> **MCAT STRATEGY >>>**
>
> You'd be surprised at just how many MCAT concepts revolve around "opposite charges attract." It is generally beneficial to keep this in mind when studying topics from ionic bonding to polar protic solvents to protein folding.

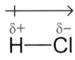

Figure 2. The polarity of a molecule of hydrochloric acid (HCl). The bond between hydrogen and chlorine is polar covalent

This polarity, termed a **dipole moment**, is often represented by an arrow with a plus sign near the atom with the δ+ charge, pointing in the direction of the electron flow towards the more electronegative atom. In molecules with multiple covalent bonds, the overall dipole is calculated by adding the dipoles of all the bonds. This, though, can lead to some traps; consider carbon tetrachloride (CCl_4), in which four polar C-Cl bonds are arranged in a tetrahedral shape. You might expect this to be a polar compound because of the large difference in electronegativity between carbon and chlorine, but their dipoles cancel out.

Bonds formed between atoms that are nearer each other have some covalent character. Carbon-hydrogen (C-H) bonds are non-polar, nitrogen-hydrogen (N-H) bonds are moderately polar, and O-H and F-H bonds are highly polar. Carbon-nitrogen bonds (single, double, or triple), are slightly polar, while carbon-oxygen (C-O or C=O) bonds are more polar.

A **coordinate covalent bond**, sometimes called a dative bond, forms when both of the shared electrons originate from a lone pair on only one of the bonded atoms. For example, when ammonia (NH_3) bonds with boron trifluoride (BF_3), the lone pair on the nitrogen atom contributes both electrons to the bond (Figure 3). This is actually a Lewis acid-base reaction, which will be discussed further in Chapter 7. A coordinate covalent bond is like any other covalent bond—the strength of the interaction depends on many factors, including those discussed next.

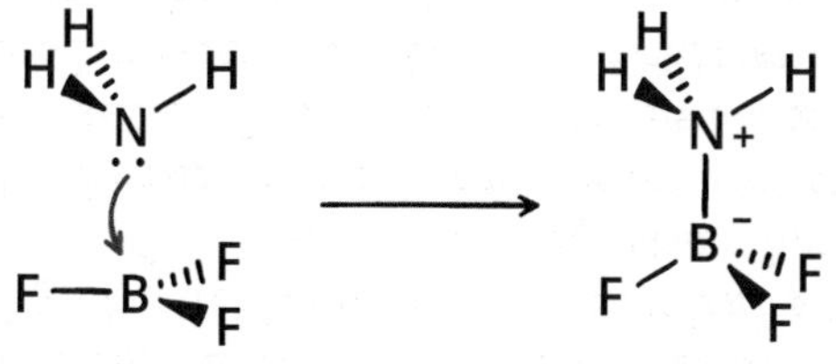

Figure 3. Coordinate covalent bond formation between NH_3 and BF_3 (with formal charges shown)

A **bond order** describes the number of bonds between two atoms. Until now, our discussion has remained centered on single bonds, which arise from the sharing of one electron pair. However, double and triple bonds can form as well: double bonds from the sharing of two electron pairs (or four total electrons) and triple bonds from the sharing of three electron pairs (or six electrons).

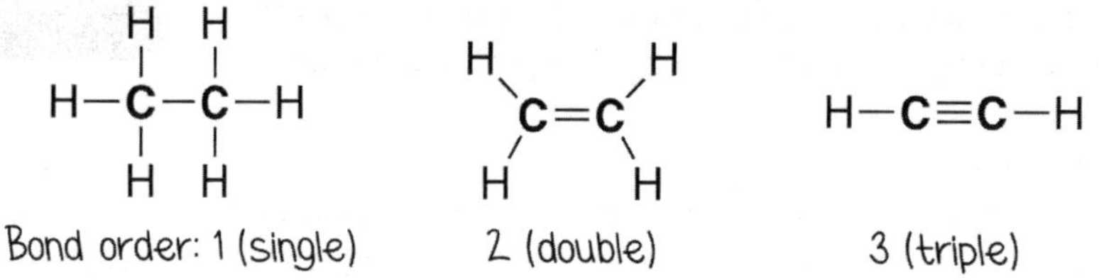

Figure 4. Examples of carbon-carbon bond order

When reading about single and multiple bonds, you may encounter the terms sigma (σ) and pi (π). These are designations used to describe the symmetry of molecular orbitals that arise from the combination of atomic orbitals in a bonded atom. A **σ bond** (σ molecular orbital), shown in Figure 5a, forms when there is an end-to-end overlap of the two atomic orbitals along the internuclear axis (Figure 5a). In contrast, a **π bond** (π molecular orbital) forms when the atomic orbitals are parallel to each other but perpendicular to the internuclear axis (Figure 5b). This is a weaker side-to-side interaction.

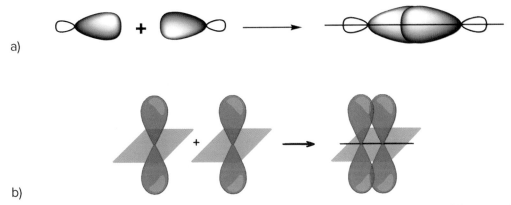

Figure 5. a) a σ bond is formed by the direct overlap of two atomic orbitals b) a π bond is formed from parallel orbitals that are pendicular to the internuclear axis

A double bond contains one σ bond along the internuclear axis and one π bond in a side-to-side interaction, while a triple bond includes one σ and two π bonds. For atoms that are not locked into position (such as they are in a cyclic structure), the σ bond allows free rotation to occur. In contrast, rotation cannot occur around double or triple bonds because doing so would break the π bond overlap.

Two other characteristics of covalent bonds are **bond length** and **bond energy**. As one would expect, bond length refers to the distance between the bonded atoms. More specifically, bond length is the average distance between the two nuclei of the bonded atoms. Bond length is inversely related to bond order; single bonds are longer than double bonds, which are longer than triple bonds. Finally, bond energy is the energy required to break the covalent bond(s) between two atoms. The higher the bond energy, the stronger the bond. Thus, bond energy increases as bond order increases.

> **>> CONNECTIONS <<**
>
> Chapter 2 of Biochemistry

Although ionic and covalent bonds are by far the most common types of intramolecular forces that you will encounter, it's also worth being aware of a final type known as **metallic bonding**. This occurs when electrons are delocalized and are attracted to multiple nuclei, producing a so-called "sea of electrons" that are free to move throughout the solid. This freedom of electron movement accounts for many familiar properties of metals, including, most notably, their ability to conduct heat and electricity. This type of bonding is weaker than ionic and covalent bonding. Electron delocalization gives metals their luster and makes them malleable (easily deformed). Consider a copper wire, for example, that can be easily shaped without breaking, and which conducts (and loses) heat readily.

3. Intermolecular Forces

Earlier, we mentioned hydrogen bonding, but we did not discuss it along with ionic and covalent bonding. You ask, "Why?" The simple answer is that hydrogen bonding is not a form of intramolecular chemical bonding, nor are hydrogen bonds actually bonds, in the classic chemical sense, at all. Instead, hydrogen bonds, along with the other main forms of intermolecular chemical forces, are attractions between positive or partially positive and negative or partially negative regions of different molecules.

Intermolecular forces are attractive forces between molecules that are notably weaker than those in intramolecular bonds. For this reason, it is typically fairly easy to disrupt these attractions with heat.

Consider two water molecules, for example. Each molecule has two O-H covalent bonds, which are intramolecular one joining the oxygen and hydrogen atoms within each molecule. However, another attractive force exists between the oxygen atom of one molecule with its partial negative charge and the hydrogen atoms of another that have partial positive charges. The attractive force is an *inter*molecular force between the oppositely charge dipoles. The partial charges exist because the bond between oxygen and hydrogen is a polar covalent bond.

The four main types of intermolecular forces in order of increasing strength are: (1) London dispersion forces (LDFs), (2) dipole-dipole interactions, (3) hydrogen bonds, and (4) ion-dipole forces. The stronger the polarity the stronger the intermolecular forces.

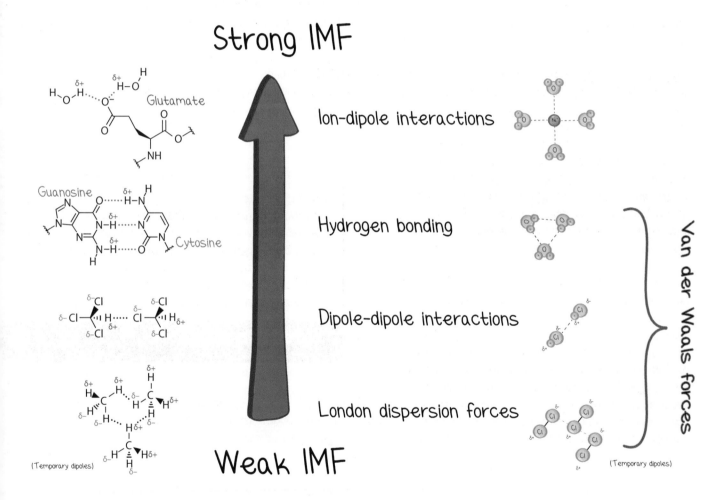

Figure 6. Major intermolecular forces sorted by strength

London dispersion forces are the weakest intermolecular force. A distinguishing feature of London dispersion forces is that they're present between *any* pair of molecules, although in molecules where stronger intermolecular forces are possible, the contribution of London dispersion forces may be so small as to make no practical difference. The reason why London dispersion forces are so ubiquitous is that they result from temporary dipoles that arise by chance. For example, let's look at two N_2 molecules that are close to each other. These molecules are completely nonpolar, as there is no electronegativity difference between the two nitrogen atoms. However, electrons move, so temporary fluctuations in electron distribution can occur. Such a fluctuation will cause a small, temporary dipole to form. This random dipole in *one* N_2 molecule can *induce* a dipole in the *other* N_2 molecule because like charges repel. This results in the formation of two dipoles: (1) a dipole caused by random electron motion, and (2) a dipole induced by that dipole. Once these two dipoles are formed, a weak attractive force will exist between the positive and negative dipoles, causing a London dispersion force. Since London dispersion forces arise from the random alignment of electrons, larger molecules are more likely to form a transient dipole at any given time, simply because they have more bonds that can form transient dipoles. Thus, because of the additive effect over a larger surface area, larger molecules have stronger London dispersion forces.

Dipole-dipole interactions are stronger than London dispersion forces. These interactions occur between molecules with *stable* dipoles (i.e., between polar molecules). In dipole-dipole interactions, an attractive force occurs between the positive end of a dipole of one polar molecule and the negative end of a dipole of another molecule. A carbonyl bond (>C=O), for example, has a stable dipole, with the partial positive charge on the more electropositive carbon atom and the partial negative charge on the more electronegative oxygen atom. The partial charges can interact with opposite charges on another carbonyl. In fact, the charge separation forms the basis of carbonyl chemistry in organic reactions.

Hydrogen bonds are stronger yet; however, they're somewhat misleadingly named, because in essence, they're just stronger versions of dipole-dipole interactions. Hydrogen bonds aren't really "bonds" in the sense of covalent or ionic bonds, which are *intra*molecular forces. More specifically, hydrogen bonding occurs when a partially positively charged hydrogen atom attached to nitrogen, oxygen, or fluorine is attracted to the lone pair of a nitrogen, oxygen, or fluorine atom on another molecule. Hydrogen-bonding only occurs with nitrogen, oxygen, and fluorine atoms because these atoms are very electronegative, and therefore they generate particularly strong dipoles when they bond with hydrogen. The weakest IMFs are collectively referred to as van der Waals forces, as labeled in Figure 6.

> **MCAT STRATEGY >>>**
>
> Intermolecular forces are a classic illustration of the principle "follow the charge!", which links a surprising amount of MCAT content, ranging from Physics to Biochemistry. As you study, always be on the lookout for how intermolecular forces (especially hydrogen bonding) affect a behavior of interest.

Ion-dipole forces occur between ions and molecules having a dipole. Since ions have a full charge, these interactions are stronger than hydrogen bonds. Be aware that in biochemistry, negatively charged areas on amino acid residues will interact strongly with positively charged regions on a receptor (the term "salt" is generally used for such interactions), but they don't form a strong ionic *bond* in the sense that we see with familiar ionic substances like NaCl.

Intermolecular forces allow us to make several predictions about how substances behave with regard to their melting and boiling points, freezing points, and other physical properties. Since melting and boiling points reflect the thermal energy required to break the attractive forces of a substance, the stronger the intermolecular forces, the higher the melting and boiling points. Both intra- and Intermolecular forces substantially affect organic and biochemical reactions, and are prominently featured on the MCAT.

4. Lewis Structures

We now return to Lewis structures to describe the relationships between atoms and their valence electrons. In a Lewis structure, valence electrons are represented by dots in pairs surrounding the element's symbol. We begin by placing a single dot on each side of a square containing the element, and then pair the dots until we have accounted for all of the valence electrons.

Figure 7. The Lewis structure of monoatomic chlorine, which has seven valence electrons

Covalent bonds are indicated by a line that represents two shared electrons connecting two atoms. Multiple lines may be used to signify double and triple bonds.

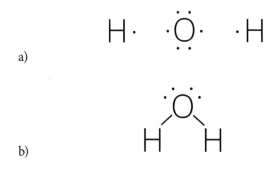

a)

b)

Figure 8. a) Lewis electron dot structures for individual O and H atoms. b) The Lewis structure of water (H_2O)

How do we count valence electrons and obtain a Lewis structure? Let's use Figure 8a as an example. We can see that each hydrogen atom (Group 1) contains a single valence electron. The oxygen atom (Group 16) has six valence electrons. In Figure 8b, the Lewis structure of water is shown, where each hydrogen contributes one electron to a covalent bond with oxygen. In turn, oxygen contributes one valence electron to each covalent bond with H. Therefore, bonding completes the valence shell for each atom: each hydrogen has a complete valence shell with 2 electrons from the covalent bond; and oxygen has a full shell with 8 electrons--four from its two lone pairs and four from its two covalent bonds.

When drawing the Lewis structure of a molecule, be certain to adhere to the following rules. We'll use carbon dioxide (CO_2) as an example, as it is a common molecule that you will see often throughout your MCAT prep.

1. Draw the atoms of the molecule in the proper positioning, placing the least electronegative atom in the center. Hydrogen atoms are terminal. For a diatomic molecule like O_2, draw two oxygen atoms next to each other. Carbon, which is less electronegative than oxygen, will be the central atom of CO_2.

2. Determine how many valence electrons must be present in the entire molecule. Remember, you can find the number of valence electrons contributed by a certain atom by the last digit of its group number in the periodic table. Here, carbon has four valence electrons, while oxygen has six, yielding a total of $(4) + (2 \times 6) = 16$ valence electrons.

3. The atoms must be connected by at least one bond, so draw single bonds to connect them.

$$O-C-O$$

4. Determine how many valence electrons are yet to be assigned. We know the compound has a total of 16; subtract two for each single bond, and we see that we need to assign an additional 12 electrons. Assign these in lone pairs to the peripheral atoms (those which are *not* the central atom), in an attempt to give each a full octet. (Recall that certain atoms can exist with an incomplete or expanded octet, as described earlier in this chapter. Carbon and oxygen cannot, so we do not need to worry about these exceptions.)

$$:\overset{..}{O}-C-\overset{..}{O}:$$

5. Uh-oh—we have a problem. Our compound has the proper number of electrons, and the two oxygen atoms have complete octets, but the central carbon atom only contains four electrons (Remember, when assessing whether an atom has an octet, you must count each single bond as two electrons). When this occurs, start erasing lone pairs on the peripheral atoms and replace each with a multiple bond to the central atom. Do this until all atoms have proper octets. The final Lewis structure of CO_2 is shown below.

$$:\overset{..}{O}=C=\overset{..}{O}:$$

Compounds that have more than one possible Lewis structure are said to have **resonance**. Resonance structures must have the same positioning and connectivity of atoms, but they differ in the distribution of electrons across the molecule. As one example, consider the nitrate, or NO_3^-, anion, below. Nitrate has three oxygen atoms, any one of which could be drawn correctly with a double bond. Therefore, nitrate can be represented by three equivalent resonance structures. The true structure of nitrate is an average of these three structures, with all three oxygens sharing the negative charge. Note that all three resonance structures have complete octets on each atom, and that the separate resonance structures are separated by a double-headed arrow, as is conventional.

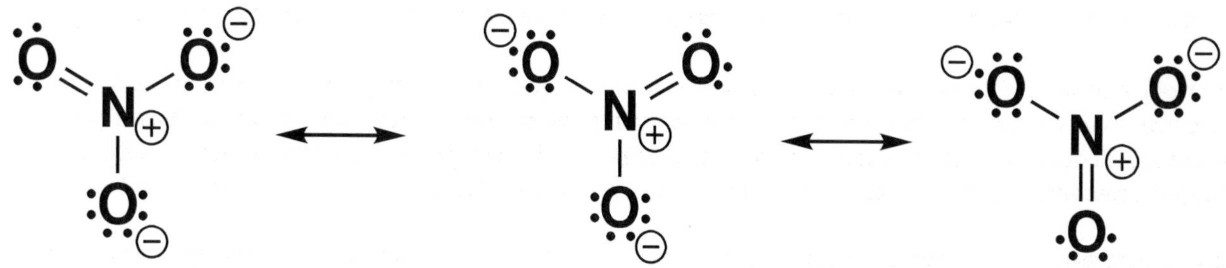

Figure 9. Resonance structures of the nitrate ion

To determine whether two structures are resonance forms of each other, be certain to clarify a few points. First, the forms must have the same number of *total* electrons, whether these are held as bonds or lone pairs. Second, when converting one resonance structure into another, shift lone pairs or π electrons to adjacent atoms, as opposed to atoms more distant on the molecule. Finally, remember that atoms themselves cannot change position if two structures are to be categorized as resonance forms.

The "true" structure of a molecule is ultimately a hybrid of all possible resonance structures. If multiple resonance structures of different stability are possible, the true structure of the molecule will most closely resemble the most stable resonance structure. For example, ozone (O_3) has two resonance structures with equal stability, so the resonance hybrid will contain two partial double bonds with an even distribution of electrons (Figure 10). The bond order of each of these bonds will be 1.5, halfway between that of a single and that of a double bond (yes, it is possible to have a bond order that is not a whole number!). Finally, note that delocalization of electrons across multiple atoms increases the stability of molecules with resonance.

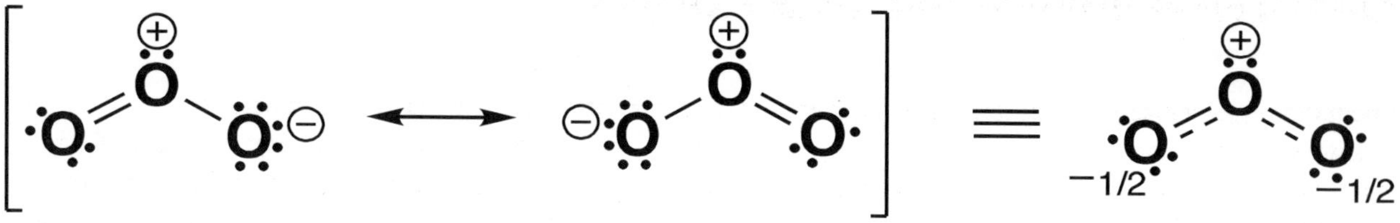

Figure 10. Resonance structures of ozone (left) and ozone's resonance hybrid (right)

If you look at the resonance forms in Figure 10, you may notice something interesting. Consider either resonance structure, and note that the central oxygen atom must have one lone pair to have a full octet. It does have one lone pair, and since each bond shares two electrons it has a full octet—so why is it positively charged instead of neutral? This brings us to the concept of formal charge, or the disparity between the number of valence electrons an atom needs to bond with in order to have an octet (according to the periodic table) and the number of bonds it actually forms in a molecule. **Formal charge** can be calculated according to Equation 1.

Equation 1. Formal charge = VE − ½ BE − LPE

>> CONNECTIONS <<

Chapter 1 of Chemistry

Here, VE refers to the number of valence electrons held by the neutral atom, according to the periodic table. BE denotes the number of bonding electrons (two per bond), and LPE refers to the number of electrons present on the atom in the form of lone pairs. Notice that VE is the number of valence electrons the atom "should" have, while the combination of ½ BE and LPE gives the number that it actually has in the molecule in question. For the central oxygen atom of ozone, the oxygen has a formal charge of 6 - ½(6) - 2 = +1.

Let's attempt another example. What is the formal charge of nitrogen in NH_3? The first step is to draw the Lewis structure of the molecule.

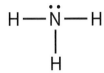

Figure 11. The Lewis structure of ammonia (NH_3)

Next, recall that formal charge = valence electrons – ½ bonding electrons – lone pair electrons. Here, then, the formal charge of the central nitrogen atom must be 5 – ½ (6) – 2 = 0. This fits with the prediction we may have made using logic, as a neutral nitrogen atom has five valence electrons and does bring five into the compound shown above. This brings up an important point about neutral atoms: a neutral hydrogen atom has one bond, oxygen has two bonds and two lone pairs, nitrogen has three bonds and one lone pair, and carbon has four bonds. We can see right away that the nitrogen and hydrogen atoms in NH_3 are neutral, so each has a formal charge of zero. The resonance structures of ozone, in contrast, show only one oxygen atom that is neutral—it has two bonds and two lone pairs. Another has three bonds and one lone pair (it has a formal charge of +1), and the other has one bond and three lone pairs (its formal charge is -1). As another example, if nitrogen has four bonds, as it does in NH_4^+, its formal charge is not zero but rather +1. Knowing the structure of the neutral atom allows you to quickly determine its formal charge without carrying out the calculation. Molecules are most stable when the sum of its formal charges is as close to zero as possible.

5. Orbital Hybridization and VSEPR Theory

In section 2 of this chapter, we briefly discussed molecular orbitals in the context of σ and π bonds. Let's dive into the details a little bit more, so we can introduce a related concept: **orbital hybridization**. First, recall from Chapter 1 that electrons occupy regions of space around a central nucleus. The subshells have characteristic shapes that become more complex in the order *s, p, d,* and *f*. The *s* orbital is spherically symmetrical, like a tennis ball. There are three *p* orbitals with dumbbell shapes, five *d* orbitals, and seven *f* orbitals. While the specific shapes of the *d* or *f* orbitals may differ, all *d* or *f* orbitals are energetically equivalent. Figure 12 shows representations of each type.

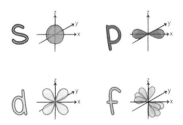

Figure 12. Examples of atomic orbital shapes. Note that *d* and *f* orbitals can take on shapes distinct from those shown here

When atoms combine to form a molecule, their atomic orbitals overlap to produce molecular orbitals. A single bond—again, consisting of two electrons—between two atoms will form a sigma (σ) bond, which has an overlapping region of electron density along the internuclear axis. Pi (π) bonds occur between two parallel *p* orbitals and are weaker than σ bonds. Double bonds consist of one π bond and one σ bond, while triple bonds include two π bonds and one σ bond.

The central carbon in methane (CH_4) has four valence electrons and would presumably have one valence *s* orbital and three *p* orbitals as shown for a neutral carbon atom in Figure 13a. In reality, however, these orbitals combine, or hybridize, to produce four energetically equivalent sp^3 orbitals. In CH_4, each of the four sp^3 orbitals overlaps with a hydrogen 1*s* orbital to form four σ bonds.

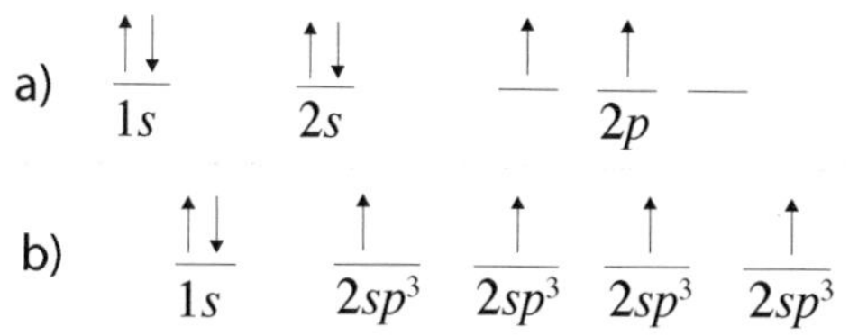

a)
$$\underset{1s}{\uparrow\downarrow} \qquad \underset{2s}{\uparrow\downarrow} \qquad \underset{2p}{\uparrow \quad \uparrow \quad \rule{0.5cm}{0.4pt}}$$

b)
$$\underset{1s}{\uparrow\downarrow} \qquad \underset{2sp^3}{\uparrow} \quad \underset{2sp^3}{\uparrow} \quad \underset{2sp^3}{\uparrow} \quad \underset{2sp^3}{\uparrow}$$

Figure 13. a) Electron configuration of a C atom. b) carbon's orbital hybridization in CH_4

Hybridization between one s orbital and two p orbitals may also occur to produce three sp^2 orbitals, or between one s orbital and one p orbital to produce two sp orbitals, as illustrated below. Notice that the number of hybrid orbitals is the same as the sum of the superscripts. So, for example, the sum of s^1p^2 gives three sp^2 hybrid orbitals. An example of sp^2 hybridization is the double-bonded carbon of ethene, which uses its three sp^2 orbitals to make σ bonds to the carbon and the two hydrogens, and the leftover p orbital to make a π bond to carbon to complete the double bond. An example of sp hybridization is the triply-bonded carbon of ethyne, which uses its two sp hybrid orbitals to form σ bonds to C and H, and its two remaining p orbitals for two π bonds to C. A quick guide to identifying the orbital hybridization of a molecule is to determine the number of groups around the atom. A group is defined as either a single, double, or triple bond, a lone pair of electrons, or even a single electron. *An empty orbital is not a group.* Two groups yields a hybridization of sp (common in cases of triple bonds or central atoms with two double bonds). Having three groups is associated with sp^2 hybridization, and having four with sp^3 hybridization.

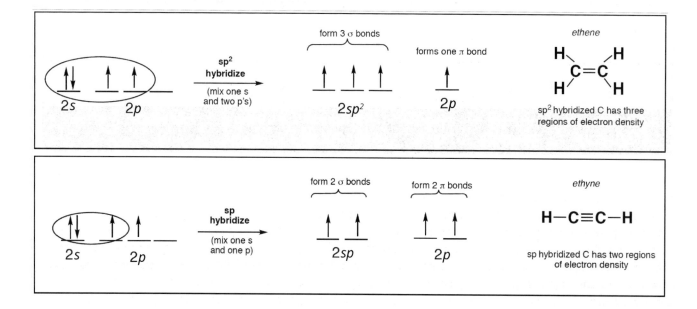

Figure 14. Orbital hybridization affects electron density

Again, let's solidify this concept by working through a simple example. Let's say we are asked to identify the orbital hybridization of the carbon atom in CO_2. To solve, we should first draw the Lewis structure of CO_2, which we have done earlier in this chapter and which is also shown below. Notice that the carbon and oxygen atoms are in neutral states, so all formal charges are zero.

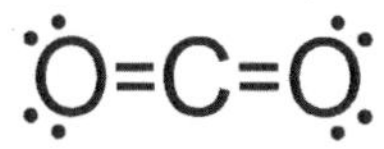

$$\ddot{O}=C=\ddot{O}$$

The central carbon atom has two groups, so it is *sp* hybridized. A carbocation has just three groups, so it is sp^2 hybridized. See—it's that easy!

Using this information we can predict molecular shapes which we were not able to do with Lewis electron structures. The **VSEPR theory** uses Lewis structures and electronic relationships to predict the shapes of molecules, assuming that the distance between groups will be maximized to reduce electrostatic repulsions. Lone pairs of electrons take up more space than bonded atoms because they are associated with only one nucleus. Thus, the number of lone pairs and bonded atoms associated with a central atom can be used to predict its bond angles and molecular shape. For example, the central carbon of CO_2 has two groups (the two double bonds), which will minimize repulsions at a bond angle of 180°, making carbon dioxide a linear molecule.

VSEPR takes into account lone pairs as well as bonded atoms when predicting shape. In contrast, **molecular geometry** (which is given in Table 1) considers only bonded atoms, although those atoms are still repelled by any lone pairs present on the central atom. Take ammonia (NH_3) as an example. Its central nitrogen atom has three bonded atoms and one lone pair, giving it four groups. As such, its electron group geometry is tetrahedral. However, its molecular geometry is trigonal pyramidal, because the lone pair of electrons is not included when determining the shape. Lone pairs do have an effect on molecular geometry, though. The N-H bond angles are slightly reduced because the lone pair of electrons occupies a larger region of space than the bonded pairs. Be aware that the MCAT expects you to know the molecular geometries!

ELECTRON-RICH REGIONS	BONDED ATOMS	LONE PAIRS	MOLECULAR SHAPE	BOND ANGLE	EXAMPLE	SHAPE
2	2	0	Linear	180°	CO_2	
3	3	0	Trigonal planar	120°	BF_3	
4	4	0	Tetrahedral	109.5°	CH_4	
4	3	1	Trigonal pyramidal	107°	NH_3	
4	2	2	Bent	104.5°	H_2O	
5	5	0	Trigonal bipyramidal	90°, 120°, 180°	PCl_5	
6	6	0	Octahedral	90°, 180°	SF_6	

Table 1. VSEPR geometries

Let's delve into a few specific molecular shapes. Tetrahedral molecular geometry is common among carbon-containing molecules, such as methane (CH_4). To maximize the separation of hydrogen atoms, the bond angle between each hydrogen atom is 109.5°.

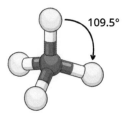

Figure 15. The bond angle between atoms in a tetrahedral molecule

Phosphine, or phosphorus trihydride (PH_3), is a molecule with three bonded atoms and one lone pair, so it also possesses four groups. Its electron group geometry is tetrahedral, whereas its molecular geometry is trigonal pyramidal. Because the lone pair generates stronger repulsive forces, the bond angle between the hydrogen atoms will be slightly smaller (107°).

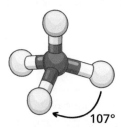

Figure 16. A trigonal pyramidal molecule, with a lone pair pushing the three bonded atoms slightly closer together than expected

Water (H_2O) also has four groups—two bonded atoms and two lone pairs so its electron group geometry is also tetrahedral. With only two bonded atoms, though, its molecular geometry is predicted to be linear. The bond angle between hydrogen atoms is even smaller due to (you guessed it!) the strong repulsive forces from both electron pairs. The bond angle between hydrogen atoms is 104.5° in the bent shape.

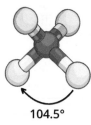

Figure 17. The bond angle between the two hydrogen atoms in water (H_2O)

Now that you have built a foundation of understanding of molecules, bonding, intermolecular forces, and VSEPR theory, you are ready to move on to the next phase of chemistry: chemical reactions and stoichiometry.

6. Must-Knows

> Molecular weight = sum of masses of individual atoms in the molecule.
> 1 mole = 6.022×10^{23} atoms or molecules (Avogadro's number).
> Valence (outermost shell) electrons participate in chemical bonding.
> The octet rule: atoms tend to prefer having eight valence electrons, and will form bonds to achieve this.
> Exceptions to the octet rule:
> — Incomplete octet: stable with < 8 valence electrons.
>   • H (max 2 electrons, 1s shell only), He (max 2, 1s shell only), Li (can be stable with 2), Be (stable with 4), B (stable with 6).
> — Expanded octet: stable with > 8 valence electrons.
>   • Elements from the third period and below.
> — Molecules with odd #s of electrons (free radicals, like NO).
> Types of intramolecular bonds.
> — Ionic (large electronegativity difference, dissociate into ions).
> — Covalent (smaller electronegativity difference, do not dissociate because atoms share electrons).
>   • Nonpolar covalent = no or virtually no electronegativity difference.
>   • Polar covalent = moderate electronegativity difference; dipole moment.
>   • Coordinate covalent = one atom donates both electrons.
> Types of intermolecular forces (weaker than intramolecular bonds).
> — Hydrogen bonding = relatively strong; requires F-H, N-H, or O-H.
> — Dipole-dipole forces = weaker than H-bonding; seen between molecules with fixed dipoles.
> — London dispersion forces = weakest; arise from instantaneous dipoles (in nonpolar molecules).
> Lewis structures: depict valence electrons/bonds/lone pairs of atoms and molecules.
> Formal charge = VE − ½ BE − LPE.
> Orbital hybridization:
> — Central atom attached to 2 groups: sp.
> — 3 groups: sp^2.
> — 4 groups: sp^3.
> VSEPR theory: uses number of bonded atoms and lone pairs to predict shape.
> Bond angles to know:
> — Bent (water): 104.5°.
> — Trigonal pyramidal: 107°.
> — Tetrahedral: 109.5°.
> — Trigonal planar: 120°.
> — Linear: 180°.

End of Chapter Practice

The best MCAT practice is realistic, with a focus on identifying steps for further improvement. For those reasons, we recommend completing practice questions in an online setting that simulates the real MCAT interface, and taking advantage of advanced analytic features to help you determine how best to move forward in your MCAT study journey.

With that in mind, online end-of-chapter questions for Biology, Biochemistry, Chemistry + Organic Chemistry, Physics, and Psychology/Sociology are available through your Blueprint MCAT account.

As a further supplement, given the importance of active learning for effective studying, we also suggest that you consult the Must-Knows as a basis for creating a study sheet, in which you list out key terms and test your ability to briefly summarize them.

This page left intentionally blank.

This page left intentionally blank.

Reactions and Stoichiometry

0. Introduction

In the previous chapter, we discussed the fundamentals of chemical bonds—what they are, which types exist, and the properties of each type. However, Chapter 2 was largely limited to describing bonds that already exist between the atoms of a molecule. How, though, did these bonds form in the first place? Can the bonds break, allowing the component atoms to form new bonds and construct new molecules? The answer to this second question is an emphatic yes. The process of breaking bonds and forming new ones to create chemically different products takes place through chemical reactions. In this chapter, we introduce empirical and molecular formulas, and then describe the various types of chemical reactions that you are likely to see on the MCAT. The chapter concludes with a discussion of stoichiometry, a form of mathematical comparison used to predict the quantity of products formed or reactants required for a chemical process to occur.

Before introducing new material, let's first briefly return to some basic concepts that were introduced in Chapter 2. Recall that a mole of any chemical substance is a quantity that contains 6.022×10^{23} particles (molecules, ions, or atoms). This value is termed **Avogadro's number** and should be committed to memory. A related concept, **molar mass**, refers to the mass of exactly one mole of a species. Molar mass has units of grams per mole (g/mol). The molar mass of a compound has the same numerical value as the compound's **molecular weight**, or the mass of one molecule in atomic mass units (amu). As an example, one molecule of diatomic hydrogen (H_2) has a mass of approximately 2.0 amu, so one mole of diatomic hydrogen gas has a molar mass of about 2.0 g/mol. Practice using the atomic weights listed on the periodic table to calculate the molar mass of larger compounds.

Stoichiometry and its related concepts are often perceived as "easy" since you likely learned about them for the first time in the early weeks of an introductory chemistry class. However, the vast majority of MCAT students harbor at least some major misconceptions about stoichiometry.

MCAT STRATEGY >>>

Note that some MCAT questions will provide molar mass values, so check before beginning any calculation. In fact, it is a good idea to double-check any relevant given information before beginning a math-heavy question. You don't want to waste time calculating a value that is already given to you in the passage text.

The MCAT tends to focus heavily on foundational concepts, so your best bet for success on Test Day is to thoroughly understand the material introduced in this chapter.

1. Chemical Formula and Percent Composition

From the very first pages of this book, you have been repeatedly presented with the terms "molecule," "compound," and "element." Recall from Chapter 1 that an **element** is matter composed of atoms that share the same number of protons, indicated by its **atomic number**. A **molecule**, then, is a species that consists of two or more atoms connected by chemical bonds. A **compound** is any substance composed of two or more different elements. A compound may consist of ions that form ionic bonds, making ionic compounds, called salts. Similarly, atoms in a compound atoms may be connected by covalent bonds, making covalent compounds, the smallest unit of which is a molecule. Note, however, that molecules can form from identical elements (like H_2) or form compounds (like CH_4).

Let's consider a simple example of a compound: sulfur hexafluoride. This compound consists of one sulfur atom attached to six fluorine atoms, so its **molecular formula** is SF_6. The molecular formula is exactly what you might expect it to be: it gives the number of atoms of each element present in a single molecule.

An alternative way to express the constitution of a compound is to use its **empirical formula**. The empirical formula consists of the ratio of atoms of each element present, simplified to the lowest whole numbers possible. In our previous example SF_6, only a single sulfur atom is present, so SF_6 already represents a simplified whole-number ratio of elements. As such, the molecular formula of SF_6 is identical to its empirical formula. For other compounds, however, these two formulas can be dramatically different. Consider glucose, one molecule of which contains six carbon atoms, twelve hydrogen atoms, and six oxygen atoms. The molecular formula of glucose is $C_6H_{12}O_6$, which directly reflects the number of each type of atom present. Contrast this with the empirical formula! Since the ratio of carbon to hydrogen to oxygen atoms in a molecule of glucose is 1:2:1, the empirical formula of glucose is CH_2O. If the ratio of atoms in the molecular formula is not already in its most reduced form, the empirical formula will differ from the molecular formula.

Another concept you will likely encounter when dealing with molecules is **percent composition** by mass. Percent composition refers to the percentage by mass of a particular element in one mole of compound. For the empirical formula of glucose, for example, which is CH_2O, the percent composition by mass of oxygen is equal to the mass contributed by oxygen divided by the total mass of the molecule. Here, using the molar masses of each of the atoms in glucose, that value would be (16 g) / (12 g + 2 g + 16 g) = about 53%.

MCAT STRATEGY >>>

Notice how we used the empirical formula rather than the molecular one? We could have calculated the same value using the molecular formula, but that would require more addition (unless we were already familiar with the molecular weight of glucose, which is approximately 180 g/mol). Becoming familiar with ways to lower your mathematical workload will help you enormously on the MCAT.

As a variation to this type of problem, we can calculate an empirical formula from percent compositions. What is the empirical formula of a compound that contains 54.5% carbon, 9.15% hydrogen, and 36.3% oxygen by mass? To solve this, note that our answer will be the same regardless of whether we have 2 grams, or 10 grams, or 1000 grams of the compound, since chemical compounds are consistent in their percent composition. The scientific principle behind this is known as the law of constant composition. The easiest way to solve this problem is to base our calculations on 100 grams of compound since we are working with percentages. Now, we need to calculate the number of moles of each element present in 100 grams of the compound.

$$\text{carbon: } \frac{54.5 \text{ g}}{12 \frac{\text{g}}{\text{mol}}} = \text{approximately 4.5 mol}$$

$$\text{hydrogen: } \frac{9.15 \text{ g}}{1 \frac{\text{g}}{\text{mol}}} = \text{approximately 9 mol}$$

$$\text{oxygen: } \frac{36.3 \text{ g}}{16 \frac{\text{g}}{\text{mol}}} = \text{approximately 2.25 mol}$$

Finally, we determine the smallest whole-number ratio of these elements. We have about twice as many moles of carbon as we do moles of oxygen, and we have twice as many moles of hydrogen as moles of carbon. Thus, carbon, hydrogen, and oxygen atoms exist in a 2:4:1 ratio, so the empirical formula must be C_2H_4O. This intuitive approach is more than sufficient for the MCAT, but you may have also heard of a slightly more formal method of working out the empirical formula. Of the three values above (4.5, 9, and 2.25), you can choose the smallest value (2.25) and divide each of the mole values by this number: 4.5 moles of carbon divided by 2.25 is 2, giving us 2 carbon atoms in the formula; and 9 moles of hydrogen divided by 2.25 is 4, which means that our empirical formula should contain 4 carbon atoms. Since, 2.25 moles of oxygen divided by 2.25 is 1, our empirical formula must be C_2H_4O—just as we found using the intuitive approach.

2. Types of Chemical Reactions

By definition, a **chemical reaction** is a process by which one or more chemical species (reactants) are converted into one or more chemically different species (products). This typically occurs via the breaking and formation of chemical bonds. In a chemical reaction, the number and types of atoms do not change; if the reactants contain only carbon and hydrogen, the products will also consist of only C and H.

> **MCAT STRATEGY >>>**
>
> As we have mentioned, you will be given a periodic table on the MCAT, but it can save time to memorize the approximate atomic weight of some common elements. In particular, the weights of hydrogen (1 g/mol), carbon (12 g/mol), and oxygen (16 g/mol) should be at the forefront of your memory.

Not *all* processes that involve a visible change to a chemical compound are chemical reactions. For example, imagine placing a block of ice on a hot sidewalk. Before long, the ice is transformed into a puddle of liquid water. Although the ice did experience a physical change from a solid to a liquid, no intramolecular bonds were broken; the H_2O molecules that formed the block of ice are still H_2O molecules in the liquid phase. Indeed, phase changes are physical processes, not chemical reactions. For the MCAT, chemical reactions can be sorted into seven reaction classes. The five basic reaction types are synthesis, decomposition, single displacement, double displacement, and combustion. More specific types of reactions to recognize are neutralization (acid-base) and oxidation-reduction (also called redox reactions). Many processes fit into multiple categories. For example, neutralization reactions are always double displacement reactions, and redox reactions may also be synthesis, decomposition, single displacement, or combustion.

> **MCAT STRATEGY >>>**
>
> One exception to the above statement is radioactive decay, in which atomic nuclei of one element can be transformed into atomic nuclei of another. This concept is discussed in detail in Chapter 10 of the Physics book.

Let's begin with **synthesis reactions**, which are also known as **combination reactions**. In a synthesis reaction, two or more reactants (elements, molecules, or ions) combine to form a single product. Most commonly, these reactions involve two reactants, but more can be involved as well. An example is the reaction of hydrogen gas and nitrogen gas to form ammonia. In the reaction below the physical state (solid, liquid, or gas) is indicated in parentheses.

$$3 H_2 (g) + N_2 (g) \rightarrow 2 NH_3 (g)$$

Decomposition reactions are the reverse of synthesis reactions. A decomposition reaction involves the breakdown of one reactant into multiple smaller products. An example is the decomposition of potassium chlorate ($2 \, KClO_3$ $(s) \rightarrow 2 \, KCl \, (s) + 3 \, O_2 \, (g)$). The breaking of chemical bonds requires the input of thermal energy. This is known as an endothermic process. As such, most decomposition reactions are endothermic overall. For example, the decomposition of potassium chlorate requires a high temperature, where the abundant thermal energy allows the decomposition to progress.

The next two reaction types are **displacement** (or "**replacement**") **reactions**, in which at least one element or group replaces another within a compound. If only one element or group is displaced, it is a single displacement reaction, whereas if two groups from different compounds exchange places the reaction is a **double displacement** reaction.

A **single displacement** reaction is shown in the example below, in which the copper (Cu) ion in copper(II) sulfate ($CuSO_4$) is displaced by elemental iron (Fe), forming iron (II) sulfate ($FeSO_4$) and elemental Cu.

$$Fe(s) + CuSO_4(aq) \rightarrow FeSO_4(aq) + Cu(s)$$

In many displacement reactions, the species that exchange places are metals; in others, a halogen may displace another halogen. The species that does the displacing (here, Fe) is typically more reactive than the species that is displaced (Cu).

MCAT STRATEGY >>>

In a biochemical context, synthesis reactions often appear as part of anabolic pathways. Anabolic processes involve the formation of larger macromolecules from multiple smaller reactants.

In double displacement reactions, both reactants are usually ionic compounds, rather than the solid metal and ionic compound typically found in a single displacement reaction. Double displacement reactions are also called metathesis reactions, since the Greek word "metathesis" means to transpose. In the double displacement reaction shown below, barium (Ba) and magnesium (Mg) cations exchange places to generate two new ionic compounds in aqueous solution (*aq*). Note that the barium sulfate product precipitates as an insoluble solid in water, making this a specific type of double displacement called a precipitation reaction.

$$BaCl_2 \, (aq) + MgSO_4 \, (aq) \rightarrow BaSO_4 \, (s) + MgCl_2 \, (aq)$$

Another type of chemical reaction is the **neutralization reaction**, in which an acid and a base react with each other to produce a salt and water. A proton from the acid reacts with the hydroxide ion from the base in a neutralization reaction that forms a molecule of H_2O. An example of an acid-base neutralization reaction between an acid (HCl) and a base (NaOH) is shown below. Acids, bases, and salts will be discussed in further detail in Chapter 7.

$$HCl \, (aq) + NaOH \, (aq) \rightarrow NaCl \, (aq) + H_2O \, (l)$$

MCAT STRATEGY >>>

In the double displacement reaction given, note that both reactants are in the aqueous phase, which means that they are dissolved in water. The barium sulfate product, however, is a solid. Keeping track of phases may seem unhelpful now, but try to do so anyway, as it will be helpful later when you review phase changes and solutions.

Combustion describes a reaction in which a compound react with elemental oxygen (O_2), producing heat and light. You have almost certainly seen these reactions many times before—for example, any time you have attended a bonfire or struck a butane lighter. Combustion reactions release a large amount of heat, which makes them *exothermic*. Although the initial reaction requires heat for bonds to break, the formation of bonds in the products releases more heat than the thermal energy required to initiate the reaction. On the MCAT as in real life, the fuel in most combustion reactions is an organic compound that contains carbon and hydrogen. The combustion of a hydrocarbon produces carbon dioxide and water, as seen below for propane (C_3H_8).

$$C_3H_8 \ (g) + 5 \ O_2 \ (g) \rightarrow 3 \ CO_2 \ (g) + 4 \ H_2O \ (g)$$

Not all combustion fuels are hydrocarbons. In chemistry class or lab, you may have observed the combustion of sulfur, a reaction which produces striking blue flames. This reaction is shown below. Again, oxygen is a reactant and a gas is produced. *Any* compound or element that reacts with oxygen to produce one or more gaseous products is a combustion reaction.

$$S \ (s) + O_2 \ (g) \rightarrow SO_2 \ (g)$$

Finally, we have **oxidation-reduction**, or **redox reactions**. We devote an entire chapter of this book (Chapter 8) to these processes, so we will discuss them here only briefly. Redox reactions involve a transfer of electrons from one species to another. The species that gives up electrons is said to be oxidized, while the species that gains electrons is reduced. Because of this transfer of electrons, there is a change in oxidation states. Note that oxidation and reduction always go hand in hand; you will never see a complete reaction where only one of the two occurs. Redox reactions are vital to our physiological function and are thus a favorite topic on the MCAT.

3. Balancing Equations and Stoichiometry

You may have noticed that some of the examples in the previous section included numbers before some or all of the species involved in the reaction. For example, the synthesis of ammonia from hydrogen and nitrogen was written as $3 \ H_2 + N_2 \rightarrow 2 \ NH_3$, *not* $H_2 + N_2 \rightarrow NH_3$. To understand why these coefficients are needed, we must understand what it means to balance a chemical reaction. A chemical reaction is balanced if the same number of each type of atom appears on both the reactant and product sides of the reaction equation.

To balance a reaction, you begin by making sure each reagent has the correct chemical formula. It is important to remember that elements can carry different charges depending on their location on the periodic table. Sodium, an alkali metal, forms the Na^+ ion through loss of an electron, oxygen usually exists as an O^{2-} ion, and so on. When ions of different charges combine to create an ionic compound, they do so in a way that makes the compound electrically neutral. The chemical formula of sodium oxide, then, is not NaO, as this would have a net charge of $(+1) + (-2) = -1$. Instead, it is Na_2O, with a net charge of $(2)(+1) + (-2) = 0$. The subscript "2" denotes the presence of two sodium ions in the compound.

If we add Na_2O to water, sodium hydroxide (NaOH) forms. We can initially write this reaction as $Na_2O \ (s) + H_2O \ (l) \rightarrow NaOH \ (aq)$. While this reaction contains the correct chemical formula for each compound, it violates an important law of chemistry and physics: the law of conservation of mass. Unless nuclear reactions are involved, elements do not change identities over the course of a reaction, so the total masses of reactants must equal the total masses of products. In the reaction above, the

> > CONNECTIONS < <

Chapter 12 of Biochemistry

MCAT STRATEGY >>>

This section of the book is a great place to start practicing finding overlap between pieces of MCAT content. Ask yourself this: which reactions can fit into multiple categories? The combustion of sulfur, for example, is also a synthesis or combination reaction, and all combustions are redox reactions. Don't just memorize discrete chunks of information; thinking actively is essential to MCAT success!

reactant side includes two sodium ions while the products include only one. We call such an equation "unbalanced," so we must **balance** the reaction.

Balancing a reaction requires that we change the coefficients so that the two sides of the reaction have the same number of each atom. For the reaction of sodium oxide, the reactant side of the unbalanced reaction has twice the sodium atoms of the product side. We can correct this by placing a coefficient of 2 in front of NaOH, as shown below.

$$Na_2O \ (s) + H_2O \ (l) \rightarrow 2 \ NaOH \ (aq)$$

Now we have two sodium atoms, two oxygen atoms, and two hydrogen atoms on each side, so we're done—the reaction is balanced! One quick note on the process: it was no accident that we began with sodium rather than oxygen. A key strategy in general chemistry is to begin with the element present in the fewest compounds. Atoms or molecules that are in elemental or diatomic form should be left for last. An example is the oxygen in a combustion reaction. By changing its coefficient last, we can finish balancing the equation without having an impact on any other species in the equation. You should be aware that on the MCAT, *you cannot assume a reaction is balanced as written!*

A properly-written chemical reaction must also be balanced with regard to charge. This stems from another law of physics: the law of conservation of charge. In an isolated system, positive and negative charges do not simply appear and disappear. As such, the *net* charge of the reactant side of a reaction should be identical to the net charge of the product side.

We now turn to *why* balancing reactions is so important. In the introduction to this chapter, we mentioned **stoichiometry**, which allows us to calculate the amounts of reactants or products in a balanced reaction. When solving problems using stoichiometry, each step relies on a basic principle: that we can begin with a piece of given information and manipulate it to find another piece using known relationships. To do this most effectively, keep track of units at all times! The main units involved in stoichiometry are grams, moles, and grams per mole (g/mol).

Suppose, for example, that 88 grams of propane (C_3H_8) are completely combusted in the presence of abundant oxygen gas. How many moles of CO_2 will be produced? First, write out the unbalanced chemical reaction. Because this is a combustion reaction, propane must react with O_2 to produce CO_2 and H_2O.

$$C_3H_8 + O_2 \rightarrow CO_2 + H_2O$$

MCAT STRATEGY >>>

Never assume a reaction is already balanced unless you are told so! The MCAT can, and will, present equations in unbalanced form, causing students who rush to miss easy points.

>> CONNECTIONS <<

Chapter 6 of Physics

Next, balance the reaction. We leave O_2 for last because it is a diatomic molecule. Both carbon and hydrogen are present in only one species on each side, so we can begin with either. Let's start with carbon, where there are three atoms on the reactant side and only one in the products. To correct this, add a coefficient of 3 before carbon dioxide:

$$C_3H_8 + O_2 \rightarrow 3 \ CO_2 + H_2O$$

Hydrogen is also unbalanced, which we can fix by placing a 4 in front of H_2O:

$$C_3H_8 + O_2 \rightarrow 3 \ CO_2 + 4 \ H_2O$$

Finally, we turn to oxygen. The reactant side contains two oxygen atoms, while the product side contains (3)(2) + (4)(1) = 10. Our reaction will be balanced if we add a coefficient of 5 in front of O_2 on the reactant side:

$$C_3H_8 + 5\,O_2 \rightarrow 3\,CO_2 + 4\,H_2O$$

We are given 88 grams of propane that reacted. The question wants us to use this value to find the amount of carbon dioxide produced. The balanced reaction tells us that for every atom of propane on the reactant side, we obtain 3 atoms of carbon dioxide on the product side. Remember, atoms directly correlate with moles, so for every *mole* of propane, we produce 3 moles of CO_2. This relationship gives us the mole ratio of 1:3. Importantly, this ratio does not carry over to grams. We cannot multiply 88 grams of propane by 3 to find grams of CO_2. Instead, we must first convert grams of propane to moles. This is a vital step in a stoichiometry procedure—after writing out the balanced reaction, you *must* convert the given mass of product or reactant to moles.

The conversion to moles is straightforward: according to the periodic table, carbon has an atomic weight of 12 amu and thus a molar mass of 12 g/mol. Hydrogen, as we should remember, has a molar mass of 1 g/mol. (Use approximate values on the MCAT to save time.) The molar mass of propane, then, is $(3)(12\text{ g/mol}) + (8)(1\text{ g/mol}) = 44$ g/mol. Units of grams cancel by setting up the equation as shown here, leaving us with moles of propane:

$$88\text{ g propane} \left(\frac{1 \text{ mol propane}}{44 \text{ g propane}} \right) = 2 \text{ mol propane}$$

Now that we have the amount of propane in moles, we can use the mole ratio from the balanced reaction to find moles of carbon dioxide produced. Recall that this ratio is 3 moles of carbon dioxide for every mole of propane, or 3:1. We cancel mol propane using this equation, leaving us with mol CO_2:

$$2\text{ mol propane} \left(\frac{3 \text{ mol } CO_2}{1 \text{ mol propane}} \right) = 6 \text{ mol } CO_2$$

This is the essence of stoichiometry: start with a quantity, progressively multiply by conversion factors to cancel unwanted units, and end with the quantity that we are asked to find.

One concept that is tested on the MCAT and that gives many students migraines is a **limiting reagent**. To define this term, let's deviate from chemistry for a moment. Imagine that you are baking cupcakes that require two cups of flour, one cup of sugar, and four tablespoons of salt per dozen. You check your kitchen and see that you have four cups of flour, two cups of sugar, and four tablespoons of salt. How many cupcakes can you bake? Looking at your flour, you have enough to make two dozen cupcakes, and the same is true of your sugar. However, four tablespoons of salt can only make one dozen. If you want to follow the recipe and not have salt-less cupcakes, then, you'll need to bake only one dozen cupcakes. Here, salt was your limiting reagent.

For all the stress it causes students, limiting reagent works just as simply with chemical reactions as it does with cupcakes. A balanced chemical reaction tells us exactly how much of each reactant we need to make a certain amount of each product. If we have enough of one reactant, but not enough of another, this latter reactant limits the amount of product we can make. The amount of product is thus solely determined by the limiting reagent. The other, non-limiting reactant is said to be in excess, and no matter how much of this excess reactant we add, we will not make any more product. For this reason, a crucial first step of any stoichiometry problem is identifying the limiting reagent. Finally, note that the concept of limiting reagent carries with it the assumption that *any* species reacts to completion. On the MCAT, unless told otherwise, assume that the limiting species reacts completely and only the excess reactants remain at the end.

Our Cr_2O_3/Al example is a good example of the impact of molar mass. We began with fewer grams of Al, and two moles of Al versus one mole of Cr_2O_3 were required to form one mole of product. With this information alone, we might think that Al was our limiting reagent. However, since Al has a much *lower* molar mass than Cr_2O_3, the amount we had constituted a much larger molar amount, leading to the formation of more product.

The safest way to identify the limiting species is to calculate the amount of product that would form from the complete reaction of each reactant. The limiting reagent is the species predicted to produce the smallest amount of product. As an example, say that 50.6 grams of chromium (III) oxide is reacted with 24.0 grams of aluminum, as shown below. Which reactant is limiting, noting that the approximate molar masses of Cr_2O_3 and Al are 152 g/mol and 27 g/mol, respectively?

$$Cr_2O_3 + 2\,Al \to 2\,Cr + Al_2O_3$$

To solve, let us compare the quantity of product generated from the complete reaction of Cr_2O_3 to that formed from the complete reaction of Al. In both equations below, the given number of grams is first converted to moles using the appropriate molar mass, then the second factor uses coefficients from the balanced equation to determine moles of Cr produced.

$$50 \text{ g } Cr_2O_3 \left(\frac{1 \text{ mol } Cr_2O_3}{152 \text{ g } Cr_2O_3}\right)\left(\frac{2 \text{ mol Cr}}{1 \text{ mol } Cr_2O_3}\right) = 0.66 \text{ mol Cr}$$

$$24 \text{ g Al} \left(\frac{1 \text{ mol Al}}{27 \text{ g Al}}\right)\left(\frac{2 \text{ mol Cr}}{2 \text{ mol Al}}\right) = 0.88 \text{ mol Cr}$$

Be sure to include units in your written-out work when completing stoichiometry problems. Cross out any units that cancel, and double-check that the units that remain are those that you want your answer to have. If your units differ from those in the answer choices, it's likely that you made a mistake.

If this math looks intimidating without a calculator, don't worry—rounding and shortcuts make it much easier. For example, for the Cr_2O_3 calculation, we know that 50 is one-third of 150, and one-third multiplied by 2 is two-thirds, or 0.66. For the Al calculation, 24/27 simplifies to 8/9, which is less than 9/10 (or 0.9), but not by much—and that is certainly larger than 0.66. Since the complete reaction of Cr_2O_3 forms the smaller molar amount of product, Cr_2O_3 is our limiting reagent and will react completely, while Al is present in excess and some will remain at the end of the reaction.

Let's review this process in order to prevent a few *extremely* common mistakes students make with the concept of limiting reagent problems. In the example above, we used both the mole ratios we obtained from the balanced reaction *and* the amount of each reactant that we actually had. Neither of these pieces of information is sufficient on its own! Many students mistakenly think, for example, that since 50.6 g of Cr_2O_3 was present and only 24 g of Al, that Al must be limiting because we have less of it. As we saw above, this is incorrect, for multiple reasons. First and foremost, we cannot compare grams of reactants directly; we can only compare moles. Even if we converted these values to moles, however, we would also need to consult the balanced reaction to find the relative molar amounts needed of each species. If 3 moles of reactant X are required to react with species Y, and we have 2 moles of X and 1 mole of Y, then X will be limiting despite its larger molar quantity, because we need *even more* of X to react with Y in the proper stoichiometric ratio.

4. Yield

Stoichiometric calculations are great at telling us what will happen if the experiment proceeds perfectly, but this virtually never happens in a real-life lab setting. Some reactant sticks to the side of the flask, a side reaction reduces the number of moles of product formed, or our starting mixture was weighed improperly due to the presence of contaminants . . . the list of ways an experiment can go wrong is a very long one. Chemists quantify the extent to which our actual results resemble the calculated predictions we make using stoichiometry. This is done by calculating the percent yield of the reaction. **Percent yield** can be obtained using Equation 1.

>> CONNECTIONS <<

Chapter 4 of Chemistry

$$percent\ yield = \frac{actual\ mass\ of\ desired\ product}{theoretical\ mass\ of\ desired\ product} \times 100\%$$

Equation 1.

Consider the reaction $2\ H_2O\ (l) \rightarrow 2\ H_2\ (g) + O_2\ (g)$, which is often performed using a technique called electrolysis, described in Chapter 8. What is the percent yield of this reaction if 1.31 grams of hydrogen gas were produced from 30 grams of water? If you are unsure where to begin, use Equation 1 as a guide. The actual mass of desired product (or actual yield) was given as 1.31 grams. In fact, the actual yield *must* be given, since we cannot possibly guess the amount of product formed in this particular experiment, based on the number of things that may have gone wrong. The only quantity left to be calculated, then, is the **theoretical yield**, which we can determine using stoichiometry:

$$theoretical\ yield = 30\ g\ H_2O\ (\frac{1\ mol\ H_2O}{18\ g\ H_2O})(\frac{2\ mol\ H_2}{2\ mol\ H_2O})(\frac{2\ g\ H_2}{1\ mol\ H_2}) = 3.33\ g\ H_2$$

Here, the given grams of H_2O reactant is first converted to moles using the molar mass of H_2O. Then, coefficients from the balanced equation are used to convert moles H_2O to moles H_2. Lastly, the molar mass of H_2 is used to convert moles H_2 to grams H_2. We now have the amount of hydrogen that would have formed if all the water had completely reacted. It is a straightforward matter to insert the two known values for actual yield (1.31 g) and theoretical yield (3.33 g) and calculate the percent yield:

$$percent\ yield = \frac{1.31\ g\ H_2}{3.33\ g\ H_2} \times 100\% = 39.3\%$$

No calculator is provided on the MCAT, so you would not need to be quite so exact in your answer. Instead, our reasoning may go something like this: 1.31 divided by 3.33 is similar to 13 divided by 33. This quantity is around 12/30, which can be reduced to 2/5, or 40%. That makes our answer somewhere around 40%, which is close enough for the MCAT. You could also simply estimate that 1.3 divided by 3.33 is slightly greater than 1/3, or 33%, which again is close enough for the MCAT.

Congratulations—now that we have covered atoms, bonding, and chemical reactions and stoichiometry, you have made it through the chemistry topics considered foundational to the MCAT. In the remaining chapters, you will be introduced to more advanced and specific topics in chemistry, so be sure you thoroughly understand the content in this chapter before moving on.

5. Must-Knows

> Chemical formulas:
  — Molecular formula: gives number of each atom present in a single molecule.
  — Empirical formula: reduces molecular formula to smallest whole-number ratio.
> Percent composition by mass = [[(mass contributed to molecule by element in question) / (total mass of molecule)] × 100.
> Chemical reactions involve one or more reactants changing into one or more products through the breaking and forming of bonds.
  — The atoms stay the same—only the bonding changes.
> Types of chemical reactions:
  — Synthesis: two or more reactants → one product.
  — Decomposition: one reactant → two or more products.
  — Single replacement: one element/group replaces another in a compound.
  — Double replacement: two elements/groups of two different compounds exchange places.
  — Neutralization: acid + base → water + salt.
  — Combustion: fuel (generally a hydrocarbon) burns in oxygen; highly exothermic.
    • For a hydrocarbon fuel: $C_?H_? + ? O_2 \rightarrow ? CO_2 + ? H_2O$ (details of coefficients depend on the hydrocarbon).
  — Oxidation-reduction (redox): involves transfer of electrons.
> Balancing reactions:
  — Law of conservation of mass: same # of each type of atom must be present on reactant and product sides.
  — Law of conservation of charge: net charge must be the same on both sides.
> Stoichiometry: allows us to use given quantities in a chemical reaction to find unknown ones.
  — One common set of steps: grams of reactant → moles of reactant → mole ratio from reaction to find moles of desired product → grams of desired product.
> Limiting reagent = the reagent that is fully used in a reaction:
  — Must take into account amount present *and* balanced reaction.
> *percent yield* $= \dfrac{\text{actual mass of desired product}}{\text{theoretical mass of desired product}}$ x 100%.
  — Measures how close results were to those predicted by calculation.

End of Chapter Practice

The best MCAT practice is realistic, with a focus on identifying steps for further improvement. For those reasons, we recommend completing practice questions in an online setting that simulates the real MCAT interface, and taking advantage of advanced analytic features to help you determine how best to move forward in your MCAT study journey.

With that in mind, online end-of-chapter questions for Biology, Biochemistry, Chemistry + Organic Chemistry, Physics, and Psychology/Sociology are available through your Blueprint MCAT account.

As a further supplement, given the importance of active learning for effective studying, we also suggest that you consult the Must-Knows as a basis for creating a study sheet, in which you list out key terms and test your ability to briefly summarize them.

This page left intentionally blank.

Equilibrium and Thermodynamics

0. Introduction

In the previous chapters, we covered the fundamentals underlying chemical reactions: atoms, ions, and molecules, and the types of reactions in which they take part. However, discussions of these basic concepts often oversimplify what *actually* happens during chemical reactions. For example, our review of stoichiometry generally assumed that the reactions involved went to completion, meaning that one or more reactant was fully converted to products. In this chapter, we will see why this is usually not the case. In doing so, you will learn about the concept of chemical equilibrium, a topic with far-reaching implications. For this reason, don't rush your review! A thorough understanding of equilibrium will help you conceptualize enzyme function and bioenergetics, described in Biochemistry Chapters 3 and 12, respectively. The other topic covered in this chapter—thermodynamics—will also give you chemistry context for the concepts you will encounter in Chapter 4 of your Physics book.

> **>> CONNECTIONS <<**
>
> Chapters 3 and 12 of
> Biochemistry and Chapter 4
> of Physics

1. Equilibrium

So if most chemical reactions do not go to completion, what happens instead? To answer this, we must introduce the concept of **reversibility**. A reversible chemical reaction is one in which products are converted to reactants and reactants are converted to products. Consider the generic reaction below, where the letters X, Y, and Z represent reactants and products, and the numbers 3, 2, and (implicitly for reactant X) 1 represent their stoichiometric coefficients:

$$X\,(g) + 3\,Y\,(g) \rightleftharpoons 2\,Z\,(g)$$

Note that the reactants and products are separated by a double-headed arrow ($\rightleftharpoons$), which denotes reversibility. Imagine that we begin with only reactants X and Y in a closed container. At first, the reaction proceeds only in the forward direction. After all, no Z is present to act as a reactant in the reverse reaction. As the process progresses, however, and some Z is made, the reverse reaction will start to take place simultaneously with the forward reaction. The rate of a chemical reaction is dependent on the concentration(s) of its reactant(s) (with the exception of zero-order reactions, which you will learn about in Chapter 6), so as X and Y are converted to Z, the reverse rate will increase as the forward rate slows. Eventually, a state will be reached in which the forward and reverse reactions

When reviewing equilibrium, be very careful to identify exactly what is taking place while avoiding making unfounded assumptions. For example, some students wrongly assume that the *concentrations* of reactants and products must be equal at equilibrium. This is not true: they can differ wildly but the composition of the system does not change! It is only the forward and reverse *rates* that must be equal.

are proceeding at the same rate, and the composition of the system doesn't change. This is termed **equilibrium**. Note that neither reaction has stopped entirely. Both continue to occur! But since the forward and reverse rates are equal, once equilibrium is reached, there will be no net change in concentrations of reactants or products. A steady-state system in which products and reactants are still interconverting is a system in dynamic equilibrium. Most reactions on the MCAT are reversible and thus reach dynamic equilibrium, although irreversible reactions (those which proceed in only one direction and fully consume the limiting reagent) do appear in the context of questions involving stoichiometry.

Let's return to our generic reversible reaction, shown again below for convenience:

$$X\,(g) + 3\,Y\,(g) \rightleftharpoons 2\,Z\,(g)$$

At equilibrium, the rate at which X and Y are converted to Z must be equal to the rate at which Z is converted to X and Y. Thus, the rate of the forward reaction must equal the rate of the reverse reaction. We can express a rate law for the forward reaction in terms of the rate forward times the concentrations of all reactants. Thus, the rate law $= k_{forward}[X][Y][Y][Y]$, or rate $= k_{forward}[X][Y]^3$. Similarly, the rate law for the reverse reaction is rate $= k_{reverse}[Z]^2$. Since the rates are equal, we can say that $k_{forward}[X][Y]^3 = k_{reverse}[Z]^2$. Rearranging this equation leads to the following relationships:

$$K_{eq} = \frac{k_{forward}}{k_{reverse}} = \frac{[Z]^2}{X[Y]^3}$$

At equilibrium the k values are constants, so we can combine them into a single constant that denotes the relative tendency for the reaction to progress forward compared to in reverse. This constant is termed the **equilibrium constant**, or K_{eq}. As shown above, K_{eq} is equal to the concentration(s) of the product(s) (each raised to the power of its respective coefficient) divided by the concentration(s) of the reactant(s) (each of which is also raised to the power of its coefficient). If we have a reaction that favors the products, which would mean that it has a numerator greater than its denominator, it will have a large K_{eq}. Meanwhile, a reaction that favors the reactants will have a small K_{eq}. Note that the concentrations used *must* be equilibrium concentrations. You cannot just substitute any concentrations into a K_{eq} expression and expect to obtain an equilibrium constant.

Solids and pure liquids or solvents should not be included in the equilibrium expression, because their concentrations are so high that they are treated as a constant and incorporated into K_{eq}. For example, if reactant X in our previous example had been in the solid phase, the denominator of the expression would have excluded [X] and included $[Y]^3$ alone.

What about the K_{eq} expression for the reverse reaction? How does it compare to the expression for the forward reaction? We can use the same example as above, only this time, we must use the reverse process: $2\,Z\,(g) \rightleftharpoons X\,(g) + 3\,Y\,(g)$. K_{eq} is still equivalent to product concentrations over reactants, with each product or reactant raised to its respective coefficient, so our $K_{eq\ reverse}$ is as follows:

$$K_{eq} = \frac{X[Y]^3}{[Z]^2}$$

You may notice that this is simply the reciprocal of the K_{eq} for the forward process. This holds true in general: K_{eq} for a reverse reaction will always be equal to $\frac{1}{K_{eq}}$ for the forward reaction. Finally, note that since concentrations (usually given in units of moles/liter, or molarity) cannot be negative, K_{eq} cannot take on a negative value. It can, however, have either a very large value (for example, 4×10^{17}, which denotes an equilibrium heavily leaning toward the product side) or a very small value (for example, 2×10^{-21}, which corresponds to a reaction in which barely any products are formed). Rather, K_{eq} is temperature-dependent; reaction rates increase with temperature, and K_{eq} is a ratio of two rates. For this reason, textbooks that give select K_{eq} values generally do so with the stipulation that the temperature is 25°C, or standard ambient (room) temperature.

Let's use what we have learned to write the K_{eq} expression for an actual chemical reaction, shown below:

$$SnO_2 \ (s) + 2 \ CO \ (g) \rightleftharpoons Sn \ (s) \ + 2 \ CO_2 \ (g)$$

> ## MCAT STRATEGY >>>
>
> Throughout this book, you will see both standard conditions (which stipulate a temperature of 25°C (298 K), among other conditions) and standard temperature and pressure, or STP (which assumes a temperature of 273 K). Do not confuse the two! Standard temperature is typically used with thermodynamic parameters, while STP is used when dealing with gases.

First, check to ensure that the reaction is balanced (an unbalanced reaction would have incorrect coefficients). The equation above is already balanced, so we can move on. Next, remember to exclude SnO_2 (s) and Sn (s) from the expression because they are solids. Now raise the concentrations of the remaining species to their respective coefficients and place products over reactants:

$$K_{eq} = \frac{[CO_2]^2}{[CO]^2}$$

Just be certain that you do not confuse *subscripts* (which denote how many of each type of atom is contained within a single molecule, like the "2" in CO_2) with *coefficients* (which give stoichiometric ratios).

Earlier, we mentioned that only equilibrium concentrations can be substituted into the K_{eq} expression. But what if the reaction is not at equilibrium? Is there a way to discern whether a reaction is at equilibrium without being explicitly told so? If we're uncertain of or do not know the equilibrium concentrations, we use the **reaction quotient** (Q) in place of K. The equation for the reaction quotient is the same as the equation used for K_{eq}, but the concentrations used can be from any moment in time, not necessarily at equilibrium. As with K_{eq}, the Q expression should not include solids, pure liquids, or solvents. For our reaction between tin oxide and carbon monoxide, the equation for the reaction quotient is as follows:

$$Q = \frac{[CO_2]^2}{[CO]^2}$$

The reactant quotient can be used to predict the direction in which the reaction will proceed to reach equilibrium. When $Q < K_{eq}$, the ratio of products to reactants is *lower* than it would be at equilibrium, so the reaction will proceed in the forward direction to increase the product concentrations and thus, move toward equilibrium. The reverse is also true: when $Q > K_{eq}$, the ratio of products to reactants is *greater* than it would be at equilibrium, so the reaction will proceed in the reverse direction to increase the reactant concentrations. Finally, if Q is equal to K_{eq}, we know our reaction must already be at equilibrium. We can thus think of Q as "where the reaction actually is" and K_{eq} as "where it wants to be." This information is summarized in Table 1.

RELATIONSHIP	DIRECTION OF REACTION PROGRESSION
$Q < K_{eq}$	The reaction will proceed forward.
$Q = K_{eq}$	The reaction is at equilibrium.
$Q > K_{eq}$	The reaction will proceed in reverse.

Table 1. Predicted reaction progress based on the relationship between Q and K_{eq}

Let's try an example. The components of the reaction shown below are present at the following concentrations: $[I_2] = 2$ M, $[H_2] = 0.1$ M, and $[HI] = 4$ M. Will the reaction proceed in the forward or reverse direction, or is it already at equilibrium? The K_{eq} of the reaction is approximately 50.

$$H_2 \ (g) + I_2 \ (g) \rightleftharpoons 2 \ HI \ (g)$$

To find the direction in which this reaction will proceed, we must first solve for Q:

$$Q = \frac{[HI]^2}{[H_2][I_2]} = \frac{[4]^2}{[0.1][2]} = \frac{16}{0.2} = 80$$

Since $Q > K_{eq}$ (80 > 50), the ratio of products to reactants is higher than at equilibrium, and the reaction will proceed in reverse to increase the concentration of reactants until $Q = K_{eq}$.

2. Le Châtelier's Principle

If a reversible reaction is allowed to reach equilibrium, it will remain in that state if reaction conditions are maintained. But what if there is a change to the reaction conditions? The results of such a change can be predicted using **Le Châtelier's principle**. The core of this principle is simple: if an equilibrium mixture is disrupted, it will shift to favor the direction of the reaction that best facilitates a return to equilibrium. As an MCAT student, you can think of this concept as simply "a reaction will shift in the direction that relieves the stress put on the system." Here, "stress" can refer to a change in reactant or product concentration, temperature, pressure, or volume.

Consider the following reaction:

$$2 \ SO_2 \ (g) + O_2 \ (g) \rightleftharpoons 2 \ SO_3 \ (g)$$

A closed vessel contains SO_2, O_2, and SO_3 gases at equilibrium. If excess SO_2 is pumped into the reaction vessel, what will happen? We began at equilibrium, so the forward rate of reaction was equal to the reverse rate. Adding SO_2, then, will disrupt the equilibrium, resulting in an increase of reactant concentration. To compensate, the system will shift to the right (toward the product side) to consume the excess SO_2 and restore equilibrium. Note that this shift will also decrease the concentration of O_2, leading to an O_2 concentration lower than we had at equilibrium. The K_{eq} for the above reaction must be equal to $\frac{[SO_3]^2}{[SO_2]^2[O_2]}$, so we can see that equilibrium can be re-established when $[SO_2]$ is increased by lowering $[O_2]$. This is the consistent with Le Châtelier's principle: the system shifts to relieve a stress and eventually regains equilibrium, albeit not necessarily with the exact same reactant and product concentrations as before the disruption. These concentrations may change in order to maintain K_{eq}.

What can we expect if we added SO_3 instead of SO_2? The system had reached equilibrium, but subsequent addition of SO_3 results in an overabundance of product. The reaction will thus shift to the left (toward the reactants) to consume the extra SO_3. In fact, whenever the concentration of a species in an equilibrium mixture is increased, the system always shifts in the opposite direction to consume the excess species.

What if we remove a reactant like O_2? Now Q > K because our "stress" has caused the system to lose reactant. The system will shift towards reactants to restore O_2 and increase our concentration of SO_2. Alternatively, the removal of a product would cause a shift toward the right to form more product.

Le Châtelier's principle can be used to maximize the yield of a chemical reaction. One common experiment that you may have done in organic chemistry lab is the synthesis of acetylsalicylic acid, commonly known as aspirin. Acetic anhydride is combined with salicylic acid to form the desired aspirin product along with acetic acid. To maximize the yield of our product, we have two options: either add one or both reactants in excess or remove products as they form. Often times, an excess of the reactant acetic anhydride is used to push the system toward the products, forming more aspirin (and acetic acid). Alternatively, aspirin can be removed as soon as it forms. This removal of a product predictably shifts our system toward the product side, maximizing aspirin production. This latter technique of product removal is often used to drive a reaction to completion.

Until now, we've only discussed the effects of changing concentration on a system at equilibrium. What happens when we change the volume or pressure? This effect is limited to gases and not to liquids and solids, because only gases are compressible. When volume increases, pressure decreases; conversely, if volume decreases, pressure will increase. This relationship is described by Boyle's law, which you will review in more depth in the next chapter of this book.

>> CONNECTIONS <<

Chapter 5 of Chemistry

Consider the previous equilibrium mixture (shown again for convenience). What will happen if we increase the volume of the container?

$$2\ SO_2\ (g) + O_2\ (g) \rightleftharpoons 2\ SO_3\ (g)$$

All three substances are in the gas phase, and gases are affected by changes in pressure or volume. An increase in volume means that less pressure will be exerted on the walls of the container. We might already be able to predict what happens next: the system will shift in such a way as to restore equilibrium by increasing the pressure. Each gas in a mixture of gases has its own partial pressure that it contributes to the total pressure of the mixture. For example, the gaseous components of air (O_2, N_2, Ar, H_2 vapor and so on) each have a partial pressure. When added together, they comprise the total pressure of air. Changing a partial pressure (the pressure of one reactant) has the same effect as changing a concentration. Decreasing the pressure inside the vessel will shift the reaction in a direction that produces more pressure, which means the reaction will shift towards the side that produces more moles of gas. For this example, this means that the reaction will shift toward the reactant side, which includes 2 + 1 = 3 moles of gas compared to the product side, where there are only 2 moles of gas.

The opposite will happen if we reduce the volume of the container, causing the pressure to increase. To relieve this stress, the system will shift toward the side with fewer moles of gas, which is the product side in the reaction above. Note that while this reaction took place entirely in the gas phase, this may not be true for other reactions on the MCAT! As a matter of habit, be certain to only count moles of gas when using Le Chatelier's Principle. Solids and liquids do not impact the direction of the shift; remember that solids, pure liquids, and solvents are not even included in the equilibrium expression.

The final variant of Le Châtelier's principle to know is the change in the temperature of an equilibrium mixture. Unlike concentration, pressure, or volume, temperature changes have results that cannot be predicted without additional information. In particular, we need to know whether the reaction is endothermic (it requires heat input, $+\Delta H$) or exothermic (it releases heat, $-\Delta H$). This will typically be given, but it may not be in the form of a direct statement ("This reaction is exothermic!"). Combustion reactions, for example, are well-known examples of exothermic processes, as are neutralization reactions.

Let's say you are given the generic reaction below, along with its ΔH value. This negative ΔH means that the reaction is exothermic. The reaction mixture is allowed to reach equilibrium, at which point the temperature is sharply increased. What will happen?

$$A\,(g) + B\,(g) \rightleftharpoons C\,(g) + D\,(g) \qquad \Delta H = -100 \text{ kJ/mol}$$

We have already reviewed the effects of changing the reactant or product concentration of an equilibrium mixture. If we treat "heat" as a reactant or product, we can follow the same rules we've already mastered. Exothermic reactions release heat, so heat should be written as a product, as shown:

$$A\,(g) + B\,(g) \rightleftharpoons C\,(g) + D\,(g) + \text{heat}$$

A sharp increase in temperature is effectively identical to increasing the concentration of a product (heat). This will shift the system toward the reactants. If this had instead been an endothermic reaction, we would have written "heat" as a reactant. An increase in temperature would shift the reaction toward products. Decreases in temperature, then, must function exactly like decreases in product or reactant concentration. Table 2 summarizes our discussion of Le Châtelier's principle.

DEVIATION FROM EQUILIBRIUM	EFFECT
Increased [reactant]	Shift toward products.
Decreased [reactant]	Shift toward reactants.
Increased [product]	Shift toward reactants.
Decreased [product]	Shift toward products.
Increased volume (↓ pressure)	Shift toward side with more gas moles.
Decreased volume (↑ pressure)	Shift toward side with fewer gas moles.
Increased temperature	If $\Delta H > 0$, shift toward products; if $\Delta H < 0$, shift toward reactants.
Decreased temperature	If $\Delta H > 0$, shift toward reactants; if $\Delta H < 0$, shift toward products.

Table 2. Direction of shifts expected after certain deviations from equilibrium

As with nearly all chemistry topics, it is also worth noting the exceptions to the rule, which here are changes that can be made to an equilibrium mixture *without* provoking a shift. The first such change is the addition of a catalyst. You may have read about enzymes, or biological catalysts, in Chapter 3 of your biochemistry book. Catalysts will be described in depth later. For now, just note that a catalyst increases the rate of both a forward and reverse reaction, causing it to reach equilibrium more quickly. When a catalyst is added to a reaction already *at* equilibrium, however, no disruption takes place. This is because catalysts do not change the relative amounts of products or reactants and thus do not promote a change in equilibrium concentrations. As a result, the system will remain at equilibrium.

>> CONNECTIONS <<

Chapter 3 of Biochemistry and Chapter 6 of Chemistry

Another example is the addition of an inert (unreactive) gas at constant volume. Let's return to our recent gas-phase example: $2 SO_2 (g) + O_2 (g) \rightleftharpoons 2 SO_3 (g)$. At equilibrium we have all three components in a 1-liter flask. What happens if we add 0.5 moles of nitrogen gas? Nitrogen does not participate in this reaction and is relatively unreactive in general. The total pressure inside the flask increases, but this occurs due to the added pressure from the nitrogen, not because of any changes in the partial pressures of the reactants or products. The inert gas does not appear in the equilibrium expression. As such, equilibrium will not be disturbed.

3. Introduction to Thermodynamics

Now that we have wrapped up our introduction to equilibrium, we can move on to the second main topic of this chapter: **thermodynamics.** Note that we call the first portion of this chapter an "introduction" to equilibrium because equilibrium is a concept that will arise countless

>> CONNECTIONS <<

Chapter 4 of Physics

times during your MCAT review. Equilibrium is closely tied to thermodynamics; thermodynamics describes the relationship among heat, work, and the energy content of a system at equilibrium. Our coverage of thermodynamics will remain rooted in general chemistry; for a review of the physics side of thermodynamics, consult Chapter 4 of your Physics book.

The first one we will describe is temperature. **Temperature** is directly proportional to the average kinetic energy of a system (something we'll discuss further in the context of gases in Chapter 5). Temperature can be measured using a thermometer using multiple distinct scales. The temperature scales most relevant to the MCAT are the Celsius and Kelvin scales. The conversion between Celsius and Kelvin temperatures is shown in Equation 1. The lowest temperature possible is 0 K, termed absolute zero, which is the temperature at which molecular energy is at a minimum.

>> CONNECTIONS <<

Chapter 5 of Chemistry

Equation 1.
$$K = {}^\circ C + 273.15$$

In contrast, **heat** refers to the transfer of energy, specifically thermal energy, between objects of different temperatures. This brings us to another foundational topic: the laws of thermodynamics. The **zeroth law of thermodynamics** describes the thermal relationship between systems. Specifically, it states that if one system (let's call it "System A") is in thermal equilibrium with another (we'll say that one is "System B"), and System B is in thermal equilibrium with a third system ("System C"), then System A must *also* be in thermal equilibrium with System C. "Thermal equilibrium" means that the systems have the same temperature. When this is the case, no heat transfer will take place between the systems. In contrast, if one system has a different temperature than another and thermal energy is allowed to move between the two, then heat transfer will take place. Imagine dropping an ice cube at −5°C into a glass of water at 25°C. Heat would immediately begin to transfer from the water to the ice.

The **first law of thermodynamics** goes beyond the discussion of heat to involve work as well. To conceptualize this law, we must first touch upon the definition of a system, which is discussed in detail in Chapter 4 of your Physics book. In scientific study, a **system** is whatever we are observing, while its surroundings consist of everything outside

MCAT STRATEGY >>>

If you are up-to-date on your knowledge of theoretical physics, you may have read about the potential of temperatures below absolute zero. This is well outside the scope of MCAT chemistry or physics. For best results, constantly remind yourself that the MCAT tests fundamentals, and avoid worrying about advanced/theoretical concepts unless told otherwise.

the system. This definition we're using may seem broad, but it allows our concept of a system to vary depending on the circumstances. For example, if a chemical reaction is occurring between two solids immersed in water, the solids may be considered the system and the water molecules part of the surroundings. In other situations, the entire contents of the container may be thought of as the system, while the surroundings would include the container and its environment. On the MCAT, you may see three types of systems: **open**, **closed**, and **isolated systems**. Open systems are those which can exchange both matter and energy with their surroundings. For example, imagine that you conduct a chemical reaction in an open beaker. Heat is free to leave the beaker, as is matter in the form of evaporated reactants or solvent molecules. In contrast, a closed system, allows energy to be exchanged with the surroundings, but not matter. This would be the case if we covered the beaker. Finally, isolated systems do not exchange matter or energy with their surroundings and are thus perfectly insulated.

The first law of thermodynamics states that for closed systems, the change in the internal energy of the system (ΔU) is equal to the heat transfer into the system (Q) minus the work performed by the system on its surroundings (W). This relationship is shown in Equation 2. One definition of work is force x distance (F x d). Thus, no work occurs if an object doesn't move.

Equation 2.

$$\Delta U = Q - W$$

It is worth spending some time thinking about the sign conventions used in this equation, as you may have seen sources differ on this topic. The sign on Q is fairly straightforward: if the system is being heated, it is positive, while if heat is being lost from the system, it is negative. Since Equation 2 subtracts work from heat, when work is done *by* the system on its surroundings, it is positive. This is true because work done by the system causes the system's internal energy to decrease. In contrast, work done *on* the system is negative in the above equation. This means that when work is done on a system, its internal energy increases, since -(-W) is a positive number.

We must wrap up our introduction to thermodynamics with a brief mention of a technique used to measure heat exchange: **calorimetry**. You may have performed this technique in chemistry lab with a coffee-cup calorimeter, which is a simple enough setup: a Styrofoam coffee cup, tightly covered, with a thermometer extending down into the cup's contents. If a chemical reaction is performed inside the cup, then the system is the reactants and products, and the surroundings include the solvent and cup. The resulting temperature change can be measured and used to calculate an estimate for the heat required or released by the reaction. We say "estimate" because calorimeters (especially simple ones made from coffee cups) are difficult to completely insulate, so some heat almost always escapes from the solution into the surroundings outside the cup, where it cannot be measured.

MCAT STRATEGY >>>

For MCAT chemistry, the most common example of work done by a system is the expansion of gas against a flexible container or piston. Predictably, then, the most common case of work done on a system is gas compression.

The equation most often used for calorimetry-related calculations is shown below in Equation 3. Here, Q represents heat, m is the mass of the substance under observation in grams, c is a substance-specific constant termed the specific heat capacity (which we'll talk more about in Chapter 5), and ΔT is the measured temperature change, which has the same value whether using the Celsius or Kelvin temperature scales (there is no need to convert between the two when using ΔT). In our calorimeter example, the ΔT is the temperature change of the solution during the reaction, m is the mass of the solution, and c is the solution's heat capacity (usually estimated by using the heat capacity of the solvent). Q is therefore the heat transferred to the solution, which is assumed to be equal to the change in temperature of the reaction with opposite sign.

Equation 3.
$$Q = mc\Delta T$$

4. Enthalpy and Entropy

We now shift our focus to enthalpy and entropy. Broadly, **enthalpy** is a thermodynamic measurement of heat, with typical units of joules (J) or kilojoules (kJ). You might notice that these are also the units for energy, and this is no accident: enthalpy is typically used to describe changes that involve the gain or loss of thermal energy. Enthalpy is described by Equation 4, where H represents enthalpy, U is the internal energy of the system, and PV is the product of pressure and volume.

Equation 4.
$$H = U + PV$$

On the MCAT, you typically will not be dealing with H or the enthalpy of a static system. Instead, you will be presented with changes in enthalpy, which are described using the term ΔH. We can easily modify Equation 4 to include this quantity, at constant pressure, the case for the majority of MCAT questions involving this topic, as shown below in Equation 5.

Equation 5.
$$\Delta H = \Delta U + P\Delta V$$

Recall from the previous section the equation we used to calculate changes in the internal energy of a system: $\Delta U = Q - W$. While work can be defined as $F \times d$, consider that the W (work) that we deal with most often in this context is pressure-volume work, which is equal to $P\Delta V$. We can thus rewrite our internal energy equation as $\Delta U = Q - P\Delta V$. If we substitute this quantity into Equation 5 for the ΔU term, we get $\Delta H = (Q - P\Delta V) + P\Delta V$, or $\Delta H = Q$. From this relation, we can clearly see that enthalpy change (ΔH) is equal to Q, which is the heat lost or gained from the system. For the MCAT, it is perfectly acceptable to think of enthalpy as an approximation of the total heat contained in a system. Since we most often deal with enthalpy change, we need terms that denote whether a ΔH value is positive or negative. You are familiar with these terms as endothermic and exothermic. Specifically, **endothermic** processes require heat input and thus have positive ΔH values. **Exothermic** processes, which release heat, are associated with negative ΔH values.

While these terms may seem straightforward, we need to be careful when using them. Let's consider an example. A reaction occurs between two aqueous reactants in water. After the reaction, the temperature of the water is 1.2°C lower than it was at the start (i.e., before the reaction). Is this reaction endothermic or exothermic? To answer questions like this, consider the temperature change of the surroundings, or the immediate environment in which the reaction takes place. Since the temperature of the surrounding water decreased, the reaction must have absorbed heat from the water to acquire the heat energy needed for the reaction to occur. As such, this reaction is endothermic.

On the MCAT, you are quite likely to see multiple variations of the ΔH term. Often, this term is presented with what looks like a degree symbol on its right side ($\Delta H°$). This symbol denotes standard conditions, which are 1 atm and 298 K (25°C).

> **>> CONNECTIONS <<**
>
> Chapter 8 of Chemistry

In addition to $\Delta H°_f$ and $\Delta H°_{rxn}$, you may see terms that relate to other specific enthalpy changes. One common example is $\Delta H°_c$, or the standard enthalpy of combustion. This represents the enthalpy change associated with the burning of a fuel, which is often an organic compound. It is helpful to understand that the more exothermic (negative) the heat of combustion, the more unstable the original reactant must have been, since it must contain a large amount of energy in its bonds.

The **standard enthalpy of formation** ($\Delta H°_f$) of a compound is the change in enthalpy associated with the formation of one mole of the compound from its component elements, under standard conditions. These elements must be in their standard states: that is, the phase they exist in at 1 atm and 298 K. For example, carbon dioxide can be formed from carbon, which exists in the solid form of graphite under standard conditions, and oxygen gas. This reaction, along with its $\Delta H°_f$, is shown below. Note that the $\Delta H°_f$ of any element in its standard state is zero; the $\Delta H°_f$ of O_2 (g) is 0 kJ. Standard enthalpy of formation is often used interchangeably with the term "**standard heat of formation.**"

$$O_2 \ (g) + C \ (graphite) \rightarrow CO_2 \ (g) \qquad \Delta H°_f = -393 \text{ kJ}$$
$$(393 \text{ kJ are released per mole } CO_2)$$

The notation $\Delta H°_f$ applies only to reactions in which a compound forms from standard-state elements, but the enthalpy change of other reactions can be calculated as well. The enthalpy change that takes place over the course of a reaction is denoted as $\Delta H°_{reaction}$, which is typically abbreviated as $\Delta H°_{rxn}$. Since the Δ term simply denotes a change, $\Delta H°_{rxn}$ can be calculated by finding the total standard enthalpy of formation of the reactants and subtracting that amount from the total standard enthalpy of formation of the products, as shown below in Equation 6.

Equation 6.
$$\Delta H°_{rxn} = \Delta H°_{products} - \Delta H°_{reactants}$$

Equation 6 aligns with the categorization of enthalpy as a **state function**, defined as the property of system that depends only on its present state, not on its history. Notice that work is not a state function: the amount of work expended is always dependent on the path taken. Let's attempt to use this equation to calculate the standard enthalpy change for the combustion of two moles of benzene (C_6H_6), given the information below.

molecule	$\Delta H°_f$
C_6H_6 (l)	49.0 kJ/mol
CO_2 (g)	–393.5 kJ/mol
H_2O (l)	–285.8 kJ/mol

$$2 \ C_6H_6 \ (l) + 15 \ O_2 \ (g) \rightarrow 12 \ CO_2 \ (g) + 6 \ H_2O \ (l)$$

Note that the enthalpy of formation of O_2 (g) is not given, but we know that this value must be zero, because oxygen is a pure element in its standard state. The remaining $\Delta H°_f$ values that we need are given, which will be the case on the MCAT as well. For this reason, don't memorize any $\Delta H°_f$ values!

$$\Delta H°_{rxn} = \Delta H°_{products} - \Delta H°_{reactants}$$

$$\Delta H°_{rxn} = [12 \ (\Delta H°_f(CO_2)) + 6 \ (\Delta H°_f(H_2O))] - [2 \ (\Delta H°_f(C_6H_6)) + 15 \ (\Delta H°_f(O_2))]$$

$$\Delta H°_{rxn} = [12 \ (-393.5 \text{ kJ}) + 6 \ (-285.8 \text{ kJ})] - [2 \ (49.0 \text{ kJ}) + 0 \text{ kJ}] = -6534.8 \text{ kJ}$$

Two things to note about this process: first, on the MCAT exam, you should use estimated values. That means we can round –393.5 to about –400, and –285.8 can round to the more workable –300. Additionally, 49.0 is already very close to 50. The estimated values yield the calculation below. Just keep in mind that how we rounded our first two numbers made them considerably more negative, so our estimated value will be more negative than the actual value.

As you can see, rounding yields a value that is within 200 kJ of the exact answer, and that's certainly close enough for the sake of the MCAT!

$$\Delta H°_{rxn} = [12\ (-400\ kJ) + 6\ (-300\ kJ)] - [2\ (50\ kJ) + 0\ kJ] = -6700\ kJ$$

The second thing to note is that this is the enthalpy change for the combustion of two moles of benzene. We know this because if we were asked to find the $\Delta H°_{rxn}$ for the combustion of *one* mole of C_6H_6, we'd need to divide our calculated value by two. Also, since our answer was negative, we know this must be an exothermic reaction. In fact, combustion reactions are usually highly exothermic, giving off large amounts of heat!

Students often confuse the $\Delta H°_{rxn} = \Delta H°_{products} - \Delta H°_{reactants}$ equation with the concept of bond dissociation energy. The bond dissociation energy is the enthalpy change when a given bond in the gaseous molecule is broken. Bond enthalpies can be used to calculate ΔH_{rxn}, but in this case, the relevant equation is slightly different, shown below in Equation 7:

Equation 7. $\Delta H_{rxn} = \Delta H$ (bonds broken) $- \Delta H$ (bonds formed)

Why do we take the bonds broken (which are associated with the reactants) and subtract the bonds formed (which are associated with the products)? After all, isn't the other enthalpy equation in the opposite order: products minus reactants? The explanation lies in the fact that the formation of bonds is by nature exothermic since the bonded species is more stable, and thus lower-energy, than the separate component atoms. Bond breakage, then, is endothermic. Thus, our "bonds broken – bonds formed" equation can be conceptualized as the energy required minus the energy released. This will yield a positive ΔH_{rxn} if the overall reaction is endothermic and a negative ΔH_{rxn} if the overall process is exothermic, which is exactly what we want.

Again, since enthalpy is a state function, its value depends only on the initial and final states rather than the path taken. However, sometimes you will be presented with multiple steps of a reaction procedure and asked to calculate ΔH for the overall process. In these cases, you can use **Hess's law**, which states that the enthalpy changes of the individual steps of a chemical reaction can be added together to equal the overall enthalpy change of the reaction. To illustrate this, we will use the reaction $A\ (s) + 2\ B_2C\ (g) \rightarrow AC_2\ (g) + 2\ B_2\ (g)$. This reaction is a combination of multiple steps. Imagine that you are given the following information:

Reaction 1. $A\ (s) + C_2\ (g) \rightarrow AC_2\ (g)$ $\Delta H = -393\ kJ$

Reaction 2. $2\ B_2\ (g) + C_2\ (g) \rightarrow 2\ B_2C\ (g)$ $\Delta H = -484\ kJ$

How can we find ΔH for the overall reaction? According to Hess's law, if we can arrange the two reactions above in a way that sums to the overall reaction, we can add the individual ΔH values to obtain the overall ΔH_{rxn}. The overall reaction includes $A\ (s)$ on the reactant side, as does the reaction we desire. For this reason, leave Reaction 1 as written. However, the bottom reaction has $2\ B_2C\ (g)$ listed on the product side, whereas it is a reactant in the desired reaction. We thus need to reverse Reaction 2. The reverse of a process will always have the same magnitude of ΔH as the forward process but with an opposite sign, as shown below:

Reaction 2$_{rev}$. $2\ B_2C\ (g) \rightarrow 2\ B_2\ (g) + C_2\ (g)$ $\Delta H = +484\ kJ$

Adding this all together yields $A\ (s) + C_2\ (g) + 2\ B_2C\ (g) \rightarrow AC_2\ (g) + 2\ B_2\ (g) + C_2\ (g)$. Now we're pretty close to the desired reaction. All that's left is to remove $C_2\ (g)$ that is present on both sides, which of the overall reaction equation gives us $A\ (s) + 2\ B_2C\ (g) \rightarrow AC_2\ (g) + 2\ B_2\ (g)$. This is the same equation as the one we desired, so we are good! Using Hess's law, we know that we must add up the known ΔH values of these two reactions obtain the overall ΔH: -393 kJ $+484$ kJ $= 91$ kJ. Note that in this example, we left one reaction as written and reversed the other. In some cases, you may need to multiply one or more reactions by an integral value to get the steps to properly sum to the overall reaction. When you do this, be certain to multiply all reactant and product coefficients as well as the ΔH value for that step by the integer in question.

A term often discussed in tandem with enthalpy is entropy, which is an important, but often misunderstood, concept in chemistry. **Entropy** is at times oversimplified as the amount of disorder present in a system. A more complete definition is that entropy is related to the number of configurations, or microstates, a system can have, and more potential microstates correspond to greater entropy. Solids, which form rigid crystalline structures, have low entropy; gases, consisting of individual molecules able to move unhindered, have higher entropy; and liquids typically fall in between. Similarly, a large compound has less entropy than it would if it consisted of multiple smaller molecules. Like enthalpy, entropy is a state function. With an understanding of entropy we can now introduce the **second law of thermodynamics**. According to this second law, the entropy of an isolated system will never decrease, and the entropy of the universe is always increasing. A reaction may decrease in entropy, provided it is paired with processes that increase in entropy so that the overall entropy of the system increases.

As with enthalpy, we generally care about the change in entropy (ΔS) rather than entropy itself. An entropy increase (+ΔS) is associated with favorable reactions, while an entropy decrease (−ΔS) is associated with less favorable ones. Despite these facts, we cannot deduce whether a reaction is favorable or unfavorable from ΔS alone, as we shall soon see. Note also that typical units for entropy are joules per Kelvin (J/K) or joules per Kelvin per mole (J/K·mol). Unsurprisingly (given our existing knowledge about enthalpy), standard entropy is described as ΔS°. The entropy of an overall reaction is given as $\Delta S°_{rxn}$, and $\Delta S°_{rxn} = \Delta S°_{products} - \Delta S°_{reactants}$. Entropy plays a very important role in nearly every chemical process. One particularly MCAT-relevant example is protein folding, which depends on the entropy differences associated with both the protein and adjacent solvent molecules in the folded versus the unfolded state.

>> CONNECTIONS <<

Chapter 2 of Biochemistry

MCAT STRATEGY >>>

Note that the units for ΔH (kJ) and those for ΔS (J/K) do not align—kilojoules are one thousand times larger than joules! Whenever you see dissimilar units for quantities of the same type (here, we see dissimilar units for energy), you must convert one to match the other. For ΔG calculations, it is often easiest to convert ΔH to units of joules.

5. Gibbs Free Energy

To conclude our discussion of thermodynamics, we must address a foundational concept that combines what we have learned so far. This concept is **Gibbs free energy**. Like enthalpy and entropy, Gibbs free energy is typically described in the form of a change, specifically the change in Gibbs free energy between products and reactants (ΔG). The change in free energy is the maximum amount of work that a system can perform on the surroundings while undergoing a change that is spontaneous at constant temperature and pressure. Enthalpy, entropy, and temperature all impact ΔG, which can be calculated using Equation 8 below. Because it is calculated from state functions, it too is a state function. Note that ΔH is typically given in units of kJ, entropy in units of J/K, and temperature in units of K (Kelvin).

Equation 8.
$$\Delta G = \Delta H - T\Delta S$$

Before attempting to perform any calculations, let us first solidify our understanding of ΔG with some visual help. In your chemistry classes, you were probably shown graphs called reaction coordinate diagrams, which depict the energy changes associated with a reaction over time. Examine the reaction coordinate displayed in Figure 1 as an example.

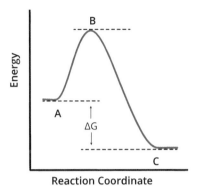

Figure 1. Reaction coordinate for the conversion of reactant A to product C

Here, the reactants are represented by the label "A," while the products are denoted by "C." The reactants begin with a certain amount of energy. For the reaction to take place, an energy barrier termed the activation energy must be overcome, a concept that will be discussed further in Chapter 6 of this book. Overcoming this barrier produces a transient species termed the transition state ("B"), which is so unstable and high-energy that it is only present instantaneously and cannot be isolated. From there, the products are formed. In Figure 1, we can clearly see that the products contain less energy than the reactants. This difference in energy, which is represented by the vertical distance between A and C along the y-axis, is the ΔG of the reaction. Notice that as a state function, this difference only corresponds to the energy of the final state—the energy of the initial state, and does not include energy associated with the pathway. Since the final state is lower than the initial state, this means that our ΔG value must be negative. A negative ΔG corresponds to a spontaneous reaction. If we were instead considering the reverse process, where C is converted back to A, the opposite would be true; ΔG would be positive, and the reaction would be nonspontaneous. Reactions with negative ΔG values are termed **exergonic**, while those with positive ΔG values are **endergonic**.

We now know how to use a reaction's ΔG value to predict whether it will proceed spontaneously. But what exactly do we mean by "spontaneous"? A **spontaneous** reaction is one that can proceed without the help of some additional, external force. Importantly, spontaneity does not relate to the rate of the reaction, or the speed at which it progresses. Rate is a kinetic parameter and is determined largely by the reaction's pathway, while spontaneity is a thermodynamic parameter and relates to ΔG, the difference in energy between products and reactants. Spontaneous reactions, then, can proceed either quickly or slowly, but they always proceed without the addition of an outside source of energy.

MCAT STRATEGY >>>

You can easily remember that a negative ΔG corresponds to a spontaneous reaction by considering the idea of stability. Stable molecules contain relatively low amounts of energy, and stability is a favorable characteristic. As such, a process in which higher-energy reactants are transformed into lower-energy products is favorable.

Some spontaneous biochemical reactions actually proceed so slowly that without help, they would not occur to any measurable extent in the body. These reactions typically need the assistance of enzymes, or biological catalysts. **Catalysts** increase the rate of reaction by lowering the activation energy. Does this alter ΔG? No! Rate refers to kinetics, not thermodynamics, so altering the activation energy does not change the value of ΔG. Remember this for your exam: adding an enzyme or other catalyst does *not* change ΔG, nor can it make a nonspontaneous reaction spontaneous.

On the MCAT, you will most often only need to discern whether, or under what conditions, a reaction is spontaneous. This means that we care about the sign of ΔG more than the actual value. Spontaneity (−ΔG) tends to be favored by exothermic (−ΔH) reactions and reactions that increase in entropy (+ ΔS). However, an endothermic (+ ΔH) reaction can be spontaneous at high temperatures if ΔS is sufficiently positive. Likewise, reactions that decrease in entropy (−ΔS) can be spontaneous at low temperatures if ΔH is negative. These guidelines are summarized in Table 3, but you can easily see the relationships based on the Gibbs free energy equation.

ΔH	ΔS	SPONTANEOUS?
+	−	Never
−	+	Always
+	+	Only at high T
−	−	Only at low T

Table 3. Signs of ΔH and ΔS and their relationship to reaction spontaneity

If we're given a reaction with ΔH = +14 kJ and ΔS = +100 J/K, how can we determine the temperature range for the reaction to be spontaneous? Since the signs given are both positive, we must substitute these values into the Gibbs free energy equation. Recall that enthalpy is given in units of kJ while entropy uses J in its numerator, so we can use either one as long as they are consistent, which means we need to do some conversions. Here we convert ΔH from +14 kJ to +14000 J so the units match. We also should set ΔG equal to 0 because temperatures above this point will make ΔG negative (spontaneous), while temperatures below this point will have a positive ΔG (nonspontaneous).

$$\Delta G = \Delta H - T\Delta S$$
$$0 = 14000 \text{ J} - (T)(100 \text{ J/K})$$
$$(100 \text{ J/K})(T) = 14000 \text{ J}$$
$$T = (14000 \text{ J}) / (100 \text{ J/K}) = 140 \text{ K}$$

Therefore, this reaction will be spontaneous at T > 140 K

MCAT STRATEGY >>>

If you don't want to have to memorize the information in Table 3, just think about the ΔG equation. In this equation, ΔS is multiplied by temperature, so the higher the temperature, the greater the effect of ΔS. If ΔS is negative (which is unfavorable) a low temperature, for instance, would minimize its effect, where a high temperature would increase that effect.

Like ΔH and ΔS, ΔG can be calculated for reactions under standard conditions (1 atm, 298 K, and 1 M concentrations of any aqueous reaction components), and can be described using ΔG° or ΔG°$_{rxn}$. The Gibbs free energy change for the formation of any compound from its standard-state elements is ΔG°$_f$, and like enthalpy, the Gibbs free energy of formation of a standard-state element is zero. Given these similarities to expressions for enthalpy, we can easily predict the equation for ΔG°$_{rxn}$, shown here in Equation 9.

Equation 9. $\Delta G°_{rxn} = \Delta G°_{products} - \Delta G°_{reactants}$

Finally, we can discuss ΔG in terms of equilibrium. Recall from earlier in this chapter that reversible chemical reactions tend to move toward equilibrium, a state in which the rates of the forward and reverse reactions are the same. This therefore means that the concentrations of reactants and products remain the same. All of this occurs because at equilibrium, the Gibbs free energy of the reaction system is at a minimum. Since the system is already in its most stable state, the concentrations of reactants and products have no impetus to change. In fact, if equilibrium concentrations of reactants and products are combined in a vessel, the reaction will simply progress in both directions at the same rate to maintain the equilibrium concentrations. Because there is no overall change in the system in this case, there is also no change in free energy, which means that the ΔG of a reaction at equilibrium is zero. Even if a reaction is not at equilibrium, we can use its ΔG to derive other useful pieces of information. Equations 10 and 11 relate ΔG to K_{eq} and Q. In these equations, R denotes the gas constant, which is 8.314 J/mol·K (0.008314 kJ/mol·K). As is typical for thermodynamic functions, T is the temperature in Kelvin.

Equation 10.
$$\Delta G_{rxn} = \Delta G°_{rxn} + RT \ln Q$$

Equation 11.
$$\Delta G°_{rxn} = -RT \ln K_{eq}$$

The "ln" term stands for the natural logarithm, and the natural logarithm of 1 is 0. The natural log of a number greater than 1 is positive, and the natural log of a number less than 1 is negative.

Let's first consider Equation 10, which relates $\Delta G°_{rxn}$ and the reaction quotient, Q, to ΔG_{rxn}. It can be used to assess a reaction under non-standard conditions. Using Equation 11, we can substitute $-RT\ln K_{eq}$ for $\Delta G°_{rxn}$ in Equation 10, so it becomes:

Equation 10a.
$$\Delta G_{rxn} = -RT \ln K_{eq} + RT \ln Q$$

Recall that if $Q < K_{eq}$, the reaction will continue in the forward direction to make more product. Thus, ΔG_{rxn} will be negative, meaning the forward reaction will be spontaneous. If $Q > K_{eq}$ the reaction will shift in the reverse direction to remove product and make more reactant. From Equation 10a, we can see that ΔG_{rxn} will always be positive in this situation, which means a nonspontaneous forward reaction (it is spontaneous in the reverse direction).

What if the reaction is at equilibrium? We already know that at equilibrium, the concentrations of reactants and products don't change; ΔG is 0, and Equation 10 becomes Equation 11, $\Delta G°_{rxn} = -RT \ln K_{eq}$.

Equation 11 defines the relationship between K_{eq} and $\Delta G°_{rxn}$. If you know that K_{eq} is equal to one, then $\Delta G°_{rxn} = -RT\ln(1) = 0$. Neither products nor reactants are favored, so reactants and products have equal free energy, and $\Delta G°_{rxn}$ must be zero. A K_{eq} greater than one means that the products are favored and $\Delta G°_{rxn}$ is negative, meaning the forward reaction is spontaneous. A K_{eq} less than one means that the reactants are favored and $\Delta G°_{rxn}$ for the forward reaction will be positive, meaning that it is not spontaneous.

To finish our discussion of ΔG, note that Gibbs free energy plays an enormous role in biochemical reactions, which are often encountered on the MCAT in the context of metabolic processes. For more information on ΔG in a biochemical context, consult Chapter 12 of your Biochemistry book.

>> CONNECTIONS <<

Chapter 12 of Biochemistry

6. Kinetic vs. Thermodynamic Control of Reactions

With our newfound understanding of thermodynamics, we may feel an urge to apply it to every additional concept we see in chemistry. However, other factors impact chemical reactions as well. For example, consider an organic reactant that can proceed through one of two different reaction pathways. We might assume that the reactant will always take the pathway that leads to the most stable product, or in other words, the pathway with the more negative ΔG. This, though, is not always the case. In such situations where one reactant can form two different products, the concept of **kinetic versus thermodynamic control** is often relevant. Chemical kinetics will be discussed in more detail later (in Chapter 6), but thermodynamic and kinetic control of reactions will be introduced here.

>> CONNECTIONS <<

Chapter 11 of Chemistry

In the reaction in Figure 2, for example, a carbonyl compound is converted to two different enolate products in a reaction that involves a base. Product 1 is more stable since its double bond is more substituted. However, the proton that is removed from the reactant to form product 2 is less sterically hindered, so product 2 is able to form more quickly.

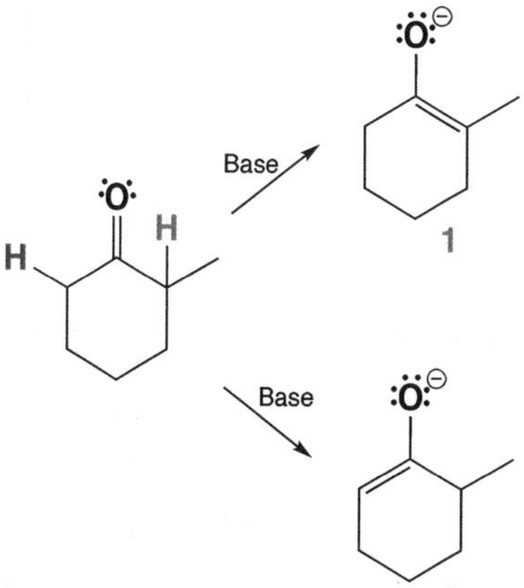

Figure 2. Thermodynamic (1) and kinetic (2) products of an organic reaction

Because product 2 is formed more quickly, it is called the kinetic product. The term "kinetic" in chemistry refers to reaction rate, and the kinetic product forms at a faster rate, even if it is the less stable product. This rapid rate is the result of a lower activation energy, E_a. Activation energy will be described further in Chapter 6, but for now, it can be thought of as the energy barrier that must be overcome for a reaction to take place. The activation energy required to make product 2, $E_{a,kinetic}$, is shown to the left on the reaction coordinate in Figure 3, where the reactant is in the center. Note how $E_{a,kinetic}$ is lower than $E_{a,thermodynamic}$ for product 1. Kinetic products like product 2 are favored at low temperatures, and have low activation barriers. They form more rapidly, but there is not enough energy in the system for the reverse reaction to occur.

Product 1 is the thermodynamic product since it is more stable. The ΔG between the reactant and product 1 is more negative than that between the reactant and the kinetic product. However, formation of the thermodynamic product is slowed by a higher activation energy in this example. Since a high activation energy must be overcome, the thermodynamic product is not favored at low temperatures. Thermodynamic products are favored at high temperatures, when sufficient energy is present to surmount both a higher $E_{a,thermodynamic}$ and reversal of the kinetic product back to the reactant. In other words, the thermodynamic and kinetic products must be in equilibrium. The kinetic product still forms faster, but the equilibrium will favor the thermodynamic product because it is more stable.

KINETIC PRODUCT	THERMODYNAMIC PRODUCT
Forms more quickly.	Forms more slowly.
Less thermodynamically stable.	More thermodynamically stable.
Lower activation energy.	Higher activation energy.
Favored at low temperatures.	Favored at high temperatures.

Table 4. Characteristics of the kinetic versus the thermodynamic product of a reaction in which the two products compete

A system at higher temperature, where the reactants and products are in equilibrium and the more stable product is favored, is said to be under thermodynamic control. A system at lower temperature, where the reactants and products are not in equilibrium and whichever product forms faster is favored, is said to be under kinetic control.

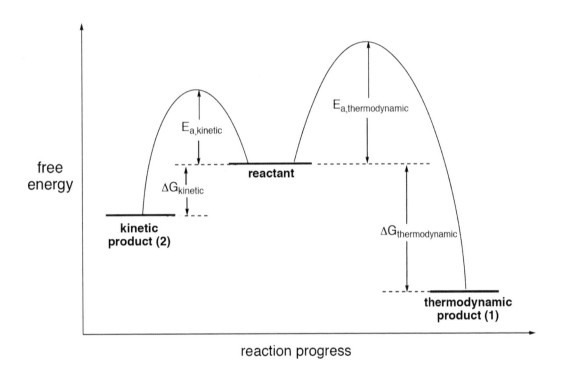

Figure 3. The reaction coordinate for a reactant that can undergo two competing pathways to give different thermodynamic and kinetic products, such as enolate products 1 and 2

7. Must-Knows

> Chemical reactions may be reversible or irreversible.
>   — Irreversible reactions go to completion (limiting reagent is entirely consumed).
>   — Reversible reactions (marked by $\rightleftharpoons$) proceed both forward and backward simultaneously and result in an equilibrium state.
> Equilibrium: a state where forward and reverse rates are equal.
> Equilibrium constant = [products]^{coefficients} / [reactants]^{coefficients}.
>   — This expression should not include solids, pure liquids, or solvents!
>   — Favors products: large K_{eq} ($K_{eq} > 1$).
>   — Favors reactants: small K_{eq} ($K_{eq} < 1$).
>   — K_{eq} = temperature-dependent; temperature at standard conditions is 298 K.
> Reaction quotient (Q) uses same equation as K_{eq} but can include non-equilibrium concentrations.
>   — $Q < K_{eq}$: reaction will proceed forward; $Q = K_{eq}$: reaction is already at equilibrium; $Q > K_{eq}$: reaction will proceed in reverse.
> Le Châtelier's principle: if disturbed, an equilibrium mixture will shift to relieve stress.
>   — Shifts can result from changing concentrations, temperature, or pressure/volume.
>   — No shift results from adding a catalyst or inert gas.
> Temperature ≠ heat; on MCAT, temperature is measured in Celsius or Kelvin (K = °C + 273.15).
> Zeroth law of thermodynamics: for thermal equilibrium, if A = B and B = C, then A = C.
> First law of thermodynamics: $\Delta U = Q - W$.
> Enthalpy (H): is usually expressed as ΔH; under constant pressure, $\Delta H = Q$.
>   — Endothermic: $+ \Delta H$, heat input is required; exothermic: $-\Delta H$, heat is released.
>   — Be familiar with standard enthalpy change ($\Delta H°$), standard enthalpy of formation ($\Delta H°_f$), and standard enthalpy of reaction ($\Delta H°_{rxn}$).
>   • $\Delta H°_{rxn} = \Delta H°_{products} - \Delta H°_{reactants}$.
>   • $\Delta H_{rxn} = \Delta H$ (bonds broken) $- \Delta H$ (bonds formed).
>   • Hess's law: enthalpies of each step in a reaction are additive.
> Entropy (S): relates to number of possible microstates, where $+\Delta S$ (increasing disorder) is favorable according to the second law of thermodynamics.
> Gibbs free energy (G): $-\Delta G$ = spontaneous (exergonic); $+ \Delta G$ = non-spontaneous (endergonic); $\Delta G = \Delta H - T\Delta S$.
> Reactants that can proceed through more than one reaction pathway may display thermodynamic vs. kinetic control.
>   — Thermodynamic: forms more stable product but may have higher E_a (and thus form more slowly); favored at high temperatures under equilibrium conditions.
>   — Kinetic: has lower E_a (and thus forms more quickly) but may be less stable; favored at low temperatures.

End of Chapter Practice

The best MCAT practice is realistic, with a focus on identifying steps for further improvement. For those reasons, we recommend completing practice questions in an online setting that simulates the real MCAT interface and taking advantage of advanced analytic features to help you determine how best to move forward in your MCAT study journey.

With that in mind, online end-of-chapter questions for Biology, Biochemistry, Chemistry + Organic Chemistry, Physics, and Psychology/Sociology are available through your Blueprint MCAT account.

As a further supplement, given the importance of active learning for effective studying, we also suggest that you consult the Must-Knows as a basis for creating a study sheet, in which you list out key terms and test your ability to briefly summarize them.

This page left intentionally blank.

Phases and Solutions

0. Introduction

Envision holding a cup of your favorite fizzy beverage and taking a sip. Imagine the heaviness of the cup in your hand, the cool liquid hitting your tongue, and the bubbles of carbon dioxide gas. The cup is formed out of a solid substance that gives it a durable shape, the liquid almost certainly contains some ions or other chemicals in solution, and the gas bubbles out into the air. This example illustrates the theme of this chapter: phases and solutions.

These are general chemistry topics that may initially seem familiar, but don't neglect them! The concept of phases has some important interconnections with thermodynamics, so developing a solid understanding of phases and phase changes is important for a successful outcome on the MCAT. The MCAT likes to go beyond 'plug and chug' equations and may test you on the theoretical assumptions underlying phase changes. Finally, solutions and solubility may not be emphasized in biochemistry textbooks, but they are still essential for understanding why our biological systems work the way they do, and therefore they are regularly tested on the MCAT.

1. Phases and Phase Changes

Let's start with **phases** and **phase changes**. There are three basic phases of matter: solid, liquid, and gas, that are tested on the MCAT. When thinking about phases and phase changes, it's important to focus your attention on **intermolecular forces**—that is, the forces that exist *between* molecules. Intermolecular forces are what help determine the phase of matter. As we will see, stronger intermolecular forces tend to be associated with solids, weak intermolecular forces with gases, and liquids are in between.

A **solid** is a structure with a rigid, tightly-packed organization of atoms, such as ice, sodium chloride (table salt), and most metals, like iron. Solids have a fixed volume, which means that they are not compressible to any significant degree, and they have a fixed shape. Solids also do not flow, although their particles do vibrate in place.

A solid may be either crystalline or amorphous in nature. Crystalline solids exhibit a regular arrangement of atoms. In solid sodium chloride (NaCl), for example, each Na^+ ion is surrounded by six Cl^- ions, and each Cl^- ion is in turn surrounded by six Na^+ ions. This structured arrangement is termed a lattice structure, as illustrated in Figure 1. The lattice is extremely difficult to disrupt, although it can be disassociated if the NaCl is dissolved in water, in which case polar H_2O molecules will "solvate" or separate and encapsulate the individual ions through ion-dipole interactions. The lattice energy of an ionic solid refers to the amount of energy required to separate the solid into its component cations and anions. As you might guess, this is typically a very large amount of energy! In contrast to crystalline solids, amorphous solids are solids that do not have a regular repeating array that produces a crystal structure. The classic example is glass, an amorphous solid typically composed of silica (SiO_2).

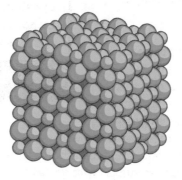

Figure 1. Lattice structure of sodium chloride

Like solids, **liquids** have a fixed volume and are considered non-compressible. Unlike solids, however, liquids do not have a fixed shape and instead assume the shape of their container. This tendency allows liquids to flow. Liquids have an associated viscosity, which is a measure of their resistance to flow. Molasses has a higher viscosity than water, for example, so it is thicker and flows much more slowly. Viscosity is discussed in more depth in Chapter 5 of the Physics textbook, which covers fluids.

The third phase of matter that we will discuss is the **gas** phase. Unlike solids and liquids, gases do not have a fixed shape and volume. They are compressible, so the density of a given gas is not constant. Rather, if the gas is forced into a smaller container, its density will increase as intermolecular forces increase.

> > **CONNECTIONS** < <

Chapter 5 of Physics

How can we predict what phase a substance will be under various conditions? How do intermolecular forces, temperature, and pressure combine to favor certain phases? Intermolecular forces, which include ionic interactions, ion-dipole interactions, hydrogen bonds, permanent dipole interactions, and London dispersion forces (in descending order of strength), determine the strength of molecular interactions. All things being equal, at a given temperature and pressure, stronger intermolecular forces will make a substance more likely to be solid rather than a liquid, or a liquid rather than a gas. Consider ethane and ethanol. Ethane only has weak London dispersion forces because it is a saturated hydrocarbon; therefore, it has a very low boiling point (–88.5°C). In contrast, ethanol has a much higher boiling point (78.37°C) because of the presence of an –OH group that can hydrogen bond. In comparing ethane and ethanol, H-bonding effects far surpass differences in molecular weight.

Higher temperatures mean that the particles in a substance will have a higher average kinetic energy and, therefore, be more likely to overcome intermolecular forces and separate. Thus, heating a solid can turn it into a liquid or a gas, and heating a liquid can turn it into a gas. In contrast, higher pressures force particles to interact with each other more closely within a confined space, so increasing the pressure can force intermolecular interactions that turn gases into liquids or solids and can turn liquids into solids.

When a substance transitions from one phase to another, there is a phase change. We can observe up to six types of phase changes, assuming that each phase can transition directly into every other phase. For the MCAT, be sure to remember all six!

1. **Melting**, or **fusion**, is the transition from solid to liquid.

2. **Freezing** is the transition from liquid to solid.

3. **Vaporization**, and **boiling**, are the transitions from liquid to gas.

4. **Condensation** is the transition from gas to liquid.

5. **Sublimation** is the transition from solid directly to gas.

6. **Deposition** is the transition from gas directly to solid.

These six types of transitions are also summarized in Figure 2.

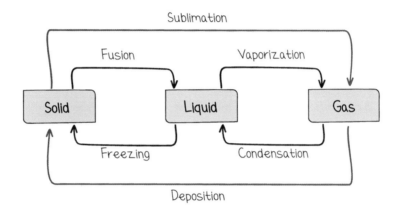

Figure 2. The six phase transitions

The endothermic phase changes—fusion, vaporization and sublimation—require a heat input ($+\Delta H$), while the exothermic phase changes—condensation, freezing, and deposition—release heat into the environment ($-\Delta H$). Endothermic processes involve breaking bonds or disrupting intermolecular forces, which require a source of energy. As you might expect, exothermic processes typically involve bond formation or an increase in intermolecular forces.

Let's now take a closer look at how heat transfer can be used to make a substance undergo phase changes. Suppose that we are heating a block of ice. At first, the heat simply raises the temperature of the ice until the temperature reaches the melting point of ice (0°C for H_2O under 1 atm of pressure). At this point, the added heat no longer increases the temperature of the ice but instead is diverted towards disrupting the intermolecular interactions holding the solid together. The added heat is associated with a phase change, not with a temperature increase, so the temperature of the system remains constant. The amount of heat that was used solely to disrupt these interactions and melt the ice at a constant temperature is the **heat of fusion**.

Once our sample is in the form of liquid water, adding heat will increase the temperature of the water until it reaches the boiling point (100°C for water at 1 atm). Again, temperature remains constant as the added the heat disrupts the intermolecular attractive forces that keep water in liquid form. The heat required to convert the

MCAT STRATEGY >>>

If you're faced with a calculation problem on your exam involving heat of fusion, heat of vaporization, or specific heat, be sure to check your units carefully! This is a common source of avoidable mistakes. In particular, watch out for units of heat energy (J, kJ, or cal) and whether the units are per mass or per mole.

liquid to gas at constant temperature is the **heat of vaporization**. Once our sample is water vapor, any additional heat will simply increase the temperature of the gas. These processes are illustrated in Figure 3.

As always, it's important to be careful about the units that we use to describe these parameters. The heat of fusion describes how much heat energy is necessary to melt a substance per unit mass or per mole, and the heat of vaporization describes how much heat energy is necessary to vaporize a substance per mole; both are generally reported in units of kJ/mol.

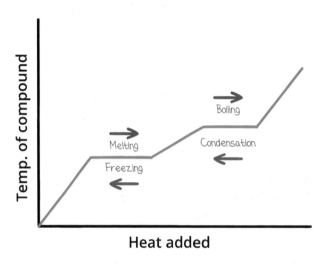

Figure 3. Phase changes as heat is added, illustrating that during a phase change the temperature is constant

You should also be aware of some specialized terminology used to describe how substances respond to the addition of heat. In particular, **specific heat capacity** is the amount of heat required to raise the temperature of one unit mass of a substance by one degree. The specific heat capacity of water is 4.184 J/g·°C. This is an unusually high heat capacity and is due to hydrogen bonding. The high specific heat capacity of water is why the temperature of the ocean does not vary much over the course of the day, even though the sand will cool at night and burn your feet under the hot sun. Because water can contain a large amount of heat without experiencing a dramatic temperature change, it is often used to cool extremely hot objects, such as a hot pan from the stove, or equipment used to contain nuclear reactions.

MCAT STRATEGY >>>

It's key to understand that adding heat to a substance does not necessarily change its temperature. At a phase change, that energy goes towards breaking intermolecular attractions, *not* to increasing the kinetic energy of the particles, which is what temperature measures.

Specific heat capacity can be used in the following equation that relates the heat applied to (or released by) a system to the temperature change.

Equation 1. $\qquad q = mc\Delta T$

In this equation, q is the heat (usually in joules) applied to or released by the system, m is mass in grams, c is the specific heat capacity of a substance (note that this value varies across different phases), and ΔT is the change in temperature. In this equation, temperature is usually measured in degrees Celsius because we are concerned with *changes* in temperature, not absolute temperature; however, for Celsius and Kelvin scales the magnitudes are identical.

Students often experience confusion about when to use which quantities and equations, so to summarize:

> At phase changes, use heat of fusion or vaporization: $q = n\Delta H$, where n is the number of moles. Units are kJ/mol. Temperature remains constant.

> Between phase changes, heat will be related to temperature change. Use $q = mc\Delta T$. Celsius and Kelvin scales give an identical value for ΔT (Fahrenheit does not, so be aware!)

Let's work through an example to illustrate this workflow in practice. Imagine that we want to take 18 g of ice from a –20°C freezer and melt it into water at 30°C under standard conditions. How much heat will this process require? We need to break it up into three steps, which you can check by referring to Figure 3. The first step is heating the ice to the melting point (0°C), the second step is applying enough heat to fully melt it into water, and the third step is to heat the water to 30°C. We will need three quantities, one for each step: the specific heat capacity of ice (c_{ice} = 2.03 J/g.°C), the heat of fusion of water (6.02 kJ/mol), and the specific heat capacity of water (c_{water} = 4.18 J/g.°C).

1. Step 1: Heating the ice. We can use $q = mc\Delta T$ and approximate c_{ice} as 2 J/g.°C and 18 g as 20 g to make the mental math easier. Thus, $q = (20\text{ g})(2\text{ J/g.°C})(20°C) = 800$ J.

2. Step 2: Melting the ice. Here, we need the heat of fusion of water. $q = (1\text{ mol})(6\text{ kJ/mol}) = 6$ kJ (Note that 18 g of ice is 18 g/(18 g/mol) = 1 mol).

3. Step 3: Heating the water. Again, we need to use $q = mc\Delta T$, and we can estimate c_{water} as 4 J/g.°C, although we should keep in mind that this will lead to underestimating the real value. Thus, $q = (20\text{ g})(4\text{ J/g.°C})(30°C) = 2400$ J.

4. Step 4: Totaling up the results. 800 J + 6 kJ + 2400 J. Notice that we have to convert our units to either joules or kilojoules. Check your answer choices to determine which you use: $q = 9.2$ kJ or 9200 J. *As always, be sure to check your units!*

The phase of a substance is affected by pressure as well as temperature. These relationships are illustrated using **phase diagrams**, which are usually drawn with pressure on the y-axis and temperature on the x-axis. A phase diagram shows the temperature and pressure conditions for phase transitions for only one substance; a typical phase diagram is shown in Figure 4a.

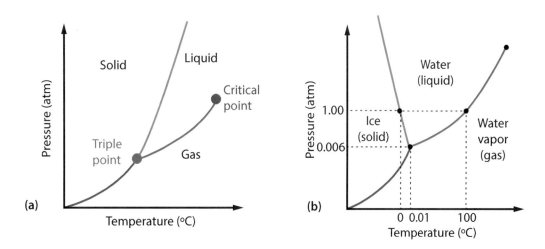

Figure 4. (a) Typical phase diagram. (b) Phase diagram for water

In phase diagrams, phase changes occur across the solid lines. An increase in pressure or decrease in temperature can convert a gas to a solid (deposition), a gas to a liquid (condensation), or a liquid to a solid (freezing), depending on the temperature. A decrease in pressure or increase in temperature can promote the opposite processes: sublimation (solid to gas), vaporization (liquid to gas), and melting (solid to liquid).

Where phase diagrams become interesting is the transition between the solid and liquid phases, depicted by green lines in Figures 4a and 4b. For most substances, the solid phase is denser than the liquid, so an increase in pressure causes liquids to form solids from an increase in intermolecular interactions, as seen Figure 4a. Ice, however, is less dense than liquid water due to its unique crystal structure. (This is how icebergs float!) Water has a maximum density at 4°C. To solidify, the molecules move apart to maximize their H-bonding interactions, thus lowering the density. This means that the temperature must be lower as pressure increases for water to freeze. Therefore, the green phase change line between solid and liquid has a negative slope for water, as shown in Figure 4b, rather than the positive slope that is characteristic of a substance such as CO_2 (Figure 4a).

As shown above, phase diagrams include a **triple point** at which solid, liquid, and gas are in equilibrium; for example, the triple point for water is 0.006 atm and 0.01°C. Each diagram also includes a **critical point**, the point that represents the end of the liquid–gas interface. Above this point, matter exists as a supercritical fluid, which possesses properties of both a liquid and a gas.

An important concept known as **vapor pressure** describes what happens when a vapor, or gas, is in contact with the liquid phase (or, theoretically, the solid phase as well). There is always some interchange between the liquid and gas phase at the boundaries of a liquid. The vapor pressure is the pressure exerted by the molecules of that substance that are in gaseous form. The equilibrium vapor pressure is reached in a closed system at a given temperature, where the number of molecules that escape into the gaseous phase equals the number of gaseous molecules condensing to the liquid phase. Vapor pressure increases with temperature as the average kinetic energy of the molecules increases. When the vapor pressure of a liquid is equal to that of the surrounding atmospheric pressure, the boiling point is reached. For example, at a pressure of 1 atm water boils at 100 °C, as indicated in Figure 4b.

Now that we've reviewed phases of matter in general, we're in a good position to focus more closely on gases and solutions.

2. Gases

The **gas phase** is particularly important for the MCAT because gases play a major role in physiology, most notably in the form of oxygen and carbon dioxide gas, which are central to the cycle of respiration. Additionally, some gases, such as nitric oxide (NO), are important signaling molecules.

Since gases are compressible, their density is affected by pressure and temperature. This means that we have to specify certain pressure and temperature conditions to compare density (or any related parameter) in a meaningful way. In general, for the MCAT, questions about gases will specify conditions of standard temperature and pressure (STP), at which the temperature is equal to 0°C (273 K), and pressure is 1 atmosphere (1 atm = 760 mmHg = 760 torr). For a more detailed discussion of pressure, including a formal definition and a review of the various units used for pressure, see Chapter 5 of the Physics textbook.

At STP, one mole of any gas has a volume of 22.4 L. In general, one mole of any gas at a given temperature and pressure will have a constant volume, as we will see in more detail in the equations presented later in this section. Thus, equal volumes of any two gases under the same conditions will always contain the same number of gas particles. This generalization is sometimes known as **Avogadro's law**, which states that the volume divided by moles is constant.

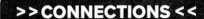

>> CONNECTIONS <<

Chapter 5 of Physics

When studying the behavior of gases, certain assumptions are used to model gases more elegantly. In particular, on the MCAT, you will generally encounter **ideal gases** unless specified otherwise. An ideal—or theoretical—gas follows the parameters of the **kinetic molecular theory**, which states that:

> Gases are made up of atoms or molecules that are in continuous, random motion.

> The average kinetic energy of gas particles is directly proportional to temperature; therefore, all gas particles will have the same kinetic energy at a given temperature.

> The gas particles have no volume (more specifically, negligible volume compared to their container).

> Gas particles do not exert attractive or repulsive forces on each other, although they do exert force on the walls of the container.

> All gas particle collisions with one another and with the walls of the container are elastic, meaning that overall kinetic energy is conserved.

In reality, no gases obey these rules. This is why they are called ideal! However, these parameters allow us to predict the behavior of gases and ascertain the extent to which a gas deviates from ideal behavior. Gases deviate from ideal behavior at high pressures and low temperatures and behave most ideally at low pressures and high temperatures.

There's an easy way to remember these relationships. Imagine cooling and compressing a gas, forcing it into liquid form. You can therefore conceptualize liquids as the "ultimate non-ideal gas" where intermolecular forces become significant. Thus, the parameters that tend to favor condensation into a liquid also favor real, non-ideal gas behavior. Conversely, the more diffuse gas molecules become—at high temperatures and low pressures—the less they interact and the more likely they are to conform to ideal behavior.

The relationships between the pressure, volume, and temperature of an ideal gas are described by several important equations called gas laws. Note that you should *always* express temperature in Kelvin for gas law equations. To convert temperature in Celsius to the Kelvin (K) scale, simply add 273. Water freezes at 0°C and 273 K, and boiling occurs at 100°C or 373 K. The weaker the intermolecular forces, the lower the freezing and boiling points. The relationship between Celsius and Fahrenheit is $°F = \frac{9}{5}°C + 32$, although you can approximate by doubling the Celsius temperature rather than multiplying by $\frac{9}{5}$. For more details about temperature scales, see Chapter 4 of the Physics textbook. As discussed in that chapter, it is more useful to be aware of the more significant Fahrenheit and Celsius values (e.g., freezing point of water = 0°C and 32°F, boiling point of water = 100°C and 212°F, body temperature = 37°C and 98.6°F, room temperature = 20-25°C or 68-77°F).

The first gas law we'll discuss is **Boyle's law**, which states that the pressure and volume of a gas are inversely proportional at a constant temperature, illustrated in equations 2A and 2B.

>> CONNECTIONS <<

Chapter 4 of Physics

Equation 2A. $\qquad$ $P_1 V_1 = P_2 V_2$

Equation 2B. $\qquad$ $PV = \text{constant}$

In Equation 2A, P_1 and V_1 represent the pressure and volume of the gas in one state, and P_2 and V_2 represent the pressure and volume in another, and the number of moles of gas and the temperature remain constant. This makes logical sense: by shrinking the volume of the container, the pressure of the gas inside will increase since gas particles must be packed more closely and will collide with the walls of the container more frequently. Alternatively, if we increase the volume of the container, the pressure will decrease as particles have more space and collide with the walls of the container less frequently. Equation 2B provides another way of thinking about this generalization: the pressure of a gas multiplied by its volume forms a constant at a given temperature. Be sure to understand that Equation 2A and 2B are two ways of formulating the same insight.

Charles's law states that the volume and temperature of a gas are directly proportional under constant pressure with the number of moles of gas also constant:

Equation 3A. $\qquad$ $\dfrac{V_1}{T_1} = \dfrac{V_2}{T_2}$

Equation 3B. $\qquad$ $\dfrac{V}{T} = \text{constant}$

As with Boyle's law, Charles's law can be written in the two equivalent forms shown in Equations 3A and 3B. Again, this relationship should make logical sense: if we heat a gas-filled balloon, the gas molecules gain kinetic energy and expand, increasing the volume of the balloon. To put it simply, increasing temperature will increase volume, and decreasing temperature will decrease volume.

Gay-Lussac's law states that at constant volume and number of moles, the pressure of a gas is proportional to its temperature.

Equation 4A. $\qquad$ $\dfrac{P_1}{T_1} = \dfrac{P_2}{T_2}$

Equation 4B. $\qquad$ $\dfrac{P}{T} = \text{constant}$

This relationship makes sense, because at higher pressure molecules collide more frequently, which produces an increase in temperature.

Synthesizing these relationships yields one of the most important equations in all of chemistry, the **ideal gas law**:

Equation 4. $\qquad$ $PV = nRT$

In this equation, n is the number of moles of a gas, and R is the universal gas constant (0.08206 L·atm/K·mol or 8.314 J/K·mol). The ideal gas law accounts for the addition or removal of molar amounts of gas. The ideal gas law can be tested on the MCAT in two major ways. One way is numerically, much like the "plug and chug" variety you may have seen in chemistry class. If you encounter such a problem on test day, you have two basic tasks. First, ensure that the units of each parameter in the ideal gas law match the units of R that you use (typically 0.0826 L·atm/K·mol), and second, you must carry out the calculation quickly and accurately, using scientific notation and/or estimations to facilitate speed and accuracy. The second way the ideal gas law can be tested is conceptually or proportionally. For example, such a problem might ask what would happen to the temperature of a gas if its volume were tripled and pressure halved.

The ideal gas law can be modified to model the behavior of non-ideal gases in a form known as the **Van der Waals equation**. We need to account for two basic factors: (1) the volume taken up by the molecules of the gas and (2) the attractive forces experienced among the gas molecules. The first factor is easy; the volume (*b*) of n moles of gas molecules is subtracted from the volume (V) of their container; the "V" term of the ideal gas law then becomes V - nb. The second factor accounts for the fact that the measured pressure is lower than the ideal pressure because of intermolecular attractive forces. This means that we must add a correction factor to simulate ideal behavior. Incorporating the modified terms for pressure and volume into the ideal gas law gives the van der Waals equation, shown in Equation 5.

MCAT STRATEGY >>>

Realistically speaking, the Van der Waals equation should not be high priority, although it is testable content. You should understand qualitatively that ideal gases are an approximation, that lower temperature and higher pressure make gases behave less ideally, and that non-ideal gas behavior can be modeled. That said, it is quite unlikely that you will be asked a question where success depends on your ability to complete a full calculation with Equation 5.

Equation 5.
$$\left(P + \frac{an^2}{V^2}\right)(V - nb) = nRT$$

All the above material on gases has been based on the assumption that we're dealing with a single gas. However, in real life, it is very common for gases to be mixed, as in the air that we breathe, which is made up of about 78% nitrogen and 21% oxygen, with small amounts of other gases and water vapor. There is some terminology relating to such situations that you need to be aware of for the MCAT. The first is the **mole fraction** (X_{gas}), which refers to the number of moles of a given gas divided by the total moles of gas in the mixture:

Equation 6.
$$x_{gas} = \frac{n_{gas}}{n_{total}}$$

Based on the previous discussion, when we have a relationship defined in terms of moles of a gas, we can relate that to other quantities, such as pressure, volume, or temperature, using the ideal gas law. Such a derivation is shown in Equation 7.

Equation 7.
$$x_{gas} = \frac{n_{gas}}{n_{total}} = \frac{P_{gas} V / RT}{P_{total} V / RT} = \frac{P_{gas}}{P_{total}}$$

This means that at constant volume and temperature, each gas in a mixture only contributes to part of the pressure of the whole. Based on this realization, we can define **partial pressure** as the pressure that a gas in a mixture would exert if it took up the same volume by itself; and corresponds to P_{gas} in Equation 7.

The relationship between the mole fraction and the partial pressure we derived in Equation 7 can be rearranged more typically as follows:

Equation 8.
$$P_{gas} = X_{gas} P_{total}$$

This equation states that the partial pressure of a gas equals the total pressure of the mixture multiplied by the mole fraction of that gas. Implicit in this is a relationship known as **Dalton's law**, which states that the total pressure of a mixture of gases equals the sum of the partial pressures of its components. Thus, for example, the total pressure of air is the sum of the partial pressures of oxygen, nitrogen, water vapor, and all other component gases.

3. Solutions and Solubility

In the final section of this chapter, we'll explore solutions. **Solutions** are homogeneous mixtures containing particles that are evenly distributed throughout the solution. Gases, liquids, solids—and even multiple phases!—can be in solution. From a theoretical point of view, this is an important point to recognize. Technically speaking, the gas mixtures we talked about in section 2 were solutions, and metallic alloys (such as steel) can be thought of as solutions made up of solids. However, on the MCAT, solutions almost always contain solids dissolved in liquids, or liquid solutions such as ethanol and water.

Dissolution occurs when solutes are dissolved in a solvent such as a liquid or gas. So how can we predict whether one substance will dissolve in another? Solute-solvent interactions are key to understanding this process. For example, hydrophilic substances are molecules that contain polar or charged groups and are capable of dissolving in water and other hydrophilic solvents, whereas hydrophobic substances are nonpolar molecules that are capable of dissolving in nonpolar, hydrophobic solvents. An easy way to remember this phenomenon is to recognize that "**like dissolves like**"—solutes will dissolve in solvents with similar properties.

As solute is added to a solvent, the solution is considered saturated when the maximum amount of solute that can be dissolved has been added. Upon heating, more solute can be dissolved in the solution, and then upon slowly cooling the solution, the same concentration of solute will remain dissolved in what is now a **supersaturated solution**. Crystals can form in supersaturated solutions with the addition of a seed crystal, which creates a nucleation site for solute to precipitate. This process is called **crystallization** when the product precipitates in crystalline form.

The concentration of a solution can be expressed in multiple ways. Solute concentrations are frequently expressed in terms of **molarity** (M), which is the number of moles of solute per liter of solution:

Equation 9.
$$\text{molarity (M)} = \frac{\text{moles of solute}}{\text{liters of solution}} = \frac{\text{mol}}{\text{L}}$$

In biological processes, it is often the case that very small amounts of a substance are present in a solution, so you may encounter millimolar (mmol), micromolar (μm), and nanomolar (nm) concentrations, which simply refer to 1×10^{-3} M, 1×10^{-6} M, and 1×10^{-9} M concentrations, respectively. In contrast, **molality** (m) is a measure of concentration that represents the number of moles of solute per kilogram of solvent:

Equation 10.
$$\text{molality (m)} = \frac{\text{moles of solute}}{\text{kilograms of solvent}} = \frac{\text{mol}}{\text{kg}}$$

Molality is less common on the MCAT than molarity, but you should be aware of it anyway. Interestingly, molality and molarity values tend to be similar for aqueous solutions with relatively small amounts of solute. This is because one liter of water weighs one kilogram, and therefore the difference between "liters of solution" and "kilograms of water" only becomes meaningful when there is enough solute present to materially affect the volume of the solution.

Other units of concentration that are important for biochemical systems are ppm and ppt. The first, ppm, is parts per million, or mg/L, whereas ppt is parts per thousand, or g/L. A normal saline solution, for example, is 9 g/L, or 9 ppt.

On a conceptually similar note, some properties of solutions are related to the total number of solute particles present in the solution (regardless of whether they are the same or different compounds). These are known as **colligative properties**. There are four colligative properties that you must be familiar with for the MCAT: (1) vapor pressure reduction, (2) boiling point elevation, (3) freezing point reduction, and (4) osmotic pressure.

The addition of solutes reduces the vapor pressure of a solvent in a relationship proportional to molal solute concentration. In other words, a nonvolatile solute decreases the concentration of solvent that exists in the gas phase because the solute reduces solvent evaporation. **Vapor pressure reduction** is expressed by **Raoult's law**:

Equation 13.
$$P = X_A P_A^{\,O}$$

In Raoult's law, P is the vapor pressure of the solution, X_A is the mole fraction of the solvent, and $P_A^{\,\circ}$ is the vapor pressure of the pure solvent. Raoult's law often feels obscure to students, but the underlying idea is fairly intuitive. Imagine the surface of an aqueous solution with a lot of solutes in it. Some of the solutes will be at the surface of the solution, and the space they take up is unavailable for the liquid-gas phase transition that is at the core of vapor pressure.

Reducing the vapor pressure of a solution is equivalent to increasing the boiling point since the boiling point is defined as the temperature at which the vapor pressure equals the atmospheric pressure. **Boiling point elevation** can therefore be calculated as follows:

Equation 14.
$$\Delta T_b = i K_b m$$

In this equation, ΔT_b is the boiling point elevation, i is the ionization factor (also known as the van 't Hoff factor); this is a measure of the number of moles of particles formed in solution per mole of solute, K_b is the boiling point elevation constant (which is specific for each solvent), and m is the molal solute concentration. A substance such as glucose has a van't Hoff factor of one in aqueous solution (it does not dissociate), whereas NaCl has a van't Hoff factor of two (one mole completely dissociates into two moles of ions in aqueous solution).

Nonvolatile solutes also decrease the freezing point of solutions. **Freezing point depression** can be calculated as follows:

Equation 15.
$$\Delta T_f = i K_f m$$

In this equation, ΔT_f is the freezing point depression, i is the van 't Hoff ionization factor, K_f is the solvent's freezing-point depression constant, and m is the molal solute concentration. A key point to note here is that the equation for freezing point depression is the same as that for boiling point elevation, with different subscripts. The formal similarity between equations 14 and 15 works in your favor to some extent, but also be sure to know that boiling point is *elevated* and freezing point is *depressed*.

Our final colligative property, **osmotic pressure**, relates to the principle of osmosis, the net flow of solvent through a semipermeable membrane from an area of higher solvent concentration to an area of lower solvent concentration. Eventually, the solution concentrations equalize. Let's consider, for example, the movement of water across a

MCAT STRATEGY >>>

It may be helpful to link boiling point elevation and freezing point depression to real-world applications, such as why salt is commonly applied to roads before it snows. If the freezing point is lower, it is more likely that the road will have liquid water instead of potentially dangerous snow or ice accumulation.

porous membrane that divides a beaker into two parts (Figure 5). If the right side contains a low concentration of solvent and the left side a high concentration, water will diffuse through the membrane from the dilute solution to the more concentrated solution on the right via osmosis.

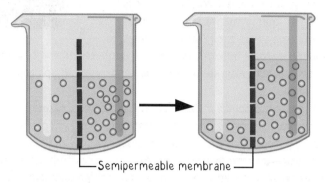

Figure 5. Osmosis through a semipermeable membrane showing the direction of solvent flow

Osmosis is important in biological contexts because the plasma membrane of eukaryotic cells is a semipermeable membrane through which osmosis can occur. The entirety of Chapter 11 in the Biochemistry textbook is dedicated to biological membranes, which reflects the importance of membranes for physiology. Osmosis is also discussed there in a context more specific to physiological functioning.

As suggested by Figure 5, at some point, the flow of water through the semipermeable membrane will stop once the concentrations of solute have become equalized and the pressure on the right side is high enough to prevent further osmosis from occurring. This pressure required to prevent osmosis is called osmotic pressure, Π, and is given by the following equation:

Equation 16. $$\Pi = iMRT$$

>> CONNECTIONS <<

Chapter 11 of Biochemistry

Equation 16 is similar to the ideal gas equation, $PV = nRT$. If you were to take the ideal gas equation and divide through by V, the (n/V) term would appear on the right side, making the equation $P = (n/V)RT$. Moles divided by volume is molarity M, so the equation becomes $P = MRT$. We then use Π to indicate that this is the *osmotic* pressure, not the pressure of a gas and use the van 't Hoff factor, i, to account for the number of dissociated ions in solution. In both the ideal gas and osmotic pressure equations, R is the ideal gas constant, and T is the absolute temperature.

At this point, we've put a fair amount of effort into thinking about what happens when we already have a solution, but we also need to explore making solutions, in particular the extent to which various substances will dissolve in a solvent. This is known as **solubility**. Solubility equilibrium occurs when a solute dissolves at the same rate as it precipitates out of solution. For instance, the dissociation reaction of solid magnesium chloride to give dissolved magnesium and chloride ions is represented by the equilibrium $MgCl_2(s) \rightleftharpoons Mg^{2+}(aq) + 2\ Cl^-(aq)$. For dissolution equilibria, we can define an equilibrium constant that is known as the solubility product constant (K_{sp}); in our example, $K_{sp} = [Mg^{2+}][Cl^-]^2$. Note that this is simply the equilibrium constant for the dissociation reaction, remembering that solids and solvents are not included in equilibrium constants.

>> CONNECTIONS <<

Chapter 4 of Chemistry

When the concentrations of the dissolved species are not known to be at equilibrium, we refer to this expression (in our example, $[Mg^{2+}][Cl^-]^2$) as the ion product Q_{sp}. Conceptually, this is the exact same idea as the reaction quotient Q_{eq} that you saw in Chapter 4—that is, we're analyzing the relative concentrations of products and reactants in the same way that we do for K_{sp} or K_{eq}, but the reaction is not at equilibrium.

A high K_{sp} value means that a substance will readily dissolve in a solution (usually water for the MCAT), while a very low K_{sp} value means that it is essentially insoluble. K_{sp} values can vary tremendously; for example, magnesium chloride ($MgCl_2$) is highly *soluble* and has a K_{sp} of nearly 740, while aluminum hydroxide, $Al(OH)_3$, a highly *insoluble* compound, is 3×10^{-34}. An important point to understand here is that solubility encompasses a wide range of values, although we often talk about compounds either as 'soluble' or 'insoluble'. The solubility product allows us to capture some important dynamics associated with solubility. One of the most important of these phenomena is known as the **common ion effect**.

Consider silver chloride, AgCl, which is only slightly soluble in water ($K_{sp} = 1.77 \times 10^{-10}$). Let's first consider what this value would imply for dissolving AgCl in pure water. We can write the solubility product as follows: $K_{sp} = 1.77\times10^{-10}$ $= [Ag^+][Cl^-]$. Then, we can substitute x for the concentration of the ions:

$$1.77 \times 10^{-10} = [x][x]$$
$$1.77 \times 10^{-10} = [x]^2$$
$$[x] = 1.3 \times 10^{-5}\,M$$

We have just found that $1.3 \times 10^{-5}\,M$ is the maximum concentration of AgCl that we can have suspended in solution before some will start to precipitate out. Now, let's imagine that we dissolve AgCl in a solution of 0.5 M NaCl. In this case, the $[Cl^-]$ term will be [0.5 M] because the amount of chloride ion that comes from AgCl is comparatively insignificant. The Ag^+ concentration can now be calculated as follows:

$$K_{sp} = 1.77 \times 10^{-10} = [Ag^+][Cl^-]$$
$$1.77 \times 10^{-10} = [x][0.5]$$
$$[x] = 3.54 \times 10^{-10}\,M$$

This shows that *dramatically* less—to be precise, 50,000 times less—AgCl will dissolve now that we have flooded the reaction environment with $[Cl^-]$. This is the common ion effect in action! Theoretically, you could drive the dissolution reaction by removing Cl^- from solution, which would push the equilibrium of the dissociation reaction to favor the dissolution of AgCl according to Le Châtelier's principle.

It is important not to confuse solubility with ionization, although it can be easy to do so because examples like the dissolution of $MgCl_2(s)$ into its component ions are very common in discussions of solubility. Such substances are called electrolytes because charged cations and anions are capable of conducting electricity in solution. The more readily a substance ionizes in solution—for example, strong acids and ionic compounds with high K_{sp} values—the stronger the electrolyte. However, it is possible for molecules composed of covalent bonds that do not readily ionize in solution to be very soluble. A classic example of this is glucose, although many biologically relevant molecules would also fall into this category. These molecules are referred to as nonelectrolytes.

To some extent, it is possible to make predictions about whether a substance will be soluble in water under various conditions. In particular, it's worth making a note of the effects of temperature and pressure. Some of the effects of temperature are familiar to anyone who's ever tried (unsuccessfully) to dissolve sugar in a cup of iced coffee—that is, higher temperatures favor the solubility of most compounds. There are some exceptions to this, though. For ionic compounds, this has to do with whether dissolution is exothermic or endothermic. Most dissolution reactions in water are endothermic, meaning that increased heat favors them, but some are exothermic, in which case the opposite effect can be expected.

> **>> CONNECTIONS <<**
>
> Chapter 4 of Chemistry

Gases, in contrast, are more soluble at lower temperatures. This is because higher temperatures provide gases with more kinetic energy that they can use to escape the solution. Additionally, higher pressure favors the solubility of gases. A way you can think about this is that the ideal storage conditions for a bottle of soda (or your carbonated beverage of choice)—that is, cold and unopened (at high pressure)—help carbon dioxide remain in solution.

Finally, some trends help us predict whether ionic compounds will be soluble in water. These are presented below in Table 1.

SOLUBLE IONIC COMPOUNDS
Alkali metals (Li^+, Na^+, K^+, Rb^+, Cs^+, Fr^+) and NH_4^+ Nitrates (NO_3^-), acetates (CH_3COO^-), and chlorates (ClO_3^-) Halides (Cl^-, Br^-, I^-) except compounds containing Ag^+, Pb^{2+}, or Hg_2^{2+} Sulfates (SO_4^{2-}) except compounds containing Ca^{2+}, Sr^{2+}, Ba^{2+}, Ag^+, or Pb^{2+}
INSOLUBLE IONIC COMPOUNDS
Carbonates (CO_3^{2-}), phosphates (PO_4^{3-}), sulfides (S^{2-}), and sulfites (SO_3^{2-}) except compounds containing alkali metals or NH_4^+ Hydroxides (OH^-) and metal oxides except compounds containing alkali metals, Ca^{2+}, Sr^{2+} or Ba^{2+}

Table 1. Solubility rules for ionic substances in water

MCAT STRATEGY >>>

The effects of temperature on the solubility of solids are yet another example of how Le Châtelier's principle appears again and again in chemistry. Recall that for endothermic reactions, heat can be thought of as a 'reactant,' while for exothermic reactions, heat is a 'product.' A hot environment can be thought of as having more heat on the reactant side, which will therefore favor endothermic reactions and disfavor exothermic reactions.

MCAT STRATEGY >>>

It is unlikely that the MCAT will test you on the details of the solubility rules, but you should familiarize yourself with some of the general trends of the table, like how alkali metals tend to form strongly soluble compounds.

4. Must-Knows

> Phases of matter: solid (fixed volume and shape), liquid (fixed volume, flows to the shape of its container), gas (variable volume, variable shape).
>> — Strong intermolecular interactions favor solids (vs. liquids) and liquids (vs. gases). High temperature and low pressure favor gases (vs. solids/liquids); low temperature and high pressure favor solids.
> Adding heat changes the phase:
>> — Heat of fusion = heat necessary to convert from solid to liquid.
>> — Heat of vaporization = heat necessary to convert from liquid to gas.
>> — At phase changes, temperature remains constant while heat is being added.
>> — Between phase changes, adding heat increases temperature ($q = mc\Delta T$).
> Phase diagrams: generally, solid → liquid → gas in clockwise order (SLUG).
>> — Triple point: solid, liquid, and gas are in equilibrium.
>> — Critical point: end of liquid-gas interface (beyond critical point matter is a supercritical fluid).
> Assumptions of kinetic molecular theory for ideal gases:
>> — (1) average KE is proportional to T.
>> — (2) particles have no volume.
>> — (3) particles exert no forces on each other. Non-ideal behavior is found at low T and high P.
> Ideal gas law: $PV = nRT$.
>> — Avogadro's law: V/n is constant (1 mole occupies 22.4 L at STP).
>> — Boyle's law: PV = constant ($P_1V_1 = P_2V_2$).
>> — Charles's law: V/T = constant ($V_1/T_1 = V_2/T_2$).
> Partial pressure: the pressure that a gas in a mixture would exert if it took up the same volume by itself.
>> — Dalton's law: partial pressures of components add up to form total pressure of a mixture; $P_{gas} = X_{gas}P_{total}$.
> Solutions: units include molarity (mol/L), molality (mol/kg$_{solv}$), ppm (mg/L), and ppt (g/L).
> Colligative properties: depend solely on number of solute particles in solution:
>> — Vapor pressure reduction: Raoult's law $P = X_aP_A^O$.
>> — Boiling point elevation: $\Delta T_b = iK_bm$.
>> — Freezing point depression: $\Delta T_f = iK_fm$.
>> — Osmotic pressure: $\Pi = iMRT$.
> Solubility constant: for AB(s) → aA(aq) + bB(aq), $K_{sp} = [A]^a[B]^b$.
>> — High solubility constant = high solubility.
>> — Solubility constant is an *equilibrium constant* (i.e., does not change, but defined relative to a given temperature); Q (ion product) is same expression when mixture is not at equilibrium.
> Common ion effect: presence of one ion already in solution will decrease the solubility of a compound containing that ion (i.e., very little AgCl will dissolve in a solution of NaCl because [Cl⁻] is already high).
> Key solubility rules:
>> — Soluble:
>>> • Alkali metals (Li⁺, Na⁺, K⁺, Rb⁺, Cs⁺, Fr⁺) and NH_4^+.
>>> • Nitrates (NO_3^-), chlorates (ClO_3^-), acetate (CH_3COO^-).
>>> • Halides (Cl⁻, Br⁻, I⁻) except compounds containing Ag⁺, Pb²⁺, or Hg_2^{2+}.
>>> • Sulfates (SO_4^{2-}) except compounds containing Ca²⁺, Sr²⁺, Ba²⁺, Ag⁺ or Pb²⁺.
>> — Insoluble:
>>> • Carbonates (CO_3^{2-}), phosphates (PO_4^{3-}), sulfide (S²⁻), and sulfites (SO_3^{2-}) except compounds containing alkali metals or NH_4^+.
>>> • Hydroxides (OH⁻) and metal oxides except compounds containing alkali metals, Ca²⁺, Sr²⁺, or Ba²⁺.

End of Chapter Practice

The best MCAT practice is realistic, with a focus on identifying steps for further improvement. For those reasons, we recommend completing practice questions in an online setting that simulates the real MCAT interface, and taking advantage of advanced analytic features to help you determine how best to move forward in your MCAT study journey.

With that in mind, online end-of-chapter questions for Biology, Biochemistry, Chemistry + Organic Chemistry, Physics, and Psychology/Sociology are available through your Blueprint MCAT account.

As a further supplement, given the importance of active learning for effective studying, we also suggest that you consult the Must-Knows as a basis for creating a study sheet, in which you list out key terms and test your ability to briefly summarize them.

This page left intentionally blank.

This page left intentionally blank.

Kinetics

0. Introduction

Kinetics is the branch of chemistry that deals with the rate of reactions, which is a biologically relevant topic because an organism must complete metabolically important reactions quickly to function. This chapter will review the mechanisms of chemical reactions, discuss the effect of catalysts, describe rates and rate laws, and compare kinetics and equilibrium, an essential distinction to master for the MCAT.

1. Mechanisms

Let's start our analysis of **kinetics** by thinking about what it means for a reaction to take place. For a reaction to occur, the reactants must collide with each other in the correct spatial orientation and with sufficient kinetic energy to overcome a threshold which is known as the **activation energy** (E_a) of a reaction. The rate of a reaction corresponds to how many such collisions take place over a given unit of time. The **Arrhenius equation**, shown below, defines k, the reaction **rate constant**, which signifies the frequency of collisions leading to a reaction.

Equation 1.
$$k = Ae^{-E_a/RT}$$

In this equation, k is the rate constant, and A is the frequency factor, corresponding to the frequency of collisions between reactants in proper spatial orientations. E_a is the activation energy, R is the ideal gas constant, and T is the temperature in kelvins. Since A is a constant, e is a mathematical constant, and R is a physical constant, the rate constant can only meaningfully be affected by the activation energy and the temperature. Larger values of E_a make $-(E_a/RT)$ more negative, demonstrating an inverse relationship between the activation energy and the reaction rate. The idea that lower activation energies correspond to faster reaction rates is fundamental for kinetics on the MCAT. In contrast, temperature directly relates to reaction rate; higher values of T make E_a/RT smaller, meaning that $-(E_a/RT)$ is less negative or larger. Chemically, higher temperatures increase the overall collision rate and the proportion of collisions with enough kinetic energy to exceed the activation energy. Thus, there are two ways to speed up a reaction: reduce the activation energy or increase the temperature. According to the Arrhenius equation, a reaction rate will double for every 10°C rise in temperature. However, the body can't raise the temperature significantly, so as we will see in physiology and biochemistry, biological systems use enzymes (biological catalysts) to regulate reaction rates by reducing the activation energy.

The Arrhenius equation, gives a reaction rate constant, other parameters can affect a reaction rate. The concentration of the reactants is directly incorporated into the rate law of a reaction. This is discussed in Section 3. Additionally, the reaction rate of gaseous reactions can be affected by pressure; higher pressures increase the reaction rate for essentially the same reason that higher temperatures do (i.e., more pressure means more effective collisions). The rate of reactions in solution can be affected by properties of the solvent, but the details vary among reactions.

Reactants that collide with sufficient energy in the proper orientation form a transient **transition complex**. For example, in the reaction $H_2(g) + Cl_2(g) \rightarrow 2HCl(g)$, there is an extremely brief period in which the covalent bonds in the reactants begin to weaken, and the bonds in the products begin to form. In organic chemistry, the five-coordinate intermediate that is characteristic of S_{N2} reactions is a transition state. The activation energy, E_a, refers to the energy necessary to reach the transition state, as shown in Figure 1. Transition complexes are not isolable and occur at the highest-energy point of the reaction.

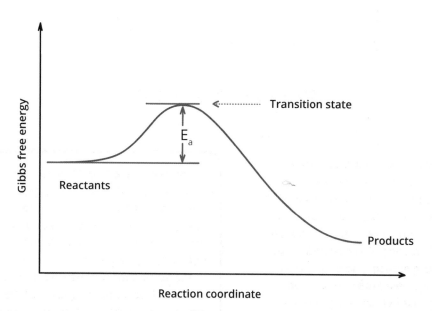

Figure 1. Transition complex.

Reactions that occur in multiple steps can be summed to give the overall reactants and products. For example, consider the reaction $NO_2(g) + CO(g) \rightarrow NO(g) + CO_2(g)$. This reaction proceeds in the following two steps, each of which is an elementary reaction:

$$\text{Step 1: } NO_2(g) + NO_2(g) \rightarrow NO(g) + NO_3(g) \qquad \text{(slow)}$$

$$\text{Step 2: } NO_3(g) + CO(g) \rightarrow CO_2(g) + NO(g) \qquad \text{(fast)}$$

Note that $NO_3(g)$ can be canceled when combining these elementary reactions. In the overall reaction, $NO_3(g)$ acts as a reaction intermediate, an isolable species that is the product of an elementary reaction and is a reactant in another. It is transformed during the reaction process. A carbocation, for example, is a reaction intermediate that can be stabilized by solvent interactions and goes on to form product. Step 1 is slow, and step 2 is fast, indicating that each step can be considered a distinct reaction with its own individual reaction rate. A reaction with multiple steps can go forward no faster than its slowest step, which means that the slowest step is referred to as the rate-limiting step of a reaction.

Reaction coordinate diagrams are used to illustrate how the energy states of a reaction proceed over time, as shown for a single-step reaction in Figure 2. The x-axis of a reaction coordinate diagram indicates time, and the y-axis indicates Gibbs free energy. The difference between the initial energy and the energy of the transition-state complex is the activation energy (E_a) of the reaction, and the difference between the free energy of the initial reactants and the final products is ΔG. In Figure 2, the products are at a lower energy state than the reactants, so ΔG is less than zero. The reaction is **exergonic**, meaning that it is spontaneous and energy is released. If $\Delta G > 0$, the reaction is **endergonic**, meaning that it is non-spontaneous and energy is absorbed. Recall that ΔG is a state function, so it is only defined by the energy of the products minus the energy of the reactants. In contrast, E_a is a kinetics quantity, which is used to determine the reaction mechanism. Only kinetics describes the stepwise mechanism of a reaction, or how a reaction occurs. In contrast, thermodynamics tells us whether or not a reaction will occur.

> **MCAT STRATEGY >>>**
>
> Be able to distinguish reaction intermediates and transition states. It may be helpful to think of transition states as theoretical constructs used to explain how a reaction proceeds. As such, they're not a "real" substance—you can't isolate them. In contrast, reaction intermediates are at least in principle isolable, although they may be quite reactive and therefore unstable.

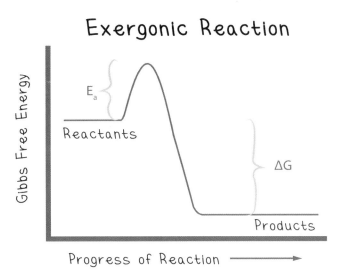

Figure 2. Single-step reaction coordinate diagram

It is crucial for the MCAT to distinguish between kinetics and thermodynamics. For instance, the oxidation of iron in air (i.e., the formation of rust) is spontaneous but occurs quite slowly.

A reaction coordinate diagram can also be used to illustrate reactions that occur in multiple steps, as shown below in Figure 3. Such reaction diagrams can be used to evaluate ΔG of the overall reaction, or be used to illustrate the kinetcs of the reaction as reflected by the presence of two transition states with two distinct E_a values. In Figure 3, the first step is the rate determining step—it has the higher E_a.

> **>> CONNECTIONS <<**
>
> Chapter 12 of Biochemistry

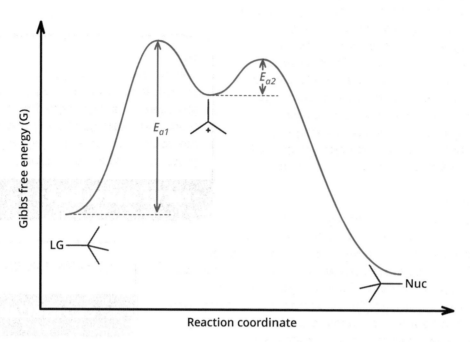

Figure 3. Two-step reaction coordinate diagram showing a carbocation intermediate which then goes on to form product

It is important to recognize that a reaction coordinate diagram can be viewed as occurring from reactants to products or from products to reactants. If viewed from products to reactants, the reaction depicted in Figure 3 is endergonic, and the highest energy barrier corresponds to the first step in the reverse process. Notice that this E_{a1} is substantially higher than E_{a1} for the forward reaction, so there is a significant energy barrier that must be overcome for the reverse reaction to occur.

2. Catalysts

Catalysts are substances that increase the rate of a reaction by reducing its activation energy.

Common physical mechanisms through which catalysts accomplish this include:

> Stabilizing the transition state
> Weakening bonds within the reactants
> Changing the orientation of the reactants to facilitate effective collisions
> Increasing the frequency of collisions
> Donating electron density to the reactants

Effectively, this means that catalysts provide an alternative reaction mechanism. The effect of a catalyst on an exergonic reaction is shown in Figure 4.

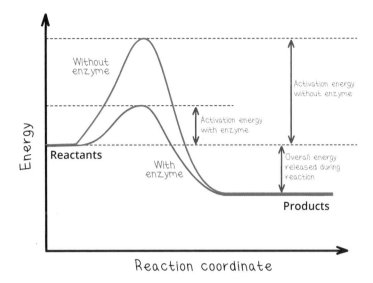

Figure 4. Reaction coordinates for a catalyzed versus uncatalyzed exergonic reaction

Catalysts do not affect any thermodynamic parameters of the overall reaction. As shown in Figure 4, the ΔG values for the catalyzed and uncatalyzed reactions are identical (as are the ΔH and ΔS terms). This means that catalysts cannot make thermodynamically unfavorable and nonspontaneous reactions favorable and spontaneous. Moreover, catalysts are not consumed in the reaction.

In heterogeneous catalysis, the catalyst is in a different phase from the reactants. Typically, the catalyst is solid, and the reactants are liquids or gases. In such cases, the reactants must adsorb onto the catalyst for it to be effective. Since this depends on the surface area of the catalyst, it may be necessary to grind it or find other ways of optimizing the surface area. An example is the Haber synthesis of ammonia ($N_2(g) + 3\,H_2(g) \rightarrow 2NH_3(g)$), which is performed in industrial contexts under high temperature and pressure with ground iron catalysts. Homogeneous catalysis occurs when the catalyst and reactants are in the same phase. Many biologically relevant reactions involve homogeneous catalysis in aqueous solution, with examples including any organic reactions in which H^+ or OH^- function as a catalyst.

The catalysis of biological reactions is crucial for the function of organisms because physiological functioning depends both on whether a reaction occurs at all and whether it occurs in a timely manner. Proteins that catalyze biological reactions are known as enzymes. Since enzymes play a fundamental role in regulating metabolic processes, they are one of the highest-yield biochemistry topics on the MCAT. Although enzymes are covered in more detail in Chapter 3 of the Biochemistry textbook, a thorough understanding of the fundamentals of kinetics is important for properly understanding enzyme function.

MCAT STRATEGY >>>

The fact that catalysts do not affect the thermodynamic parameters of a reaction is a perennial MCAT favorite. No matter how a question is phrased, the *only* correct thing about the effects of a catalyst is that it increases the reaction rate by reducing the activation energy of the reaction. Anything else is a trap.

>> CONNECTIONS <<

Chapter 3 of Biochemistry

MCAT STRATEGY >>>

Since enzymes are biological catalysts, all the points we made about MCAT strategy regarding catalysts apply to enzymes too. Enzymes never affect the thermodynamic constants of a reaction and can never turn a nonspontaneous reaction into a spontaneous one.

3. Rates and Rate Laws

A reaction rate describes how fast reactants are consumed and how fast products form. This is an experimentally determined value that is expressed in terms of the appearance or disappearance of a concentration per unit time. The reaction of sucrose with water to produce ethanol and carbon dioxide illustrates the process for determining a reaction rate:

$$C_{12}H_{22}O_{11} \, (aq) + H_2O \, (l) \rightarrow 4C_2H_5OH \, (aq) + 4CO_2(g)$$

The reaction rate can be expressed in terms of the disappearance of sucrose or water, or of the appearance of ethanol or CO_2. Concentrations that decrease with time are negative, and those that increase are positive. Concentrations are normalized to a molecular or molar level by dividing the concentration by its stoichiometric coefficient. Units are M/s unless otherwise specified. Here are expressions for the reaction rate of the reaction described:

$$\text{rate} = \frac{-\Delta[\text{sucrose}]}{\Delta t} = \frac{-\Delta[H_2O]}{\Delta t} = \frac{1/4\Delta[\text{EtOH}]}{\Delta t} = \frac{1/4\Delta[CO_2]}{\Delta t}$$

The **rate law** of a reaction is given as a function of the rate constant, which does not change under a given set of conditions and is k discussed above (see Equation 1 for the Arrhenius equation), and the concentration of reactants other than solids and solvents. It is an expression that describes the relationships between reactant rates and reactant concentrations in a chemical reaction. A rate law can be directly written from an elementary step, but otherwise it is determined experimentally. The rate law of a general reaction of the form $aA + bB \rightarrow cC + dD$ is given in Equation 2.

Equation 2. $\qquad\qquad\qquad\qquad \text{rate} = k[A]^x[B]^y$

The rate itself has units of M/s or mol/L·s unless otherwise indicated. In the health sciences, for example, a rate might have units of M/min. [A] and [B] are concentrations of the reactants in units of M or mol/L. The exponents x and y must be experimentally determined; they do *not* correspond to the stoichiometric coefficients a and b in the reaction formula. The **order of a reaction** is defined by the sum of the exponents in the rate law; here, these are given as x and y, although a third reactant $[C]^z$ could theoretically be present but have no impact on the rate. If the exponents sum to zero, the reaction is **zero-order**. If the exponents of the reactants sum to 1, the reaction is **first-order**. If they sum to 2, it is **second-order**. If they sum to 3, it is **third-order**, and so on. In principle, non-integer values are possible, as well as negative values for individual components of the rate law; however, in practice, the MCAT emphasizes zero-order, first-order, and second-order reactions, so just be aware of third- or higher-order rates as a possibility.

The rate law can be determined experimentally using the method of initial rates. In this method, multiple trials are run with variations in the concentration of individual reactants. The initial rate is then measured to identify how changes in the concentration of a reactant affect the rate. An example is given for the hypothetical reaction $A + B \rightarrow C + D$.

Trial	Initial rate (mol/L·s or M/s)	Initial concentration of A (mol/L or M)	Initial concentration of B (mol/L or M)
1	1.0×10^{-5}	0.2	0.2
2	2.0×10^{-5}	0.4	0.2
3	4.0×10^{-5}	0.2	0.4
4	3.0×10^{-5}	0.6	0.2

Table 1. Method of initial rates

A systematic approach is key for analyzing a table like this. First, make sure your exponents in your initial rates are consistent so you can easily identify changes. In this series of experiments, all exponents are the same (10^{-5}). Next, determine the effects of changing the concentration of A by looking for pairs of trials in which the concentration of A changes while the concentration of B remains constant. In this table, that is the case for Trials 1 and 2 and Trials 1 and 4. Using Trial 1 as a baseline, we see that in Trial 2 [A] was doubled, and the initial rate was doubled, while in Trial 4 [A] was tripled and the rate tripled. This means that in the rate law for this reaction, the term for [A] is $[A]^1$ and that this reaction is first-order with respect to A. Turning to B, we again use Trial 1 as a baseline and observe that in Trial 3, only the concentration of B was changed. In this trial, doubling [B] quadrupled the reaction rate, meaning that the term for [B] in the rate law of this reaction is $[B]^2$ and that this reaction is second-order with respect to B. Therefore, the rate law for this reaction is rate = $k[A][B]^2$, meaning that it is third-order overall. In circumstances where the rate does not change with a change in concentration, the reaction is zeroeth order with respect to that species.

MCAT STRATEGY >>>

The math in this example was as nice as it could be, making it easier to follow the logic of the process. However, on the exam, you could be given a table with more challenging math. Trial 1 might not be the baseline trial, and the values could be given in more complex scientific notation, requiring you to recognize, for instance, that 3.59×10^{-3} is 6 times 5.99×10^{-4}. Alternatively, you could be asked to explore the effects of tripling or quadrupling reactant concentrations. These possibilities emphasize the importance of constant practice with scientific notation and estimation and of using a systematic approach to tackle these questions.

The rate constant k can be calculated from any of the trials in Table 1 after the exponents of the rate law have been established, and the units of k can be derived once those exponents are known. Given the general rate law equation of rate = $k[A]^x[B]^y$, the algebraic logic for calculating k, either numerically or in units, is presented in Equation 3.

Equation 3.
$$k = \frac{rate}{[A]^x[B]^y}$$

For this reaction, we can find the units of k as follows:

$$\frac{M}{s} = k(M)(M^2)$$

$$k = \frac{1}{M^2 \cdot s}$$

An important point to note about the units of k is that while the units of M (alternatively expressible as mol/L) vary according to the overall order of the reaction, the units of k must always involve inverse seconds. The units of k for the reaction orders most commonly encountered on the MCAT are presented in Table 2, but it is important to understand that they can easily be derived and presented in different ways depending on whether units of molarity or moles per liter are used, and whether inverse units are represented using a fraction or a negative exponent.

Order	Units of k (molarity, negative exponents)	Units of k (molarity, fractions)	Units of k (mol/L, negative exponents)	Units of k (mol/L, fractions)
Zero	$M \cdot s^{-1}$	M/s	$mol \cdot L^{-1} \cdot s^{-1}$	mol/(L·s)
First	s^{-1}	1/s	s^{-1}	1/s
Second	$M^{-1} \cdot s^{-1}$	1/(M·s)	$mol^{-1} \cdot L \cdot s^{-1}$	L/(mol·s)
Third	$M^{-2} \cdot s^{-1}$	$1/(M^2 \cdot s)$	$mol^{-2} \cdot L^2 \cdot s^{-1}$	$L^2/(mol^2 \cdot s)$

Table 2. Reaction order and the rate constant k

MCAT STRATEGY >>>

Do not memorize Table 2. Instead, make sure you understand the algebra and dimensional analysis necessary to interconvert between these various ways of representing the units of k and review how they can be derived from the underlying rate law. MCAT questions about k can seem intimidating, but they are very doable if you invest the time in understanding the fundamentals because there are only so many ways they can ask the question.

>>CONNECTIONS <<

Chapter 11 of Chemistry

Because the units of the rate constants for different reaction orders are different, we cannot compare the magnitudes of rate constants for reactions that have different orders. If reactions are of the same order, however, the one with the higher rate constant is the faster reaction.

Physiologically, zero-order reactions are exemplified by enzyme-catalyzed reactions in which the enzyme is saturated—that is, when concentrations of the reactant far exceed the available active sites on enzymes. In such a situation, catalysis is the rate-limiting step, and the concentration of the reactant is irrelevant. First-order reactions are exemplified by radioactive decay and S_N1 reactions that are dependent on carbocation formation. Second-order reactions physically involve collisions between two reactant molecules, as in S_N2 reactions.

The rate law formula tested on the MCAT refers to the initial rate of the reaction. It is also possible to plot the concentration of reactants over time as the reaction progresses. The shape of such a graph differs depending on the order of the reaction. It is linear for zero-order reactions because the rate of the reaction never changes based on the concentration of the reactants. For a first-order reaction, such a graph is non-linear, but transforming the graph to be a plot of the natural logarithm of the reactant as a function of time results in a linear plot. For a second-order reaction in which the rate is dependent on one reactant (i.e., rate = $k[A]^2$), a graph of [A] versus time is again non-linear, but transforming the graph to 1/[A] versus time results in a linear graph.

4. Must-Knows

> Activation energy refers to the energy necessary to reach the transition state.
> The rate of a reaction can be increased by increasing temperature or decreasing the activation energy (E_a).
> $\Delta G < 0 \rightarrow$ exergonic and spontaneous. $\Delta G > 0 \rightarrow$ endergonic and nonspontaneous.
> Be able to read a reaction coordinate diagram and identify the following features:
>   — ΔG.
>   — E_a.
>   — Transition state(s).
>   — Intermediate(s).
>   — The spontaneity of the reaction.
> ΔG, ΔH, and ΔS are thermodynamic properties independent of rate.
> Catalysts increase reaction rate by reducing E_a.
> Enzymes are biological catalysts made of proteins.
> Catalysts (and therefore enzymes) *cannot* turn a nonspontaneous reaction into a spontaneous one or change any thermodynamic parameters of a reaction (ΔG, ΔH, or ΔS).
> A reaction rate is how fast reactants are consumed and how fast products are formed. It is expressed as a decrease (-) or increase (+) in concentration per unit time, each concentration divided by the stoichiometric coefficient.
> The rate law of aA + bB $\rightarrow$ cC + dD is rate = $k[A]^x[B]^y$.
>   — The exponents x and y must be experimentally determined. They do not reflect the stoichiometric coefficients a and b.
>   — This rate law reflects the initial rate.
>   — The units of the rate constant k can be determined algebraically. Rate is in M/s unless otherwise indicated, and concentration is in M.
>   — The overall order of this reaction is the sum of the exponents x and y.
> Be able to use the method of initial rates to determine the order of a reaction.
>   — Compare two trials where the concentration of only one reactant is changed and see how that change affects the rate. If doubling the reactant concentration doubles the rate, the reaction is first-order for that reactant. If doing so quadruples it, it is second-order for that reaction, etc.
>   — Repeat for all reactants.

End of Chapter Practice

The best MCAT practice is realistic, with a focus on identifying steps for further improvement. For those reasons, we recommend completing practice questions in an online setting that simulates the real MCAT interface, and taking advantage of advanced analytic features to help you determine how best to move forward in your MCAT study journey.

With that in mind, online end-of-chapter questions for Biology, Biochemistry, Chemistry + Organic Chemistry, Physics, and Psychology/Sociology are available through your Blueprint MCAT account.

As a further supplement, given the importance of active learning for effective studying, we also suggest that you consult the Must-Knows as a basis for creating a study sheet, in which you list out key terms and test your ability to briefly summarize them.

This page left intentionally blank.

This page left intentionally blank.

Acid-Base Chemistry

0. Introduction

In this chapter, we discuss acid-base chemistry. It's underlying principles connect chemistry, organic chemistry, biochemistry, and biology. For example, in biochemistry, the acidic or basic nature of amino acid side chains impact their behavior and function. Also within the field of biochemistry and detailed in Chapter 5 of the Biochemistry textbook, recall isoelectric focusing, a procedure that uses charge differences to separate amino acids or proteins along a pH gradient. And later in this book, we discuss organic functional groups and their acidic or basic tendencies. These examples all highlight the importance of concepts and relationships.

Throughout this chapter, keep in mind both stability and charge. The stability of a compound and its ionic form(s) directly impact its tendency to act as an acid or a base, and a compound's charge can be altered through protonation and deprotonation. In turn, charge affects other fundamentals, such as solubility in water or organic solvents and the ability to easily diffuse through a cell membrane.

> **>>CONNECTIONS<<**
>
> Chapters 2 and 5 of Biochemistry and Chapter 10 of Chemistry

1. Definitions and Nomenclature

First, what is an **acid**, and what is a **base**? There are several answers to this question dependent on different definitions. For the MCAT, you are required to know three different systems that define acids and bases, however some systems are more modern and relevant than others.

The earliest of the three systems is the **Arrhenius definition of acids and bases** and is the least relevant for the MCAT. In 1884, Svante Arrhenius proposed that acids and bases dissociate in aqueous solution to form ions or charged species. In particular, acids dissociate in a manner that increases the concentration of protons (H^+ ions) in solution, while a base increases the concentration of hydroxide (OH^-) ions. Arrhenius acids contain H^+, so examples include HBr, H_2CO_3, and H_3PO_4. Arrhenius bases, conversely, contain OH^-, and include $NaOH$, KOH, and $Ba(OH)_2$. In modern science, this definition is considered too limiting for general use as acidic and basic compounds may break the narrow Arrhenis definition. For example, ammonia (NH_3) is a common base that does not contain hydroxide.

Our next system addressed this limitation. The **Brønsted-Lowry** defines an acid as a proton donor, or in other words, a compound that can donate a proton to another compound or solution. This follows the Arrhenius definiton, but where the Brønsted-Lowry system differs is in its definition of a base. A Brønsted-Lowry base is a proton *acceptor.* Remember ammonia, which violated the Arrhenius definition? Ammonia, or NH_3, can gain a proton to yield ammon*ium* or NH_4^+. As such, ammonia is a classic Brønsted-Lowry base. As the Brønsted-Lowry system categorizes some compounds as bases even though they do not contain the hydroxide ion, it is broader than the Arrhenius system.

MCAT STRATEGY >>>

Unless you are told otherwise, assume the MCAT is using the Brønsted-Lowry definition of acids and bases. We will thus focus a great deal on proton donation and acceptance in the rest of this chapter.

Before moving on to our final system, let us outline two major concepts from the Brønsted-Lowry scheme. Recall that a Brønsted-Lowry acid is a proton donor. After an acid has lost its proton, the resulting species is a *conjugate base* of the original acid. A base accepts the proton, forming a conjugate acid in the products. This means that for every acid-base reaction, there are two conjugate acid-base pairs. Figure 1 shows an example of acid-base conjugates pairs in the context of an organic reaction. Notice that each acid-base conjugate pair differs by a single proton, which makes them easily identifiable.

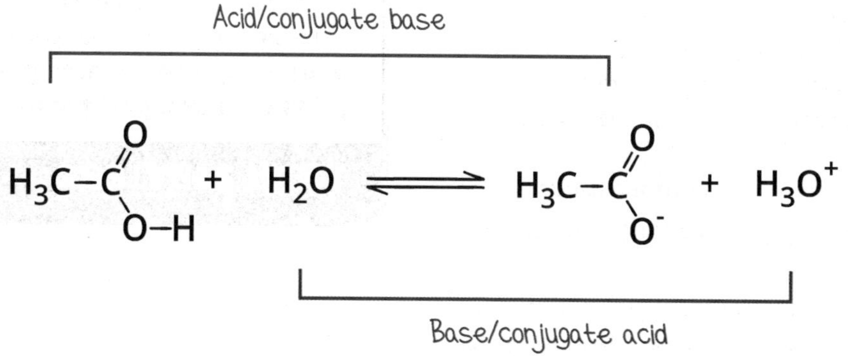

Figure 1. The reaction of acetic acid (the acid) with water (the base) to form acetate (the conjugate base) and hydronium (the conjugate acid)

However, the broadest acid-base classification scheme is the **Lewis system**. Lewis proposed that acids are electron acceptors, while bases are electron donors. For example, in the reaction shown in Figure 2, the lone pair of electrons on NH_3 attacks the empty *p* orbital of the central boron atom in BF_3 (recall that boron is electron deficient). Therefore, in this reaction NH_3 serves as an electron donor (or Lewis base), while BF_3 acts as an electron acceptor (or Lewis acid). From this example alone, we see the key advantage of the Lewis definition. Under either Arrhenius or Brønsted-Lowry, BF_3 would never be considered an acid, as because it contains no hydrogen ions to donate. However, BF_3 *does* react with the basic NH_3. The Lewis system addresses this deficiency by defining acids and bases in terms of electron transfer, which helps us tie acid-base behavior to the important ideas of oxidation and reduction. The fact that the Lewis definitions are more universal means that a Brønsted-Lowry base is also a Lewis base, but a Lewis base is not necessarily a Brønsted-Lowry base.

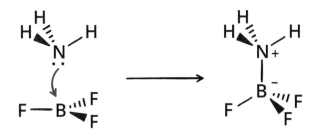

Figure 2. Acid-base reaction between BF_3 (a Lewis acid) and NH_3 (a Lewis base with formal charges shown)

Some compounds can act as either an acid or a base, depending on the other reactants present. These compounds are characterized as **amphoteric**. These species can either accept or donate a proton (as such, they are given the more specific descriptor of "**amphiprotic**."). Common examples include water, which can either gain a proton to become H_3O^+ or lose one to become OH^-. Other examples include amino acids. Polyprotic anions, such as $H_2PO_4^-$ are also amphoteric.

Acids can be named using a few simple guidelines. Acids that lack oxygen are named by combining the prefix *hydro-*, the root of the parent anion, and the suffix *-ic acid*.

Cl^-	Chloride	HCl	Hydrochloric acid
F^-	Fluoride	HF	Hydrofluoric acid

Oxyacids—acids that contain oxygen atoms—use a slightly more complex nomenclature system (Note that the term "oxyacid" typically refers to inorganic oxygen-containing acids. Organic acids, which contain -COOH, are generally not termed "oxyacids," even though they do contain oxygen. The naming of organic acids will be discussed in Chapter 10 of this book).

Pay attention to the prefix and suffix of each oxyanion. We've outlined what is by far the most MCAT-relevant example of this naming convention below: the chlorine-containing oxyacids.

ClO^-	**Hypo**chlor**ite**	HClO	**Hypo**chlor**ous** acid
ClO_2^-	Chlor*ite*	$HClO_2$	Chlor**ous** acid
ClO_3^-	Chlor**ate**	$HClO_3$	Chlor**ic** acid
ClO_4^-	**Per**chlor**ate**	$HClO_4$	**Per**chlor**ic** acid

2. Acid and Base Equilibria

Chemical reactions typically do not proceed to completion—that is, 100% of reactant molecules are not converted to products. Instead, most reactions reach a state known as **equilibrium**, where the rate of conversion of reactants to products is equal to the rate of conversion of products to reactants. Acid-base reactions are no different. Therefore, in this section, we will discuss equilibria of reactions in which protons are gained and lost. First, we must clarify one key point of confusion: with say "protons," you may initially think of H^+ cations, but H^+ does not exist on its own in aqueous solution. Instead, in water it produces H_3O^+, the hydronium cation. For the remainder of this chapter, in aqueous solution the terms "hydronium" and "proton," as well as the species H^+ and H_3O^+, are functionally equivalent.

>> CONNECTIONS <<

Chapters 4 and 5 of Chemistry

Recall that the equilibrium constant (K_{eq}) denotes the relative concentration of products and reactants at equilibrium. K_{eq} is a general term for this constant, but know that all equilibrium constants are expressed in the same way: the concentrations of products, each raised to a power corresponding to their coefficient, divided by the concentration of reactants, each also raised to a power that is the coefficient. Solids and pure liquids are not included in the expression for any K. The first specific type of equilibrium constant is K_w, the constant for the **autoionization** of water (H_2O). The reaction is shown here:

$$H_2O\ (l) + H_2O\ (l) \rightleftharpoons H_3O^+\ (aq) + OH^-\ (aq)$$

In a solution of pure water, the vast majority of species present are H_2O molecules, but a small proportion of H_3O^+ and OH^- ions also exist, formed through the autoionization reaction above. The concentrations of H_3O^+ and OH^- are equal, resulting in a neutral solution. We can write out the equilibrium expression for this process, shown below. Remember, pure liquids are not included in the expression!

$$K_w = [H_3O^+]\,[OH^-]$$

The value of K_w at standard (room) temperature (25°C, or 298.15 K) is 1.0×10^{-14}. Note that this is only true at standard temperature! Like all equilibrium constants, K_w is temperature-dependent; water ionizes more readily at high temperatures, yielding a larger value for K_w. Since $[H_3O^+] = [OH^-]$, we can set both concentrations as equal to x.

$$K_w = [x][x]$$

$$1.0 \times 10^{-14} = x^2$$

$$x = [H_3O^+] = [OH^-] = 1.0 \times 10^{-7} M$$

As long as the hydronium and hydroxide ion concentrations are equal, the solution is neutral. Pure water is thus neutral at any temperature.

MCAT STRATEGY >>>

When finding the square root of a number written in scientific notation, simply *square root the coefficient* and *cut the exponent in half*. Here, the square root of 1.0 is 1.0, and half of −14 is −7.

Let's now widen our discussion beyond water and discuss acidic and basic solutions in a general manner. Like water, acids and bases ionize in solution, and as such, they have their own equilibrium constants. Each acid has its own **acid dissociation constant**, or K_a, while each base has a **base dissociation constant** (K_b). The dissociation of a generic acid is shown below. In this process, the acid reacts with water to yield a hydronium ion and the conjugate base of the acid, A⁻.

$$HA\ (aq) + H_2O\ (l) \rightleftharpoons H_3O^+\ (aq) + A^-\ (aq)$$

For example, consider hydrofluoric acid (HF), a weak acid that dissociates in water, as shown below.

$$HF\ (aq) + H_2O\ (l) \rightleftharpoons H_3O^+\ (aq) + F^-\ (aq)$$

The equilibrium expression for this reaction is $K_a = \dfrac{[H_3O^+][F^-]}{[HF]}$. A high K_a must therefore correspond to an acid that dissociates more readily, while a low K_a corresponds to an acid that does not dissociate to a large degree.

Base dissociation reactions follow the same principles. The dissociation of a generic base in water is shown below. Here, B denotes a weak base.

$$B\ (aq) + H_2O\ (l) \rightleftharpoons BH^+\ (aq) + OH^-\ (aq)$$

The base accepts a proton from a water molecule to yield a hydroxide ion and its conjugate acid, BH^+. From this reaction, we can write the K_b expression for this same generic base.

$$K_b = \frac{[BH^+][OH^-]}{[B]}$$

As in our K_a expression, the constant K_b represents a ratio of products to reactants. The greater the degree of dissociation, the larger the K_b, and vice versa.

3. Acid Strength and the pH Scale

We know from the previous section that acids that dissociate to a large extent have high K_a values, while those that dissociate less have low K_a values. Thus, acids vary enormously in their level of dissociation. On one end of this spectrum lies a small number of acids that dissociate fully—that is, virtually all of their molecules ionize when placed in water. These acids are termed **"strong"** acids and have extremely large K_a values, reflecting that their products greatly outnumber reactants at equilibrium. For example, strong acid, hydroiodic acid, or HI has a K_a of 3.2 $\times\ 10^9$. Strong acids are characterized by having K_a values > 1.

In contrast, any acid that does *not* fully dissociate is a **weak acid**. When a weak acid is placed in water, most of its molecules remain intact, with only a few dissociating to form the conjugate base and hydronium ions. Since the weak acid equilibrium favors the reactants, its K_a will be small (for example, hydrofluoric acid, which we mentioned earlier, has a K_a of only 6.6 $\times\ 10^{-4}$). The products are heavily favored when a strong acid dissociates ($K_a > 1$), while dissociation of a weak acid significantly favors the reactants ($K_a < 1$).

When dealing with acid strength, resist the urge to call an acid strong, unless you know for certain that it fully dissociates in solution. This is a rare phenomenon, and as such, there are only a handful of strong acids you must memorize for the MCAT. Table 1 lists these strong acids, along with the strong bases that you must know, which we will discuss next.

STRONG ACIDS	STRONG BASES
Hydrochloric acid (HCl)	Lithium hydroxide (LiOH)
Hydrobromic acid (HBr)	Sodium hydroxide (NaOH)
Hydroiodic acid (HI)	Potassium hydroxide (KOH)
Chloric acid ($HClO_3$)	Cesium hydroxide (CsOH)
Perchloric acid ($HClO_4$)	Calcium hydroxide ($CaOH_2$)
Sulfuric acid (H_2SO_4)	Strontium hydroxide ($SrOH_2$)
Nitric acid (HNO_3)	Barium hydroxide ($BaOH_2$)

Table 1. Strong acids and bases to know for the MCAT

MCAT STRATEGY >>>

When memorizing lists, look for patterns. Here, for example, the strong bases are in Groups 1 and 2. Also, it can be helpful to focus not only on the terms that are included but also on what is *not* included. For example, the common acids hydrofluoric acid (HF), carbonic acid (H_2CO_3), and phosphoric acid (H_3PO_4) are not strong acids. Remembering this can help you avoid traps into which many students have fallen before!

While the seven strong acids listed above are the only ones you will need to remember for the MCAT, **strong bases** are not so simple. For general chemistry, be sure to know the eight listed above (all of which are hydroxides of alkali or alkaline earth metals). In organic chemistry, however, you may encounter others, including NH_2^- (the conjugate base of ammonia, or NH_3), the hydride anion (H^-), and methoxide (CH_3O^-), ethoxide ($CH_3CH_2O^-$), and *tert*-butoxide (($CH_3)_3CO^-$).

Like a strong acid, a strong base fully dissociates in water. Thus, a 2 M solution of hydrobromic acid (HBr) will produce a 2 M solution of H_3O^+ upon dissociation, while a 0.75 M solution of KOH will produce a final solution with an [OH^-] concentration of 0.75 M.

The **pH scale** is commonly used to describe the concentration of a weak acid, along with its counterpart, pOH. The pH scale is logarithmic, making it particularly effective at describing a wide range of concentrations using a narrower interval of more relatable numbers. The relationships are shown in the equations for pH and pOH below.

Equation 1.
$$pH = -\log[H_3O^+]$$

Equation 2.
$$pOH = -\log[OH^-]$$

As an example, an aqueous solution of 1 mol hydrochloric acid in 10 L of water has a molar concentration of (1 mol)/(10 L), or 0.1 M HCl. Since HCl is a strong acid, it fully dissociates to yield 0.1 M H^+. Its pH is calculated as follows:

$$pH = -\log [H^+] = -\log 0.1 = -\log (1 \times 10^{-1})$$

The logarithm of this value is equal to its exponent (–1), meaning that the *negative* logarithm of 1×10^{-1} is –(–1) or 1. What if the coefficient is something other than 1? Answer choices on the MCAT are sufficiently far apart, to use estimation. For example, let's say you are asked to find the value of $-\log (9 \times 10^{-8})$. 9×10^{-8} falls between 1×10^{-8} and 10×10^{-8}, or 1×10^{-7} (the 9 is between 1 and 10). Our answer, then, must fall between 8 and 7. To be even more specific, since 9×10^{-8} is much closer to 1×10^{-7} than to 1×10^{-8}, our answer must be closer to 7, perhaps around 7.1. An alternative to this method uses this trick:

1. Take the positive value of the exponent (8).
2. Take the coefficient (9) and move its decimal place one position to the left to make it 0.9.
3. Subtract 0.9 from 8 to yield 7.1.

This trick works well enough for the MCAT, although it does not always yield a perfectly accurate answer.

The concepts of pH and pOH are intricately related to K_a, K_b, and K_w, which we discussed in the previous section. Recall the equilibrium expression below for K_w, the autoionization constant of water.

$$K_w = [H_3O^+][OH^-] = 1 \times 10^{-14} \text{ at } 25\ °C$$

If we take the negative logarithm of both sides, we get the following:

$$-\log(K_w) = -\log([H_3O^+][OH^-])$$

Terms that are multiplied together within a log expression can be separated into individual logarithms, as shown below:

$$-\log(K_w) = -\log([H_3O^+]) + -\log([OH^-])$$

Since K_w is equal to 1×10^{-14} at standard temperature, pK_w is equal to 14 under the same conditions.

Equation 3 (standard temperature). $pK_w = -\log (K_w) = 14$

Equation 4 (standard temperature). $pH + pOH = 14$

Equation 4 makes it simple to find pOH if you are given pH or vice versa. For example, under standard conditions, a solution with a pH of 3 must have a pOH of 11. Be careful, though: some students mistakenly interpret Equation 4 as implying that the pH and pOH scales range from 0 to 14. In reality, values lower than 0 and higher than 14 are possible. For example, a 10 M solution of HCl, is synonymous with a concentration of 1×10^1 M protons. The negative logarithm of 1×10^1 M is -1, meaning that the pH of this acidic solution is negative.

Just as pK_w is the negative logarithm of K_w, pK_a and pK_b are the negative logarithms of K_a and K_b. Here, the negative sign has a significant impact. If you recall from the previous section, high values for K_a and K_b denote strong acids and bases, respectively. High values for pK_a corresponds to *weak* acids; that is, there is a reverse relationship between K_a or K_b and pK_a or pK_b. As pK_a increases, for example, K_a decreases. Moreover, just like pH and pOH, pK_a and pK_b can be negative. In fact, the strong acid H_2SO_4 has a pK_a of -3 for its first proton. In keeping with the fact that weaker acids have higher pK_a values, the pK_a of carbonic acid—a weak acid—is around 6.3, and the pK_a of a virtually neutral generic alkane is approximately 50.

Now that we have introduced pK_a and pK_b and the mathematical relationships in Equations 3 and 4, let us outline some additional relationships you should be aware of.

MCAT STRATEGY >>>

You can remember that a small pK_a corresponds to a stronger acid by relating pK_a to pH, which looks similar. Small pH values correspond to more acidic solutions.

Equation 5.

$$K_a \cdot K_b = [H_3O^+][OH^-] = 1 \times 10^{-14} \text{ at } 25\,°C$$

>> CONNECTIONS <<

Chapter 2 of Biochemistry

Note that K_a and K_b here refer to an acid and *its conjugate base*, not an acid and some random other base, and certainly not the exact same species. For example, at standard conditions, the K_a of HCO_3^- and the K_b of CO_3^{2-} must multiply to yield 1×10^{-14}. The larger the K_a of the acid, the smaller the K_b of the corresponding conjugate base, meaning that the stronger an acid, the weaker its conjugate base, and vice versa. This does NOT mean that all weak acids have strong conjugate bases or that all weak bases have strong conjugate acids! It only means that if Acid A is stronger than Acid B, the conjugate base of Acid A must be weaker than the conjugate base of Acid B. Also know that acid-base reactions favor the direction that forms the weaker acid and base, as you might expect. In Figure 1, acetic acid, a weak acid, reacts with water, a weak base, to form acetate, a strong conjugate base, and hydronium ion, a strong conjugate acid. This reaction favors the formation of acetic acid and water, the weaker acid and base, so dissociation is low. We see this reflected in the pK_a, which is 4.75.

Earlier in this section, we calculated the pH of a solution of strong acid, which is fairly simple because strong acids and bases fully dissociate. pH calculations become more complex when they involve weak acids or bases. Since weak species dissociate very little, we cannot consider the concentration of the original acid or base to be equal to the concentration of H_3O^+ or OH^- at equilibrium. Instead, we must use the K_a or K_b to predict the extent of dissociation. The good news is that the MCAT does not expect you to memorize K_a or K_b values for random acids or bases. Instead, they will give these values directly when needed or give their analogous pK_a or pK_b values.

Let's try this out with an example, using the weak organic acid, benzoic acid ($C_7H_6O_2$). What is the pH of a 0.1 M solution of benzoic acid in distilled water at 25°C ($K_a = 6.3 \times 10^{-5}$)? To solve, we must first determine the concentration of each species at equilibrium. This is often accomplished using an **ICE table**, where the initial (I) concentration, change (C) in concentration, and equilibrium (E) concentration of each species is listed.

$$C_7H_6O_2 \leftrightarrow H_3O^+ + C_7H_5O_2^-$$

	$C_7H_6O_2$	H_3O^+	$C_7H_5O_2^-$
I	0.1 M	0 M	0 M
C	-x	+x	+x
E	0.1–x	x	x

As shown above, we set the amount of benzoic acid that dissociates equal to x. For each benzoic acid molecule that dissociates, exactly one H_3O^+ and one $C_7H_5O_2^-$ ion is produced, so we can call each of those concentrations x. We can use the final equilibrium expressions and substitute them into the equilibrium expression for the dissociation of benzoic acid to find the final concentrations.

$$K_a = \frac{[H_3O^+][C_7H_5O_2^-]}{[C_7H_6O_2]} = \frac{(x)(x)}{(0.1 - x)} = 6.3 \times 10^{-5}$$

For the MCAT assume there is little dissociation, so you can drop the x term in the denominator, and estimate:

$$\frac{x^2}{0.1} = 6.3 \times 10^{-5}$$

$$x^2 \sim (6 \times 10^{-5})(0.1) = 6 \times 10^{-6}$$

$$x = [H_3O^+] = 2.5 \times 10^{-3}$$

$$pH = -\log (2.5 \times 10^{-3}) = 2.6$$

4. Buffers

Physiologically, it is desirable to avoid the large shifts in pH that can result from fluctuations in acid or base concentrations. For example, our blood is kept at a pH of approximately 7.4, with a range of 7.35-7.45, depending on various factors. Deviation from this range can cause extreme sickness, failure of body systems, and even death. Such deviation does not need to be large—a blood pH of 6.7 would almost certainly result in fatal acidosis (acidic plasma), while a pH of 7.9 would constitute

> **>> CONNECTIONS <<**
>
> Chapter 9 of Biology

fatal alkalosis (alkaline or basic plasma). However, conditions ranging from heavy exercise to irregular respiration can impact the pH of our blood plasma. How do our bodies ensure that this pH remains at a physiologically optimal level?

The answer to this question lies in the concept of **buffers**. A buffer is a solution that resists changes in pH upon the addition of acid or base. While buffers cannot protect against the addition of large amounts of acid/base, they are highly effective at maintaining a pH when small to moderate quantities are added. Let's discuss how these solutions work using the example of the **bicarbonate buffer system**, an important physiological example of how the blood protects against dramatic changes in pH. A buffer must contain either a weak acid and its conjugate base or a weak base and its conjugate acid. In the body, carbon dioxide and water form carbonic acid or H_2CO_3, which dissociates to form bicarbonate or HCO_3^-, and hydrogen ions. Carbonic acid is the weak acid, and bicarbonate is a conjugate weak base. This reaction is reversible (it is an equilibrium reaction), which allows the body to compensate for changes in pH, making it a good buffering system.

The pH of a buffer solution can be calculated using the **Henderson-Hasselbalch equation** (Equation 7), where HA refers to a generic weak acid and A^- refers to its conjugate weak base. For the fraction part of this equation, we can substitute in either moles or concentration for both species since it is a ratio, and both acid and conjugate base are held in the same volume of solution.

Equation 7.

$$pH = pK_a + \log \frac{[A^-]}{[HA]}$$

We can solidify our understanding of this equation through an example. How many moles of sodium acetate (CH_3COONa) must be added to 100 mL of a 0.05 M solution of acetic acid (CH_3COOH) to produce a buffer with a pH of 6.74 (pK_a acetic acid = 4.74)? Recognize that sodium acetate is a salt that completely dissociates in water.

$$pH = pK_a + \log \frac{[A^-]}{[HA]}$$

$$6.74 = 4.74 + \log \frac{[A^-]}{0.1 \times 0.05}$$

$$2 = \log \frac{[A^-]}{0.005}$$

calculation continued on next page

$$\frac{[A^-]}{0.005} = 10^2$$

$$[A^-] = 0.5 \text{ mol } CH_3COO^-$$

More simply put, since we wanted our final pH to be 2 units higher than the pK_a of acetic acid, and since pH is on a logarithmic scale, we needed to include 100 (or 10^2) times more conjugate base than conjugate acid. This would not be a very effective buffer, as buffer efficacy is highest when the concentrations of conjugate species are close to equal. If the concentrations between HA and A^- are equal in a buffer solution, then pH = pK_a because the log of 1 is 0. Buffers work well when their pH = pK_a because they can counteract changes in pH when additional acid or base is added. When selecting an acid-base pair that would serve as a good buffer, try to choose one where the acid has a pK_a close to the desired pH of the buffered solution. In summary, when using the Henderson-Hasselbalch equation if $[A^-]/[HA] < 1$, a negative number is added to the pK_a and pH < pK_a. If the ratio = 1 then pH = pK_a, and if the ratio >1 then a positive number is added to pK_a, so the pH > pK_a.

MCAT STRATEGY >>>

When asked to calculate the pH of a solution, first ask yourself whether the solution contains a strong acid (or base) alone, a weak acid (or base) alone, or a buffer. Knowing this from the beginning can speed up calculations.

The above discussion of buffers includes the full scope of content required for the MCAT on this topic. However, MCAT questions can still trip up even those students who understand buffer chemistry. One such point of confusion stems from what we have termed "hidden buffer" questions. Envision a situation in which 1 mole of HBr is added to 2 moles of NH_3 to form 1 L of solution. Many MCAT students become stumped here—it doesn't appear to be a buffer, but this solution *is* a buffer! 1 mole of HBr will neutralize exactly 1 mole of NH_3, leaving 1 mole of NH_3 remaining. Thus, the neutralized ammonia will now exist in the form of 1 mole of NH_4^+. Our final solution has equal concentrations of the weakly basic ammonia and its conjugate, ammonium, making it an effective buffer.

5. Titrations

>> CONNECTIONS <<

Chapter 3 of Chemistry

Our final section of this chapter deals with **titrations**, a procedure that you likely conducted in the lab. In broad terms, titration is a technique used to determine the concentration of a solution of unknown molarity. To accomplish this, a solution of *known* concentration is added until an endpoint is reached. This endpoint usually coincides with a color change, and the amount of known solution required to reach the endpoint can be used to determine the concentration of the unknown reactant. In a titration, the solution of unknown concentration is termed the analyte, while the known-concentration solution is called the titrant. Multiple types of titration exist, but the two most MCAT-relevant are acid-base titrations and oxidation-reduction titrations. In this chapter, we will focus on acid-base titrations. Oxidation-reduction reactions will be covered in the next chapter of this book.

>> CONNECTIONS <<

Chapter 8 of Chemistry

The endpoint of an acid-base titration, alternatively termed the **equivalence point**, occurs when the added base or acid has fully neutralized the original acid or base in solution.

The language we have used so far assumes that the acid in question contains only one acidic proton, as is true for species such as HCl and HCN. Such acids are categorized as monoprotic. However, other acids are diprotic, such as H_2SO_4, and some are even triprotic, like H_3PO_4 (Figure 3) (Note that acids that can lose more than one H^+ ion are often lumped together under the heading of "polyprotic."). For **polyprotic acids**, a complete titration involves neutralizing multiple protons. Loss of the first proton proceeds smoothly, but the second and subsequent protons are being removed from a negatively charged species. The likelihood that a proton will be lost diminishes with an increase in negative charge. This means that a 1 molar solution of H3PO4 will not produce a 3 molar solution of H^+. The second proton is removed from $H_2PO_4^{1}$, and the third from HPO_4^{2-}; as the negative charge increases from 0 to -1 to -2, the extent of dissociation goes down.

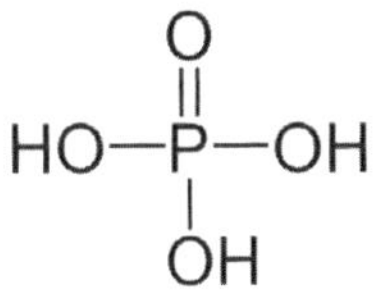

$$
\begin{array}{c}
\text{O} \\
\parallel \\
\text{HO—P—OH} \\
\mid \\
\text{OH}
\end{array}
$$

Figure 3. Phosphoric acid, a triprotic acid

The amount of base (or acid) required to neutralize acid (or base) is given by Equation 8, where a and b represent the number of dissociable protons or hydroxide ions, respectively.

Equation 8. $$a M_a V_a = b M_b V_b$$

In a titration, complete neutralization occurs at a position termed the **equivalence point**. **Indicators** are weak acids or weak bases that change color depending on their protonation state. For example, phenolphthalein (Figure 4) is colorless when protonated and pink when deprotonated. The solution is initially colorless when protonated, but after enough base is added its pH nears and exceeds the pK_a of the indicator and the solution turns pink. The initial color change signifies the equivalence point. A general rule of thumb when choosing an indicator is that the pK_a of the indicator should be as close as possible to the predicted pH of the solution at its equivalence point.

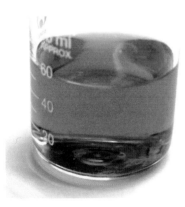

Figure 4. A solution turned pink by phenolphthalein, indicating a basic solution

MCAT STRATEGY >>>

If Equation 8 looks familiar, it probably is. A very similar equation is used for dilutions, in which water is added to a solution to weaken its concentration. You may have seen this equation as $M_1V_1 = M_2V_2$, or $moles_1 = moles_2$. Finding relationships between different equations can help you understand the fundamentals.

A graphical representation of a titration is known as a titration curve. These include another important position: the *half*-equivalence point, which marks the position where half of the volume of titrant required to reach the equivalence point has been added. As we add more base, we reach the half-equivalence point where the concentration of the original weak acid equals the concentration of its conjugate base. Half of the original acid molecules have been neutralized, and the pH equals the pK_a. The pH of the solution changes minimally in this region, so the solution can also act as an effective buffer.

Table 2 outlines the differences between the equivalence and half-equivalence points, which you should be sure to master by test day. Again, for the sake of simplicity, this table describes the titration of a monoprotic acid.

EQUIVALENCE POINT	HALF-EQUIVALENCE POINT
Represents full neutralization.	Represents half-neutralization.
Moles acid = moles base added.	Moles acid = moles conjugate base.
Solution has virtually no buffering ability.	Solution acts as a relatively effective buffer.
Located in the middle of a steep part of the titration curve.	Located in the middle of a plateau on the titration curve.

Table 2. Equivalence vs. half-equivalence point

Let's finally look at some titration curves corresponding to different scenarios. The appearance of these curves can vary based on the identity of the analyte (acid or base) and the strengths of the species involved. For example, when a strong acid is titrated with a strong base, the pH increases steeply and passes through the equivalence point. Beyond this point, OH^- will predominate in solution, and the pH will become increasingly basic. The entirety of this titration procedure is depicted in Figure 5. At the equivalence point $[H^+] = [OH^-]$ so the pH of the solution is 7. This is true of all strong acid/strong base titrations.

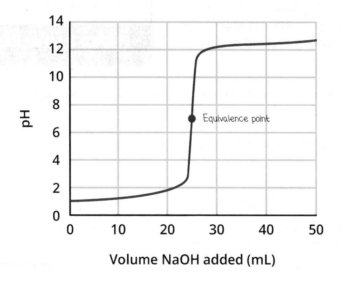

Figure 5. The titration curve for 50 mL of 0.1 M HCl titrated with 0.2 M NaOH

Next, let's examine the titration curve for a weak acid titrated with a strong base (Figure 6). Notice that the initial pH and the equivalence point are higher than the previous strong acid/strong base titration curve. The equivalence point for a weak acid/strong base titration is always > 7 under standard conditions. To explain this, we again turn to the products present at the *end* of the neutralization: here, H_2O and CH_3COONa, or sodium acetate. Water and sodium are neutral, but the acetate anion is the conjugate base of the weak acid, acetic acid. Since acetic acid is weak, and acetate is moderately basic, the solution will be basic overall.

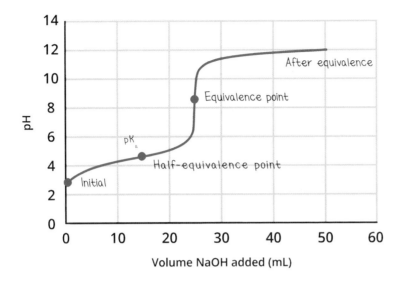

Figure 6. Titration curve for 50 mL 0.1 M CH_3COOH titrated with 0.2 M NaOH

Notice in Figure 6 that the half-equivalence point (or halfway to the equivalence point along the x-axis) falls between 4.5 and 5. The pK_a of acetic acid is approximately 4.8, where there is the strongest resistance to a change in pH. This is the buffer region.

The final type of titration is a strong acid/weak base titration. Predictably, the equivalence point of such a titration has a pH of less than 7 under standard conditions. For example, consider the titration of HNO_3 with NH_3. At the equivalence point, only H_2O and NH_4NO_3 will remain; NH_4^+ is a weak acid, while NO_3^- (the conjugate base of a strong acid) is functionally neutral. As such, the equivalence point will fall at an acidic pH.

Until now, we have discussed the titration of an acid analyte with a basic titrant. We can just as easily conduct the titration of a basic analyte with an acid titrant; the only difference will be the starting point of this titration, which will correspond to a basic pH. The curve will then slope downward instead of upward. Otherwise, the fundamental principles are the same.

> ## CONNECTIONS <<
>
> Chapter 2 of Biochemistry

MCAT STRATEGY >>>

We have seen how strong acid/strong base titrations differ from weak acid/strong base titrations in the pH of their equivalence points. However, a common misconception is that they also differ in the *quantity of base required* to reach this point. In reality, it does *not* require more moles of base to titrate a strong acid than a weak one. If this seems confusing, think about stoichiometry. For example, NaOH and the weak acid HF react in a 1:1 ratio, similar to NaOH and the strong acid HBr.

What about polyprotic titrations, or those in which more than one proton is neutralized? As we mentioned before, phosphoric acid (H_3PO_4) is a polyprotic acid that can undergo multiple ionization steps. As described earlier, the first proton is lost the most readily and corresponds to the largest K_a value. The second proton is more difficult to lose, as it must be lost from an anion, to which it is electrostatically attracted. The third proton is even harder to lose and has the smallest of the three K_a values.

$$H_3PO_4 \leftrightarrow H_2PO_4^- + H^+ \qquad K_{a1} = 7.3 \times 10^{-3}$$
$$H_2PO_4^- \leftrightarrow HPO_4^{2-} + H^+ \qquad K_{a2} = 6.3 \times 10^{-8}$$
$$HPO_4^{2-} \leftrightarrow PO_4^{3-} + H^+ \qquad K_{a3} = 4.0 \times 10^{-13}$$

Since the dissociation of each proton is associated with a unique K_a, there must also be three relevant pK_a values and thus three half-equivalence points. Since each proton must be fully neutralized, three equivalence points will also be present. This is a helpful general rule: the number of acidic protons is always equal to the number of equivalence points *and* half-equivalence points on the titration curve. The curve for H_3PO_4 is shown in Figure 7.

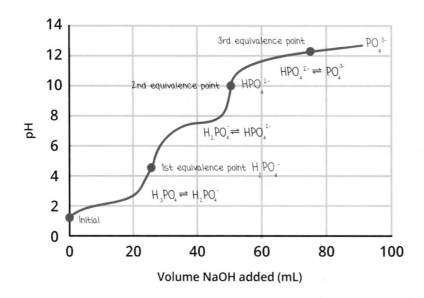

Figure 7. Titration curve for H_3PO_4. Note that the third proton is only very weakly acidic, so the third equivalence point is not in the middle of a steep curve like most equivalence points

Before the first half-equivalence point is reached, the predominant species in solution is H_3PO_4. At the first half-equivalence point, $[H_3PO_4] = [H_2PO_4^-]$; between this position and the first equivalence point, the $H_2PO_4^-$ concentration exceeds the H_3PO_4 concentration until the first proton has been entirely neutralized at the first equivalence point. Similarly, the second equivalence point marks the full neutralization of the second proton (leaving only HPO_4^{2-} in solution), and the final equivalence point denotes the full neutralization of the third and final proton, yielding PO_4^{3-}.

The MCAT commonly tests polyprotic titrations in the form of titrations of **amino acids**. Nonpolar amino acids, like alanine and valine, have only two equivalence points corresponding to their carboxyl and amino terminal groups. Acidic and basic amino acids, such as glutamic acid and lysine, display three equivalence points. As in a typical titration, each *half*-equivalence point corresponds to the pK_a of the relevant group, whether carboxyl terminal, amino terminal, acidic, or basic side chain. Take lysine, for example, held in a solution of pH 1 and titrated with NaOH. Lysine has pK_a values of approximately 2.2, 9.0, and 10.8, where 10.8 is the pK_a of its side chain. Initially, lysine will be protonated at every possible position, yielding a net charge of + 2 (0 for the carboxyl terminal, + 1 for the amino terminal, and + 1 for the basic side chain). Once its first equivalence point is reached, its -COOH terminal will have been fully deprotonated, giving it a net charge of + 1. Its second equivalence point denotes the deprotonation of its amino terminal, yielding a charge of 0, and its final equivalence point represents the deprotonation of its side chain. An important value associated with amino acids is the **isoelectric point** (pI), which refers to the pH at which the amino acid carries a net charge of 0. Lysine is uncharged at its second equivalence point, which falls exactly halfway between its second half-equivalence point (pH = pK_{a2} = 9.0) and its third half-equivalence point (pH = pK_{a3} = 10.8). The pI of lysine, then, is the average of its two highest pK_a values, or about 9.9.

6. Must-Knows

> Acid-base definitions:
>> — Arrhenius: acid donates H^+, base donates OH^-.
>> — Brønsted-Lowry: acid donates H^+, base accepts H^+.
>>> • When a B-L acid loses H^+, it becomes its conjugate base.
>>> • When a B-L base gains H^+, it becomes its conjugate acid.
>> — Lewis: acid accepts electron pair, base donates electron pair.
> Acid nomenclature:
>> — For acids that do not contain oxygen, use prefix "hydro-" and suffix "-ic acid".
>> — For inorganic oxyacids: named as follows, depending on number of oxygen atoms.
>>> • Per____ic acid, ____ic acid, ____ous acid, hypo____ous acid
> Rules for chemical equilibria apply to acid-base reactions!
> K_w = autoionization constant for water.
>> — $K_w = [H_3O^+][OH^-] = 1 \times 10^{-14}$ at 25°C.
>> — $[H_3O^+] = [OH^-] = 1 \times 10^{-7}$ at 25°C.
>> — K_w is temperature-dependent, but $[H_3O^+] = [OH^-]$ in pure water.
> K_a = equilibrium constant for acid dissociation; high K_a corresponds to greater dissociation/stronger acid.
>> — "Strong" acids = acids that fully dissociate in water to produce H_3O^+. $K_a > 1$.
>>> • HI, HBr, HCl, HNO_3, H_2SO_4, $HClO_4$, $HClO_3$
> K_b = equilibrium constant for base dissociation; high K_b corresponds to greater dissociation/stronger base.
>> — "Strong" bases = bases that fully ionize in water to produce OH^-. $K_b > 1$.
>>> • Hydroxides of alkali and alkali earth metals.
> $pH = -\log[H_3O^+]$; $pOH = -\log[OH^-]$.
> $pK_w = pH + pOH = -\log K_w = 14$ at 25°C.
> $K_a \times K_b = K_w = 1 \times 10^{-14}$ at 25°C; $pK_a + pK_b = pK_w = 14$ at 25°C.
> Buffers: solutions that resist large changes in pH.
>> — Include weak acid + its conjugate base (or weak base + its conjugate acid).
>> — Follow Henderson-Hasselbalch equation: $pH = pK_a + \log\dfrac{[A^-]}{[HA]}$
>> — Physiological example: bicarbonate buffer system (H_2CO_3 and HCO_3^-).
> Polyprotic acids: contain more than one H^+ (example: H_2SO_4).
> Titrations: concentration of unknown solution (analyte) is found using known solution (titrant).
>> — Equivalence point = "endpoint" = full neutralization:
>>> • $aM_aV_a = bM_bV_b$
>>> • Moles H^+ = moles OH^-; found on steep segment of curve.
>>> • Indicator changes color (ideal pK_a of indicator = pH range of equivalence point).
>> — Half-equivalence point = half of volume required for full neutralization:
>>> • Moles acid = moles conjugate base; $pH = pK_a$; found on flat segment of curve (plateau).

End of Chapter Practice

The best MCAT practice is realistic, with a focus on identifying steps for further improvement. For those reasons, we recommend completing practice questions in an online setting that simulates the real MCAT interface, and taking advantage of advanced analytic features to help you determine how best to move forward in your MCAT study journey.

With that in mind, online end-of-chapter questions for Biology, Biochemistry, Chemistry + Organic Chemistry, Physics, and Psychology/Sociology are available through your Blueprint MCAT account.

As a further supplement, given the importance of active learning for effective studying, we also suggest that you consult the Must-Knows as a basis for creating a study sheet, in which you list out key terms and test your ability to briefly summarize them.

This page left intentionally blank.

This page left intentionally blank.

Redox Reactions and Electrochemistry

CHAPTER 8

0. Introduction

This chapter covers oxidation-reduction (redox) reactions and electrochemistry. These topics are closely-related and track, in essence, the movement of electrons. These topics are intimately related, and the essence of both involves closely tracking the movement of electrons.

One of the challenges of studying redox chemistry for the MCAT is to thoroughly master definitions that at first glance may seem counterintuitive. For this reason, the first section of this chapter will deal with important redox definitions and how to set up and analyze simple redox reactions. We will then proceed to the topic of reduction potentials, which are, commonly tested on the MCAT. Next, we will explore how galvanic and electrolytic cells work. This corresponds to the core content of redox chemistry and electrochemistry, but there are a few other interconnections that can come up on the MCAT. Consequently, in the last part of the chapter, we will discuss redox titrations and the relationship to electrochemistry and thermodynamics, which have useful applications in biochemistry.

> **> > CONNECTIONS < <**
>
> Chapters 1 and 2 of Chemistry and Chapter 10 of Physics

1. Redox Definitions and Redox Reactions

We'll start this chapter by presenting the most important fact you need to know for the MCAT: **oxidation** means *losing* electrons, and **reduction** means *gaining* electrons.

Redox reactions are reactions in which electrons are transferred between atoms such that one atom gains one or more electrons while another atom loses one or more electrons. Stepping back for a minute, we can note that this isn't the case for many reactions. Consider, for instance, nucleophilic substitution reactions. These are discussed in more depth in Chapter 11, but for our purposes, it suffices to note that the central carbon atom exchanges one substituent for another. It's still sharing the same number of electrons, so it does not count as a redox reaction. We summarize this reasoning by saying that a redox reaction is one in which oxidation states change. In fact, in any redox process, electrons flow from one chemical substance to another. One substance is oxidized and one substance is reduced.

Oxidation state (measured using **oxidation numbers**) keeps track of how electrons have been gained or lost. The tendency to gain or lose electrons is based on electronegativity values, ionization energies, electron affinities, and other periodic properties described in Chapter 1 of this book. Each atom within a molecule or ion has its own oxidation state, and the rules for how those oxidation states are summed together correspond to the overall charge of the molecule or ion. The rules are summarized below:

> Pure elements in their standard state have an oxidation state of zero. This also applies to diatomic molecules, such as O_2 or F_2.

> The oxidation state of monoatomic ions is equal to their charge. Thus, the Fe^{2+} ion has an oxidation state of + 2, and the chloride anion (Cl^-) has an oxidation state of –1.

> The sum of the oxidation states is equal to the overall charge of the molecule or ion (zero for neutral molecules and some integral value for polyatomic ions).

Rules for assigning oxidation states to individual atoms within a compound are summarized below and are in order of priority:

> The oxidation state of F is –1 because it is the most electronegative element.
> — Other halogens will usually have an oxidation state of –1 unless they are bonded to a more electronegative halogen, N, or O. In that case, their oxidation state may be + 1, + 3, + 4 (for Br), + 5, or even + 7. (This scenario is not common on the MCAT, but you should be aware of the possibility. For example, the oxidation state of chlorine in $HClO_4$ is + 7.)

> The oxidation state of H is + 1, except when it is bonded to a more electropositive element, such as with elements in Groups 1 and 2 in which case it will be –1. The examples you are most likely to encounter on the MCAT are the reducing agents NaH, $NaBH_4$, and $LiAlH_4$.

> The oxidation state of O is usually –2, with some important exceptions, such as peroxides (recognized by the -O-O- bond), which are –1.

> Recall from Chapter 1 that elements want to attain a noble gas configuration, so the oxidation state of alkali metals (Group 1) is + 1, and that of alkaline earth metals (Group 2) is + 2.

Once you apply these rules, you can use simple algebra to figure out the oxidation state of the other atoms in a compound. Let's take the example of carbon in a carboxylic acid functional group (CH_3–COOH). This species is neutral, so the overall oxidation states have to sum up to zero. The C–C bond doesn't affect the oxidation state of the –COOH carbon, so we don't have to include it. We have one hydrogen with an oxidation state of + 1 and two oxygen atoms, each with an oxidation state of –2. This sums to an oxidation state of –3. For the overall oxidation state to sum to 0, the oxidation state of the carbon has to be + 3.

Next, let's see what happens in a carboxylate ion (CH_3–COO⁻). The oxidation state of the ions needs to sum up to –1, due to the overall –1 charge. As in the previous example, we don't include the C–C bond. According to our rules, the oxidation state of oxygen is –2, so the two oxygen atoms add up to –4. The carbon must have an oxidation state of + 3 for the overall compound to have an oxidation state of –1. Notably, this is the same value we calculated in the previous example! This may seem surprising at first, but it makes sense. Deprotonating oxygen shouldn't do anything to the distribution of valence electrons around carbon.

Let's work through one other example containing carbon that illustrates a few useful points. What about the carbon in a molecule of methane (CH_4)? We can analyze this molecule fairly quickly. The overall oxidation state is zero, and the H atoms all have oxidation states of + 1, resulting in a total of + 4. The only way to balance the charges is for carbon to have an oxidation state of –4. Note that carbon can have various oxidation states depending on the compound.

Let's look at a few ionic compounds, the most common type of compound encountered in electrochemistry. The first example is calcium oxide (CaO). The oxidation states will sum to zero, and our rules tell us that the oxidation state of O is –2 and that of Ca (an alkaline earth metal) is + 2. You can think of the oxidation states as representing the charges on the two components of the ionic compound, since ionic bonds are defined by complete electron transfer. Now let's look at a slightly more complicated example: Fe_2O_3. For an uncharged molecule, the oxidation states of its constituents must add up to zero. The three oxygen atoms each have an oxidation state of –2, resulting in a total of –6. The two Fe atoms must balance this out, so each must have an oxidation state of (+ 6/2) = + 3. Fe_2O_3 or iron(III) oxide distinguishes it from compounds such as iron(II) oxide (FeO), where iron has a + 2 oxidation state. Next, let's consider an ionic compound in which one of the components is a polyatomic ion, such as the oxidizing agent $KMnO_4$. The oxidation states of the four oxygen molecules add up to –8. According to our rules, K must have a + 1 oxidation state, so the oxidation state of Mn is + 7.

Now that we've covered the definition of oxidation states and how you can calculate them, we can move on to redox reactions.

> Non-redox reactions. Many interesting things may be happen, but the oxidation states don't change because the overall distribution of electrons remains the same.

— *Acid-base chemistry*: the oxidation state does not change in common proton transfer reactions (see the example above comparing –COOH and –COO⁻ carbons) or in classic neutralization reactions (e.g., HCl + NaOH → NaCl + H_2O).

— *Precipitation reactions*: an example is KCl (*aq*) + $AgNO_3$ (*aq*) → AgCl (*s*) + KNO_3 (*aq*). The ions are rearranged, and some bind tightly with each other to fall out of solution, but no electron transfer occurs, and the oxidation states of the ions do not change.

— *Many substitution reactions*: consider an example of nucleophilic substitution chemistry, in which OH⁻ + CH_3Br → CH_3OH+ Br⁻. On both sides of the reaction, the oxidation state of O is –2, Br is –1, H is + 1, and C is –2.

— *Many double displacement reactions*: in double displacement reactions, ions switch places. Acid-base neutralization reactions and precipitation reactions are just specialized examples of this more general category.

> Redox reactions. In addition to 'classic' redox reactions, which are mostly single displacement reactions, a surprising amount of biologically relevant reactions are redox reactions. Some noteworthy examples of redox reactions include:

— *'Classic' redox (single displacement reactions)*: in these reactions, a free element displaces one element of an ionic compound, liberating it as another free element. An example includes $Cu + 2\ AgNO_3 \rightarrow Cu(NO_3)_2 + 2\ Ag$. Copper begins with an oxidation state of 0 and then oxidizes to + 2. Silver starts with an oxidation state of + 1 and reduces to an oxidation state of + 0.

— *Combustion*: combustion is often neglected as a type of redox reaction, but it is an important example! Consider the combustion of methane: $CH_4 + 2\ O_2 \rightarrow CO_2 + 2\ H_2O$. The oxidation state of the carbon in methane is −4, but becomes + 4 in carbon dioxide. Correspondingly, oxygen reduces. The oxidation state of O_2 is zero because it is a free element, while the oxidation state of oxygen in both water and carbon dioxide is −2.

— *Combination reactions*: in combination reactions, free elements combine to form a molecule. A classic example is the formation of ammonia from hydrogen and nitrogen gas: $3\ H_2 + N_2 \rightarrow 2\ NH_3$. By definition, the oxidation state of free elements is zero, so such reactions are redox reactions.

— *Many metabolic reactions*: glycolysis is a net redox reaction. Glucose ($C_6H_{12}O_6$) is oxidized in to two pyruvate molecules ($C_3H_3O_3^-$). Moreover, redox reactions appear in both the citric acid cycle and the electron transport chain and metabolism, such as the beta-oxidation of fatty acids.

Any redox reaction can be separated into two half-reactions. Consider, for instance, the reaction $2\ AgNO_3 + Zn \rightarrow 2\ Ag + Zn(NO_3)_2$. Nothing is happening to the nitrate ion in terms of redox chemistry, so it is referred to as a spectator ion and we can neglect it. The two half-reactions are: the reduction half-reaction for silver ($Ag^+ + e^- \rightarrow Ag$) and the oxidation half-reaction for zinc ($Zn \rightarrow Zn^{2+} + 2e^-$). In any redox process the number of electrons lost must equal the number of electrons gained, so we must multiply the reduction half-reaction by 2. Summing the two half-reactions and canceling electrons gives us the overall redox reaction: $2Ag^+\ (aq) + Zn\ (s) \rightarrow 2Ag\ (s) + Zn^{2+}\ (aq)$.

Next, let's review how to **balance redox reactions**. The principle of conserving mass and charge carries over from balancing reactions in general. Let's illustrate this with an example: how do we balance the reaction $MnO_4^- + H_2C_2O_4 \rightarrow Mn^{2+} + CO_2$ in acidic conditions?

1. Split into half-reactions:

   Reduced: $MnO_4^- \rightarrow Mn^{2+}$ Oxidized: $H_2C_2O_4 \rightarrow CO_2$

2. Assign oxidation states. In this reaction, the oxidation state of Mn will change from + 7 to + 2, and that of C will change from + 3 to + 4. Therefore, Mn is reduced, and C is oxidized.

3. <u>Balance the reaction (except hydrogen and oxygen).</u> Focus on balancing non-oxygen and non-hydrogen atoms. We have an unbalanced carbon in $H_2C_2O_4 \rightarrow CO_2$, so adjust this to $H_2C_2O_4 \rightarrow 2\,CO_2$.

4. <u>Balance the oxygens.</u> Balance oxygens by adding H_2O. Our half-reaction with carbon has balanced oxygens (four on each side), but we need to add oxygens to the Mn half-reaction. Doing so, we get $MnO_4^- \rightarrow Mn^{2+} + 4\,H_2O$.

5. <u>Balance the hydrogens.</u> In an acidic environment, add H^+ as needed. This results in (1) $8\,H^+ + MnO_4^- \rightarrow Mn^{2+} + 4\,H_2O$ and (2) $H_2C_2O_4 \rightarrow 2\,CO_2 + 2\,H^+$.

6. <u>Add electrons to balance the charge.</u> Charge must be conserved, so we must add electrons to ensure that charge is balanced. In $8\,H^+ + MnO_4^- \rightarrow Mn^{2+} + 4\,H_2O$, there is a $+7$ charge on the reactant side and a $+2$ charge on the product side, so we need to add 5 electrons to the reactant side. Likewise, in $H_2C_2O_4 \rightarrow 2\,CO_2 + 2\,H^+$, we have a 0 charge on the reactant side and a $+2$ charge on the product side, so we need to add 2 electrons to the product side to balance it out. This results in (1) $5\,e^- + 8\,H^+ + MnO_4^- \rightarrow Mn^{2+} + 4\,H_2O$ and (2) $H_2C_2O_4 \rightarrow 2\,CO_2 + 2\,H^+ + 2\,e^-$.

7. <u>Multiply so that both half-reactions have the same number of electrons.</u> We need to multiply the Mn half-reaction by 2 and the C half-reaction by 5 to do so, resulting in:

   Reduced: $10\,e^- + 16\,H^+ + 2\,MnO_4^- \rightarrow 2\,Mn^{2+} + 8\,H_2O$
   Oxidized: $5\,H_2C_2O_4 \rightarrow 10\,CO_2 + 10\,H^+ + 10\,e^-$

8. <u>Combine and cancel like terms.</u> If the same item is present on both sides of the reaction, we can add and cancel them, resulting in our final equation:

   $6\,H^+ + 2\,MnO_4^- + 5\,H_2C_2O_4 \rightarrow 2\,Mn^{2+} + 8\,H_2O + 10\,CO_2$

> > **CONNECTIONS** < <

Chapters 1, 7, and 8 of Biochemistry

MCAT STRATEGY >>>

Balancing redox reactions is testable content for the MCAT, so you should be aware of the process and remember that elimination is a useful technique for multiple-choice questions. If you're ever faced with an equation-balancing question (redox or non-redox), a first step might be to skim the answer choices and eliminate anything that makes an obvious error, like failing to conserve atoms or charge.

MCAT STRATEGY >>>

This may be a useful place to go back to review the definition of voltage (electric potential). Much like gravitational potential, voltage is defined as the difference in electric potential between two points. The fact that reduction potentials are comparative is a reflection of the nature of electric potential itself.

The procedure above was specific for acidic conditions. In basic conditions, we slightly modify step 5. We add the hydrogen atoms as usual. We then add an equal amount of OH^- to both sides of the equation. Combine H^+ and OH^- to form H_2O. Finally, cancel out the H_2O on both sides of the equation.

We need to cover one final point before moving on: **oxidizing agents** and **reducing agents**. An oxidizing agent is a substance added to a reaction mixture that oxidizes another substance, and a reducing agent is a substance that reduces another substance. Oxidizing agents are themselves reduced, and reducing agents are themselves oxidized. The terms come from what they do to the other species.

A useful application of oxidizing and reducing agents is to predict a reaction outcome on the MCAT. Oxidizing agents generally contain metals in high oxidation states. Common examples you may see in MCAT organic chemistry include CrO_3, $Na_2Cr_2O_7$, $KMnO_4$, and pyridinium chlorochromate (PCC which contains Cr^{6+}). Reducing agents, in contrast, tend to be hydrogen, neutral transition metals, or hydrides. Common examples including $NaBH_4$ and $LiAlH_4$.

2. Reduction Potentials

Given a mix of ions that could participate in redox reactions, how do we predict which will be reduced and which will be oxidized? The tendency to gain or lose electrons is measured using standard reduction potential.

The electric potential is symbolized as E, measured in volts. $E°$ is under standard conditions (1 M, 1atm, 298 K) and is a measure of the driving force of the reaction. Potentials are defined relative to the standard hydrogen electrode, which is assigned a value of 0 V and corresponds to the reaction $2 H^+ (aq) + 2 e^- \rightarrow H_2 (g)$. Potentials are tabulated, and by convention are always written as reduction potentials. Because we are measuring the driving force of a reaction, stoichiometric coefficients do not affect $E°$ values. This is an important point that is generally tested on the MCAT.

A negative reduction potential indicates a substance that is more easily oxidized, and a positive $E°$ one that is more easily reduced. The greater the magnitude of the potential the more easily the substance is either oxidized or reduced. Fluorine, for example, the most electronegative element on the periodic table, has a tabulated reduction reaction of $F_2 + 2e^- \rightarrow 2F^-$ and has a very positive reduction potential (+2.87 V). In contrast, Li has a strong tendency to lose an electron, so the tabulated reduction reaction, $Li^+ + e^- \rightarrow Li$, has a very negative reduction potential (-3.05 V).

Another way to understand tabulated reduction values is to recognize that a negative reduction potential means that the substance donates electrons and is oxidized, whereas a positive value means that it accepts electrons and is reduced. This means that negative values correspond to reductants, and positive values to oxidants.

Table 1 below presents some selected reduction potentials that we can use as examples. You are *not* expected to memorize any reduction potentials for the MCAT (that the standard hydrogen electrode is defined as 0V).

REDUCTION HALF-REACTION	$E°$ (V)
$F_2(g) + 2\ e^- \rightarrow 2\ F^-(aq)$	+ 2.87
$O_2(g) + 4\ H^+(aq) + 4\ e^- \rightarrow 2\ H_2O(l)$	+ 1.23
$Cu^{2+}(aq) + 2\ e^- \rightarrow Cu(s)$	+ 0.34
$S(s) + 2\ H^+(aq) + 2\ e^- \rightarrow H_2S(g)$	+ 0.14
$2\ H^+(aq) + 2\ e^- \rightarrow H_2(g)$	0.00
$Zn^{2+}(aq) + 2\ e^- \rightarrow Zn(s)$	−0.76
$Li^+(aq) + e^- \rightarrow Li(s)$	−3.05

Table 1. Selected reduction potentials (for aqueous solution)

Now, let's imagine that we have a reaction mixture containing two of the species from Table 1. When solid Zn is placed in a solution of $CuSO_4$, this spontaneous reaction occurs:

$$Zn\ (s) + Cu^{2+}\ (aq) \rightarrow Zn^{2+}\ (aq) + Cu\ (s)$$

The solid Zn begins to dissolve and Cu begins to plate out from the solution. In this reaction Zn is oxidized and Cu is reduced. The oxidation half-reaction is $Zn\ (s) \rightarrow Zn^{2+}\ (aq) + 2e^-$ and the reduction half-reaction is $Cu^{2+}\ (aq) + 2e^- \rightarrow Cu\ (s)$. Adding the half-reactions gives us the overall reaction. As you can see from the table, Cu^{2+} has a tendency to be reduced (it has a positive potential). Zn^{2+} has a negative potential, so Zn, like Li, has a tendency to be oxidized. This is consistent with the spontaneous reaction that occurs. In all cases, if we reverse a reaction the sign of $E°$ must be reversed.

MCAT STRATEGY >>>

The mnemonic *AN OX* (<u>an</u>ode = <u>ox</u>idation) and *RED CAT* (<u>red</u>uction = <u>cat</u>hode) are often used to remember which electrode is which.

3. Galvanic and Electrolytic Cells

If we carry out redox reactions, we can either generate chemical energy from spontaneous reactions or apply electrical energy to a nonspontaneous reaction. All **electrochemical cells** must have two electrodes, which are the site of redox half-reactions. By definition, the electrode where oxidation occurs is known as the **anode**, while the electrode where reduction happens is known as the **cathode**. In our reaction of Zn + and Cu^{2+}, Zn is oxidized at the anode and Cu^{2+} is reduced at the cathode. The anode will lose mass and the cathode will gain mass. The flow of electrons is from anode to cathode.

>> CONNECTIONS <<

Chapters 6 and 7 of Physics

In a **galvanic cell** (also known as a **voltaic cell**), a spontaneous redox reaction generates a positive potential difference that can drive current. The total standard potential generated by a cell, $E°_{cell}$, can be calculated from the tabulated standard reduction potentials of the half-reactions. The simplest way of defining $E°_{cell}$ is presented below:

Equation 1.
$$E°_{cell} = E°_{cathode} - E°_{anode}$$

Since this is an important calculation that is frequently tested on the MCAT, let's work through how to approach it systematically. You may be given a table of standard reduction potentials and asked to calculate the potential of the galvanic cell using two specific half-reactions. Here's how to tackle that problem:

> Identify which substance is oxidized and which is reduced. Oxidation occurs at the anode, and reduction occurs at the cathode.

> Substitute tabulated values into the equation $E°_{cell} = E°_{cathode} - E°_{anode}$.

> A positive $E°_{cell}$ indicates a spontaneous reaction, which is characteristic of a galvanic, or voltaic, cell. If $E°_{cell}$ is negative, the reaction is non-spontaneous, which means that it spontaneous in the reverse direction.

The **Nernst equation** helps us account for how the electrical potential of a cell is affected by conditions including temperature and the concentration of reactants. You may encounter the Nernst equation in two different forms. The first is the more theoretically general one:

Equation 2A.
$$E'_{cell} = E°_{cell} - \frac{RT}{nF} \ln Q$$

In this equation, E'_{cell} refers to the actual cell potential under a given set of conditions, $E°_{cell}$ is the standard cell potential, R is the ideal gas constant, T is the temperature (in Kelvin), n is the number of moles of electrons transferred, F is the Faraday constant (a measure of charge per mole of electrons, defined as 1×10^5 C/mol e⁻), and Q is the reaction quotient (i.e., the concentration of products divided by the concentration of reactants, with each product or reactant raised to the power of its stoichiometric coefficient). In physiology, a simplified version of this equation that uses base-10 logs assumes physiological temperature and can be used to calculate cellular potential:

Equation 2B.
$$E'_{cell} = E°_{cell} - \frac{0.059}{n} \log_{10} Q$$

Understanding the basic definition of a galvanic cell and how the cell potential can be predicted is often all you need to succeed on MCAT questions about this topic, but it is nonetheless useful to invest some time into understanding the physical setup of galvanic cells. The most common example you will see is known as a **Daniell cell**. This type of cell clearly illustrates the principles of a galvanic cell. That said, although the battery of—for instance—your remote control can be thought of as a galvanic battery in general terms, don't make the mistake of thinking that batteries used in modern electrical and industrial applications are just scaled-down Daniell cells. The crucial point, though, is that for the MCAT, the Daniell cell is the prototype of a galvanic cell and uses the same principles.

In a Daniell cell, the half-reactions are carried out in two physically separated half-cells. A conductive wire connects the electrodes. A salt bridge also connects the half-cells—typically containing a salt such as KNO_3 or KCl that will not interfere with the intended redox reaction and prevents a strong charge gradient from building and hindering the progress of the reaction. A Daniel cell for the redox reaction involving zinc and copper is shown below in Figure 1.

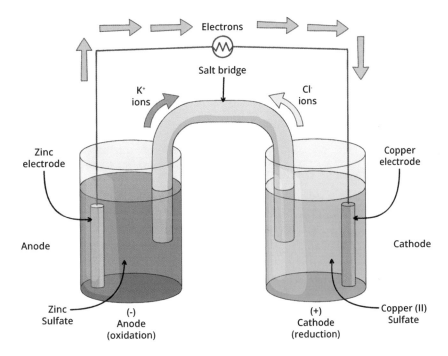

Figure 1. A Daniell cell

As described previously, the full redox reaction taking place is $Zn(s) + Cu^{2+} (aq) \rightarrow Zn^{2+} (aq) + Cu(s)$. We can predict this from the fact that the reduction potential for $Zn^{2+} (aq) + 2e^- \rightarrow Zn (s)$ is -0.76 V and that of $Cu^{2+} (aq) + 2e^- \rightarrow Cu (s)$ is $+ 0.34$ V. Therefore, zinc is oxidized and therefore is the anode and copper in solution is reduced, so copper is the cathode. The total E_{cell} is 0.34 V $-$ (-0.76 V), which indicates a spontaneous process. The zinc electrode will dissolve, while the copper electrode will gain mass. This accumulation onto the cathode is known as plating. The salt bridge serves to preserve electrical neutrality. Can you predict which direction these ions must move? Since electrons are traveling along the wire from anode to cathode, the nitrate ions must travel the opposite direction—from cathode to anode—to prevent the anode from becoming excessively positive. Without the salt bridge the electrochemical reaction will stop. Be careful, though. If the ions in the salt bridge cause a precipitate to form, electrical neutrality can no longer be maintained and the reaction will stop. It will also stop is those ions participate in the electrochemical process.

A common shorthand is used for these cells, in which the anode and the anode solution are specified on the left-hand side of a pair of double bars ($\|$), and the cathode solution and cathode are specified on the right-hand side. Given 1 M concentrations of the solutions, we can represent the cell as this: $Zn(s) \mid Zn^{2+} (aq)$ (1 M) $\| Cu^{2+} (aq)$ (1 M) $\mid Cu(s)$. You may see this notation on test day, but as always, since the MCAT is a standardized test, you will not have to produce it independently yourself. The most important thing is recognizing that the anode is on the left and the cathode is on the right—if you notice that, you can save some time and effort. Knowing which half-reaction occurs at the anode and which at the cathode allows you to use tabulated reduction values to calculate $E°_{cell}$.

MCAT STRATEGY >>>

As you're studying redox chemistry, get in the habit of always calculating the oxidation states for the atoms in examples or practice problems. If you can turn oxidation state calculations into a reflex, you will easily be able to double-check which species is being reduced and which is being oxidized, potentially avoiding errors on your exam. Additionally, you'll find that building this skill will help you understand electrochemistry better in general.

By convention, the anode of a galvanic cell is negative because it is the source of electrons, while the cathode is a positive because it is where electrons are taken out of solution via a reduction reaction.

In the Daniell cell, the two half-reactions are physically separated, but it is possible to create a galvanic cell in which the two half-reactions occur in the same chamber. Such cells are known as **concentration cells**. They must satisfy two conditions: first, there needs to be a concentration difference between two regions of the cell, and second, the electrodes need to be made out of the same material. The reduction half-reaction will then take place at one electrode, and the oxidation half-reaction will take place at another electrode. The concentration difference of the species participating in the redox reactions means that there will be an electric potential difference measured in volts, and current will flow as a result until the concentrations are equalized. The cell with the higher concentration of ions corresponds to the reduction half-reaction (at the cathode), and the one with a lower concentration of ions to the oxidation half-reaction (at the anode). Once the concentrations equalize the potential will be zero.

Concentration cells have a few interesting applications. One that you may have come across in chemistry labs is a pH sensor. One end of the pH sensor is an electrode where a redox reaction takes place. The AgCl wire is placed in a solution filled with KCl at a pH of 7. On the other end, there is a reference sensor with a known concentration. When the pH sensor comes in contact with a solution of unknown pH, there is a potential difference. The electrical reaction between the AgCl and the hydrogen ions from the unknown solution is used to measure the pH. Therefore, a high potential difference indicates a high hydrogen ion concentration corresponding with an acidic solution. Biological membranes are another common example. The concentrations of various ions (predominantly Na^+, K^+, and Cl^-) on each side of the cell membrane are tightly regulated, and the difference in those concentrations sets up a potential difference, known as the resting membrane potential (usually about -70 mV for neurons).

In an **electrolytic cell**, energy is *applied* to the system to drive a non-spontaneous reaction. To take the example that we used in Figure 1, instead of $Zn(s) + Cu^{2+}(aq) \rightarrow Zn^{2+}(aq) + Cu(s)$ (the spontaneous reaction shown in that figure), by applying a current we'll reverse it, to get $Zn^{2+}(aq) + Cu(s) \rightarrow Zn(s) + Cu^{2+}(aq)$.

A classic example of this is the electrolysis of water into hydrogen and oxygen gas. Another application is known as electroplating; in this process, a nonspontaneous reduction reaction of a metal ion in solution is driven via electrical current, resulting in the deposition of solid metal onto the electrode. Copper pennies, for example, are created through electrolysis in a technique called electroplating. A Zn pellet forms the cathode, and Cu is the anode. Copper ions are plated out onto the Zn pellet, creating a smooth copper surface, and the copper ions in solution are replenished at the Cu anode. Because we are forcing a non-spontaneous reaction to occur by applying a current, the anode is + and the cathode is − (recall that in a galvanic cell, the anode is - and the cathode is +).

Let's take a look at the electrolysis of water. Our overall reaction in this process will be $2 H_2O(l) \rightarrow 2 H_2(g) + O_2(g)$. Our first step is to determine what is being reduced and what is being oxidized. In H_2O, the hydrogen atoms each have an oxidation state of $+ 1$, while the oxidation state of H_2 is zero by definition. Since the oxidation state of hydrogen is changing from $+ 1$ to 0, it is being reduced, and reduction occurs at the cathode. In contrast, the oxidation state of oxygen in water is -2, while that of O_2 is zero by definition. Since its oxidation state is increasing, oxygen is being oxidized, and oxidation occurs at the anode.

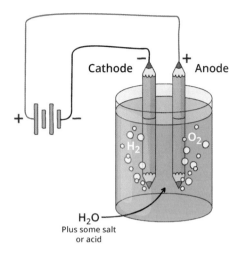

Figure 2. Electrolysis of water

There's nothing special about the makeup of the electrodes in a cell for the electrolysis of water; usually, they are just composed of a conductive metal that will not engage in unwanted side reactions, such as stainless steel. However, once current is applied, each half-reaction will take place at a different electrode.

The charge convention used for an electrolytic cell is the same as that used for electrophoretic biochemical procedures like SDS-PAGE and isoelectric focusing. For these techniques, remember: the cathode is negative, while the anode is positive, because a voltage source is used to drive the reaction in the nonspontaneous direction!

If we are using an electrolytic cell to carry out electroplating, it turns out that we can predict the amount of metal that will be deposited. As with the copper penny, the mechanism of electroplating involves the reduction of metal ions in solution. Schematically, we can represent this as $M^{n+} + n\,e^- \rightarrow M(s)$, where M is a metal and n represents the oxidation state of the metal ion. We can relate the amount of metal formed to the amount and duration of current provided to the cell.

This topic is frequently challenging for MCAT students, so let's take a look at an example. First, remember that the unit for charge is the coulomb (C) and that current is charge per unit time. If we're given a current in amperes ($1\text{ A} = 1\frac{C}{s}$), we can multiply current by time to obtain a value in coulombs.

> **MCAT STRATEGY >>>**
>
> The charge conventions change between galvanic/voltaic and electrolytic cells, but the definitions of anode and cathode (as sites of oxidation and reduction, respectively) do *not*. Those definitions, and their corresponding mnemonic (AN OX and RED CAT), are universally applicable.

To convert between units of charge and moles of electrons, we need to use the **Faraday constant (F)**. The Faraday constant is just a simple dimensional conversion process. By definition, 6.02×10^{23} electrons are in a mole, and each electron has a charge of 1.6×10^{-19} C. Therefore, to get a measure of charge per mole, we can derive the Faraday constant as follows:

Equation 3.
$$F = \frac{1.6 \times 10^{-19}\,C}{e^-} \times \frac{6.02 \times 10^{23}\,e^-}{e^-} \approx 1 \times 10^5\ \frac{C}{mol\ e^-}$$

This gives us the following equation for electroplating:

Equation 4.
$$\text{moles of metal} = \frac{I \times t}{n F}$$

In this equation, I is current in amperes, t is time in seconds, n is the number of moles of electrons needed to reduce the metal ion to its elemental state, and F is the Faraday constant.

The same logic can be applied to electrolytic processes involving the production of gas (as in our example of the hydrolysis of water). You would solve the problem the same way; the only difference is whether the products are solids or gases.

So far, we've been treating galvanic (voltaic) and electrolytic cells as two completely separate devices, but they can be combined. This is what happens in the rechargeable batteries that we use every day! For the MCAT, you should be aware of a few main types of rechargeable batteries. However, you certainly don't need to delve into the engineering intricacies that allow them to reliably power tiny devices. The basic principle of a rechargeable battery is the design of a physical setup that can both discharge spontaneously (acting as a galvanic cell that produces current) and recharge (acting as an electrolytic cell) that needs to be plugged in and recharged.

The first type of rechargeable battery developed, which is still used in various applications, including car batteries and cell phone towers, is a lead storage battery or a lead-acid battery. Lead-acid batteries have a relatively low energy density, which means that a heavier battery is needed for a given amount of output than other battery designs. In its charged state, a lead storage battery has a lead oxide electrode and a lead electrode, separated by an area that contains concentrated H_2SO_4, as shown in Figure 3.

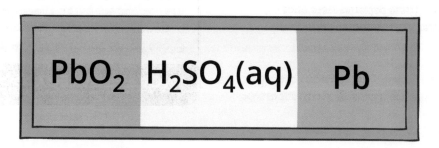

Figure 3. Charged form of lead-acid battery

Two redox half-reactions take place during discharge. The oxidation half-reaction occurs at the Pb electrode, and can be summarized as this:

$$Pb(s) + SO_4^{2-}\ (aq) \rightarrow PbSO_4(s) + 2e^-$$

$$E° = -0.36 \text{ V}$$

Pb(s) has an oxidation state of 0, while the Pb in $PbSO_4(aq)$ has an oxidation state of + 2. The oxidation state of lead increased, so this is the oxidation half-reaction and occurs at the anode. The reduction half-reaction is:

$$PbO_2(s) + SO_4^-\ (aq) + 4H^+\ (aq) + 2e^- \rightarrow PbSO_4(s) + 2\ H_2O(l)$$

$$E° = 1.69 \text{ V}$$

In this half-reaction, the oxidation state of Pb goes from + 4 in PbO_2 to + 2 in $PbSO_4$(s), so it occurs at the cathode. There are two important things to note about this cell: (1) $PbSO_4$(s) is the product of *both* half-reactions, and (2) $PbSO_4$(s) is *solid* because it is very poorly soluble in water. The tabulated reduction potentials indicate that $E°_{cell}$ = 2.04 V, so for a 12 V battery there must be six cells. Notice that this is a spontaneous reaction, because it has a positive $E°_{cell}$. Consequently, when the galvanic cell proceeds to completion, we're left with a coating of $PbSO_4$(s) and some dilute H_2SO_4, as shown in Figure 4.

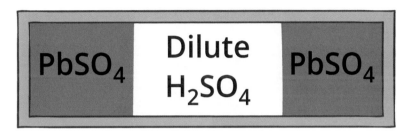

Figure 4. Discharged form of lead-acid battery

Once the lead-acid battery is discharged, current can be applied to recharge it, reversing the reactions described above.

Nickel-cadmium batteries are another example of rechargeable batteries. These batteries were once commonly used for personal electronic devices but have been supplanted by other, more environmentally friendly battery designs. Nonetheless, you are expected to be aware of the basics of nickel-cadmium batteries for the MCAT. As the name suggests, they have one cathode containing nickel (more precisely, nickel oxide-hydroxide [NiO(OH)]) and one anode containing cadmium. When discharging, the oxidation half-reaction is Cd *(s)* + 2 OH⁻ *(aq)* →
Cd(OH)₂ *(s)* + 2 e⁻, and the reduction half-reaction is 2 NiO(OH) *(s)* + 2 H_2O *(l)* + 2 e⁻ → 2 Ni(OH)₂ *(s)* + 2 OH⁻ *(aq)*. As with lead-acid batteries, during recharging, the reactions in nickel-cadmium batteries are reversed.

> **MCAT STRATEGY >>>**
>
> Focus on the principle of how the lead-acid battery works, not primarily on memorizing the constituent parts. The MCAT is highly unlikely to ask you exactly which strong acid is generally used in these batteries (for example); instead, you should understand the mechanism and be able to answer questions about it if given diagrams like Figures 3 and 4.

As spontaneous reactions are discharging, the resulting potential difference (corresponding to the cell potential of the battery can be utilized to drive current through a conductive wire. This is the setup for direct circuits, which are discussed in Chapter 7 of the Physics textbook. The potential difference that drives current is sometimes known as the electromotive force, or emf. Therefore, we can measure the 'strength' of a battery in voltage and/or emf. An example is a 9-volt battery, commonly used in applications like powering smoke and carbon monoxide detectors. It's important to avoid confusion, though: the emf is *not a force*. This is misleading terminology leftover from earlier eras of research and reflects the intuitive idea that voltage 'drives' current through a conductor.

> **>> CONNECTIONS <<**
>
> Chapter 7 of Physics

4. Titrations

Just as we can use titrations to monitor the progress of acid-base reactions, we can use them to monitor oxidation-reduction reactions. Transition metals often have different colors corresponding to different oxidation states. One example is Mn. The polyatomic MnO_4^- ion, in which Mn has an oxidation state of + 7, is purple in aqueous solution, whereas Mn^{2+} is colorless. MnO_4^- is also a strong oxidizing agent, so it is likely to participate in redox reactions with other species in solution.

With this in mind, let's consider a situation in which we have an unknown concentration of Sn^{2+} in aqueous solution. The MnO_4^- will readily oxidize Sn^{2+} to Sn^{4+} in the following redox reaction: $16 H^+ + 2 MnO_4^- + 5 Sn^{2+} \rightarrow 2 Mn^{2+} + 5 Sn^{4+} + 8 H_2O$. As we begin the titration, we add purple-colored MnO_4^- dropwise. As the MnO_4^- drops contact the solution of Sn^{2+}, they will immediately oxidize Sn^{2+}, and the solution will remain clear. As soon as some purple color from the MnO_4^- remains in the reaction mixture, we have reached the equivalence point; there is no more Sn^{2+} for the MnO_4^- to react with.

If we know the concentration of MnO_4^-, the amount added to get to the equivalence point, and the volume of the Sn^{2+} solution, we can calculate the concentration of Sn^{2+}. The equations we use are the same as for any other titration:

>> CONNECTIONS <<

Chapter 7 of Chemistry

MCAT STRATEGY >>>

If you have any uncertainty about the mechanism of *how* titration works to determine the concentration of an analyte in solution, review the information about acid-base titrations presented in Chapter 7. In the context of the MCAT, redox titrations should be thought of as an extension of the principle of acid-base titrations to a new context where we're focusing on electron flow rather than protonation/deprotonation, so make sure your acid/base fundamentals are solid.

Equation 5A.

$$n_1 M_1 V_1 = n_2 M_2 V_2$$

Five electrons are transferred with Mn, (because its oxidation state goes from + 7 to + 2) and two for Sn (because its oxidation state goes from + 2 to + 4).

Given 200 mL of Sn^{2+} that it took 40 mL of 0.20 M MnO_4^- to reach the equivalence point, we can use Equation 5 and substitute values to obtain the concentration of Sn^{2+} as follows:

$$n_1 M_1 V_1 = n_2 M_2 V_2$$

$$(5)(0.20 \text{ M } MnO_4^-)(40 \text{ mL}) = (2)(x)(200 \text{ mL})$$

$$\frac{(5)(0.20)(40)}{(2)(200)} = x$$

$$x = 0.10 \text{ M } Sn^{2+}$$

Redox titrations have many applications. One well-known example in biochemistry is the use of **Benedict's reagent** to test for reducing sugars, which after heating, reduce Cu^{2+} to Cu^+, causing a color change. You may have also experimented with **iodometric titrations** in chemistry labs, which take advantage of the fact that the iodide ion readily participates in redox reactions and that iodine combined with starch produces a vivid dark blue color.

In **potentiometric titrations**, the potential difference in volts is measured between a reference electrode that is insensitive to the properties of the solution. A detector electrode is immersed in the analyte (that is, the solution being analyzed). pH sensors work using a slightly adapted version of this principle.

5. Connections with Thermodynamics

We've been talking about spontaneous versus nonspontaneous reactions in galvanic/voltaic and electrolytic cells throughout this chapter. As a general rule of thumb, whenever you hear the word "spontaneous," you should immediately think of thermodynamics, because whether or not a reaction is spontaneous is determined by whether or not it is exergonic. More specifically, recall that reactions with a $\Delta G < 0$ are spontaneous, whereas those with a $\Delta G > 0$ are nonspontaneous.

The $\Delta G°$ of a redox reaction turns out to be directly connected with the value of $E°_{cell}$, as given in the following equation:

> **MCAT STRATEGY >>>**
>
> As with acid-base titrations, you don't need to be intimately familiar with every possible configuration for redox titrations, but you do need to understand the principle clearly. A useful exercise for yourself would be to explain verbally to a study partner what the similarities and differences are between acid-base titration problems and redox titration problems.

Equation 6.
$$\Delta G° = -nFE°_{cell}$$

In this equation, $\Delta G°$ is the standard Gibbs free energy change of a reaction, and $E°_{cell}$ is the standard cell reduction potential. The additional variables n and F refer to the moles of electrons exchanged in the reaction and Faraday's constant, respectively. Note that $\Delta G°$ will have to be expressed in joules, not kilojoules and that a coulomb (C) is definable as a joule divided by a volt (J/V).

If there are more products than reactants at equilibrium, the reaction is spontaneous and $K_{eq} > 1$, while if there are more reactants than products at equilibrium, the reaction as a whole is nonspontaneous and $K_{eq} < 1$. The relationship between $\Delta G°$ and K_{eq} can be defined as follows:

Equation 7.
$$\Delta G° = -RT\ln K_{eq}$$

Combining Equation 6 and Equation 7, we get an expression linking $E°_{cell}$ to K_{eq}:

Equation 8.
$$nFE°_{cell} = RT\ln K_{eq}$$

It is possible that you would be asked to perform a calculation with this equation, although it would almost certainly be set up in a way that would minimize the likelihood that you would have to do calculations by hand involving the natural logarithm (ln). However, it is essential that you master the conceptual relationships among the parameters of ΔG, $E°_{cell}$, and K_{eq} and how they relate to spontaneity, as shown on the next page in Table 2.

	SPONTANEOUS	NONSPONTANEOUS
ΔG	< 0	> 0
$E°_{cell}$	> 0	< 0
K_{eq}	> 1	< 1

Table 2. Spontaneity and ΔG, $E°_{cell}$, and K_{eq}

6. Must-Knows

> Oxidation = losing electrons; reduction = gaining electrons.
>> — Mnemonics: *OIL RIG* (<u>o</u>xidation <u>i</u>s <u>l</u>oss, <u>r</u>eduction <u>i</u>s <u>g</u>ain) and *LEO* the lion goes *GER* (<u>l</u>ose <u>e</u>lectrons = <u>o</u>xidation, <u>g</u>ain <u>e</u>lectrons = <u>r</u>eduction).
>> — Know the definitions of oxidation and reduction.
> Oxidation state: basis for defining oxidation-reduction (redox) reactions:
>> — Pure elements: oxidation state of 0; ions: overall oxidation state = charge.
>> — Oxidation state rules for atoms within compounds:
>>> • F: −1, most other halogens usually −1 as well, unless bonded to a more electronegative atom.
>>> • H: + 1, unless bonded to a more electropositive element (e.g., NaH).
>>> • O: −2, except −1 in peroxides.
>>> • Alkali metals (Group 1): + 1, alkaline earth metals (Group 2): + 2.
>>> • Other atoms: calculated as needed to reach overall oxidation state.
> Reduction potentials: for a given reduction half-reaction, $E°$ (in V) measures the driving force for a reaction. By convention these are tabulated as reduction potentials. More positive = reduction is more likely.
> Galvanic/voltaic cells: the reaction is spontaneous, creating a potential difference that can be used to drive current.
>> — $E°_{cell} = E°_{cathode} - E°_{anode}$
>> — By definition, oxidation occurs at the anode, reduction occurs at the cathode.
>> — Equations that reflect how actual potential is affected by non-standard conditions:
>>> • $E'_{cell} = E°_{cell} - \frac{RT}{nF} \ln Q$
>>> • $E'_{cell} = E°_{cell} - \frac{0.05916}{n} \log_{10} Q$
> Concentration cells: electrodes made of the same material. At the beginning, concentration differences drive the redox reaction as the potential goes to zero concentration equalizes.
> Electrolytic cells: current is supplied to drive nonspontaneous redox reaction.
>> — Electroplating given a current *I* for a time *t*: *moles of metal* $= \frac{I \times t}{nF}$
>> — F = Faraday constant (1×10^5 C/mol) measures how much charge is carried by a mole of electrons.
> Rechargeable batteries combine galvanic/voltaic and electrolytic functionality; examples include lead-acid and nickel-cadmium batteries. Voltage of a battery, which drives current, is sometimes called electromotive force (emf), but this is not a force.
> Redox titrations: indicators that change color between oxidized and reduced forms, or potentiometric titrations that measure changes in potential difference. Same basic principle as acid-base titrations but measure electron transfer instead of (de)protonation.
> Thermodynamics:
>> — $\Delta G° = -nFE°_{cell}$.
>> — $nFE°_{cell} = RT \ln K_{eq}$ because $\Delta G° = -RT \ln K_{eq}$.
>> — Spontaneous: $\Delta G < 0$, $E°_{cell} > 0$, $K_{eq} > 1$.
>> — Nonspontaneous: $\Delta G > 0$, $E°_{cell} < 0$, $K_{eq} < 1$.

End of Chapter Practice

The best MCAT practice is realistic, with a focus on identifying steps for further improvement. For those reasons, we recommend completing practice questions in an online setting that simulates the real MCAT interface, and taking advantage of advanced analytic features to help you determine how best to move forward in your MCAT study journey.

With that in mind, online end-of-chapter questions for Biology, Biochemistry, Chemistry + Organic Chemistry, Physics, and Psychology/Sociology are available through your Blueprint MCAT account.

As a further supplement, given the importance of active learning for effective studying, we also suggest that you consult the Must-Knows as a basis for creating a study sheet, in which you list out key terms and test your ability to briefly summarize them.

This page left intentionally blank.

This page left intentionally blank.

Organic Chemistry Basics

0. Introduction

In this chapter, we move from general chemistry to organic chemistry, which studies the carbon-containing compounds that make up the basis of all life. Carbon's ability to form chains of single, double, and triple bonds with itself provides it with the flexibility to become the chemical scaffold of life.

It may surprise you to know that organic chemistry is not an especially large component of the science content tested on the MCAT. On average, it will make up approximately 15% of the content tested in the Chemical and Physical Foundations and 5% of the content tested in the Biological and Biochemical Foundations section, corresponding to 10% of the content in the 'core' science sections and 5% of the exam overall, including CARS and Psychological/Social/Biological Foundations.

The MCAT *is* focused on ensuring that you have a solid understanding of the basic principles of organic chemistry, with a special focus on factors that help predict biologically/pharmacologically relevant properties of compounds. This translates into the following core areas that we will explore in this chapter and the remaining chapters of this textbook:

> Nomenclature: You must have a solid foundation in the rules used to systematically name chemical compounds.

> Structure and Behavior: How the structure of organic molecules contributes to their physical and chemical behavior is an important topic that includes resonance stabilization and functional groups.

> Key Reactions: Reactivity is a topic that is tested in less breadth and depth than in most college-level organic chemistry courses, but it is nonetheless important.

> Lab Techniques: Topics such as separation methods are of considerable practical importance in pharmacology and in laboratory procedures in general.

In this chapter, we'll discuss nomenclature and structure, with a particular focus on stereochemistry. The next chapter (Chapter 10) will provide a comprehensive overview of the functional groups that you need to know for the MCAT, including their key reactions. Chapter 11 is a deep dive into some of the reaction mechanisms that you should be familiar with for the MCAT, and Chapter 12 describes key laboratory techniques.

As you're studying organic chemistry for the MCAT, there are three principles to keep in mind that will help you focus your study time as you prepare for test day.

1. <u>Don't neglect the simple stuff</u>. The MCAT can and does ask straightforward questions about topics like stereochemistry that are often covered in early organic chemistry material. These early topics lay the foundation for more complex material. Don't rush through the basics! Invest time in building a solid foundation.

2. <u>Visualize things in space</u>. If you have an old molecular model kit from your previous coursework, now is the time to dust it off—and if you don't, you might think about investing in one. Alternatively, you can draw out structures and reactions on paper or use gestures and/or objects at hand in your study space to illustrate concepts.

3. <u>Follow the charge!</u> This advice applies to biochemistry as well as organic chemistry. Charge-based interactions are at the heart of both the chemical and physical properties of molecules and reaction mechanisms. These interactions affect the strengths of intermolecular forces, which contribute to overall chemical and physical behavior. The localization of electrons affects reaction mechanisms and contributes to an understanding of electron delocalization and molecular stability.

With all of the above in mind, let's get started!

1. Nomenclature and Structure

Given the vast number of known organic compounds, it is fundamental for practical purposes to develop a system of unambiguously describing their structure. **IUPAC nomenclature** is the accepted standard, but be aware that many organic molecules are identified by their common names. This section describes how IUPAC nomenclature applies to hydrocarbons—the simplest examples of organic molecules made up only of carbon and hydrogen atoms—and then extends those principles to more complicated molecules.

Alkanes are the simplest of hydrocarbons. They have only single bonds between carbon atoms. Each carbon completes its octet by forming bonds to *other* carbon atoms or to hydrogen. Generally, a carbon skeleton is used to depict organic compounds in what is known as **bond-line notation** or **skeletal diagrams**. In this system, the only atoms explicitly shown are those other than carbon atoms, which form the framework, or hydrogen atoms bound to the carbon framework. Recall that carbon forms four bonds and hydrogen only one. Each vertex in the framework is a carbon atom, and the hydrogen atoms bound to the framework are not shown. Figure 1 illustrates bond line notation for two simple compounds.

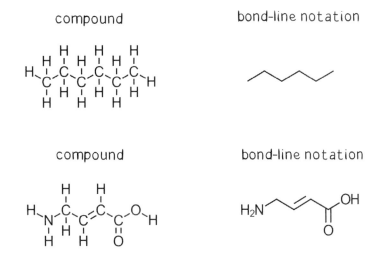

Figure 1. Examples of bond-line notation

Alkanes are named using the following steps:

1. Identify and name the longest chain of carbons. If the alkane has an unbranched chain, it is an *n*-alkane.

Unbranched Hydrocarbons (*n*-Alkanes)

1	CH_4	Methane	6	$CH_3(CH_2)_4CH_3$	Hexane
2	CH_3CH_3	Ethane	7	$CH_3(CH_2)_5CH_3$	Heptane
3	$CH_3CH_2CH_3$	Propane	8	$CH_3(CH_2)_6CH_3$	Octane
4	$CH_3(CH_2)_2CH_3$	Butane	9	$CH_3(CH_2)_7CH_3$	Nonane
5	$CH_3(CH_2)_3CH_3$	Pentane	10	$CH_3(CH_2)_8CH_3$	Decane

2. Label each carbon so that the substituents, those groups of atoms that replace one or more hydrogens, have the lowest possible numbers along the chain.

3. Identify and assign a number to each substituent. The general rule for naming alkane substituents is to use -yl as the suffix rather than -ane. Di-, tri-, and tetra- are used when two, three, and four of the same substituent is present, respectively. Common names are often used and shown next to the IUPAC name. The isopropyl group, for example, contains a single methyl branch at a carbon atom next to the end of the chain. The structures of *sec*-butyl and *tert*-butyl are indicated.

Methyl H_3C-R Isopropyl

Ethyl R

Propyl R *sec*-Butyl

Butyl R *tert*-Butyl

4. Name the compound by placing the substituents in alphabetical order before the name of the parent molecule. Prefixes such as di-, tri-, *sec-*, *tert-*, etc., should be ignored for alphabetical ordering.

Let's work through an example of the alkane shown below.

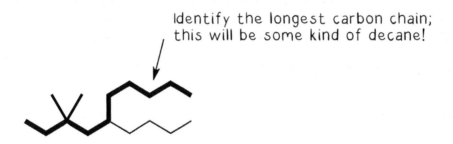

Our first task is to identify the longest carbon chain. While it might be tempting to see this molecule as a modification of the straight-chain alkane that runs across the bottom of the image, it turns out that this is not the case. The correct identification of the longest carbon chain is shown here.

Identify the longest carbon chain;
this will be some kind of decane!

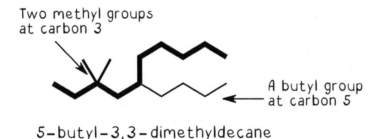

The next step is to identify and name the substituents, taking care to number the carbons such that the substituents have the smallest possible numbers.

Two methyl groups
at carbon 3

A butyl group
at carbon 5

5-butyl-3,3-dimethyldecane

We then arrange the substituents in alphabetical order, so the IUPAC name is 5-butyl-3,3-dimethyldecane.

Our next task is to describe more complicated molecules. For this we need to be able to indicate a **functional group**. This is a specific group of atoms/bonds within a molecule responsible for a characteristic set of behaviors. In the example above, the butyl and two methyl groups are functional groups. You do need to be familiar with biochemically relevant functional groups for the MCAT; their properties and key reactions are presented in more detail in Chapter 10. In this section, we will briefly present functional groups and their nomenclature.

Common functional groups include hydroxyl groups (–OH), which form compounds known as **alcohols**, and amine groups (–NR_3, where R is an H or a C atom), which form compounds known as **amines**. Figure 2 shows some simple alcohols and amines, some with additional alkyl substituents.

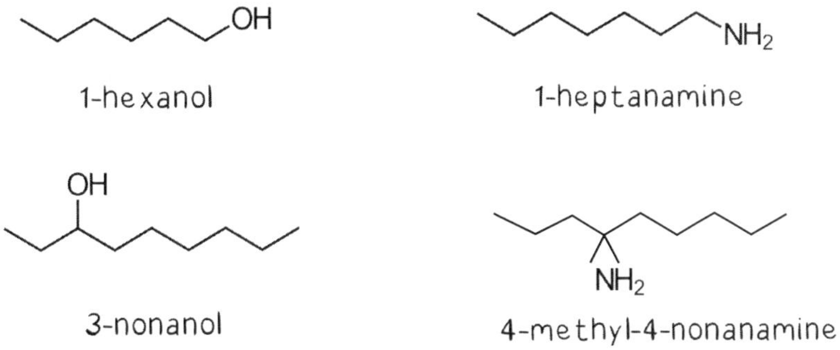

1-hexanol

1-heptanamine

3-nonanol

4-methyl-4-nonanamine

Figure 2. Alcohols and amines

Again, we need to specify the location of any functional group. Be aware that by convention, 'hexanol' is assumed to mean 1-hexanol.

What if we have *both* an amine group and a hydroxyl group on a molecule? We need to have some way of determining which functional group takes priority when naming the compound. In the case of amines and alcohols, by convention, the hydroxyl group takes priority. This means that the molecules shown in Figure 3, which have both –OH and –NH$_2$ groups, are considered to be substituted hexanols. This is true regardless of where the –OH and –NH$_2$ groups are located in the molecule; the molecule on the right, 6-amino-3-methyl-2-hexanol, is still considered a hexanol, although at first glance it might appear to be an amine.

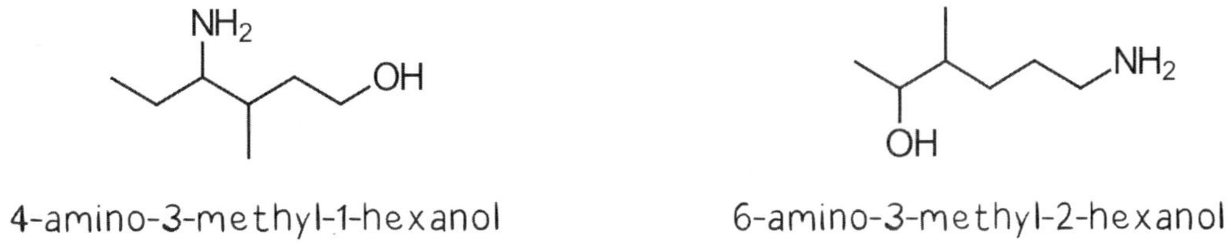

4-amino-3-methyl-1-hexanol

6-amino-3-methyl-2-hexanol

Figure 3. Two compounds with –OH and –NH$_2$ groups

IUPAC has defined a hierarchy of priority for functional groups, as shown below in Table 1. Notice that more oxidized carbons have higher priority. The oxidation and reduction of organic compounds is discussed in more detail in Chapter 10, but for now, be aware that in order of priority, Table 1 can be summarized as follows: carboxylic acids > carboxylic acid derivatives > other carbonyl-containing compounds > sulfur-containing functional groups > nitrogen-containing functional groups > hydrocarbons.

GROUP	SUFFIX	STRUCTURE	PRIORITY
Carboxylic acid	-oic acid		High
Ester	-oate		
Acyl chloride	-oyl halide		
Amide	-amide		
Aldehyde	-al		
Ketone	-one		
Alcohol	-ol		
Thiol	-thiol		
Amine	-amine		
Alkyne	-yne	$R-C{\equiv}C-R'$	
Alkene	-ene		
Alkane	-ane		Low

Table 1. Functional groups by priority

In addition to the functional groups listed in Table 1, a few functional groups have a lower priority than alkanes. The most common examples of this are the haloalkanes (also known as alkyl halides)—that is, alkanes that have one or more halogen substituents, such as 2-bromopentane. Another example is ethers, which have an oxygen bonded to two alkyl groups (C–O–C). A simple ether with a methane and an ethane group attached would be referred to as methoxyethane.

We'll now move away from nomenclature and turn to a discussion of two important topics for the MCAT, resonance and electron delocalization.

Resonance was introduced in Chapter 2 as a way to draw equivalent Lewis structures for a given molecule. Figure 4 below shows resonance structures for carboxylate anions and peptide bonds, two of the most common you will encounter on the MCAT. Carboxylate anions are deprotonated carboxylic acids (–COOH). Peptide, or amide, bonds connect amino acid residues that form the backbone of proteins.

MCAT STRATEGY >>>

IUPAC nomenclature is fair game on the MCAT, but remember that this isn't organic chemistry class, where your professor might give you some ridiculously complicated molecule, ask you to name it, and then deduct points because you put the comma in the wrong place or because you misspelled *mercapto-*. Many MCAT questions will test nomenclature indirectly by making nomenclature a prerequisite to tackling a question correctly. However, if you put in the effort to understand the principles of nomenclature and apply them carefully, it should more or less give you a free point.

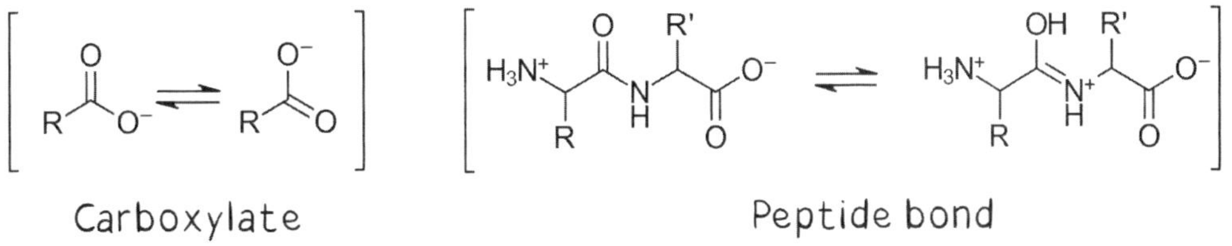

Figure 4. Resonance in carboxylate anions and peptide bonds

Resonance structures represent equivalent structures in which the electrons are delocalized. **Electron delocalization** can significantly affect the chemical properties of a compound and contribute to its stability. For example, the resonance in the carboxylate anion provides a way of stabilizing the negative charge, so the anion is said to be resonance stabilized compared to other ions containing an $-O^-$ anionic group. Resonance stabilization through loss of hydrogen means that carboxylic acids are acidic compounds. Likewise, peptide bonds are resonance stabilized.

A special case of resonance is known as **conjugation**, which occurs when three or more adjacent *p*-orbitals are aligned with each other, forming not just a π bond but a *π system*. Electrons can delocalize throughout that π system. For the MCAT, you should associate conjugation with structures containing alternating single and double bonds in carbon chains. Figure 5 shows you an example of such a molecule (retinal).

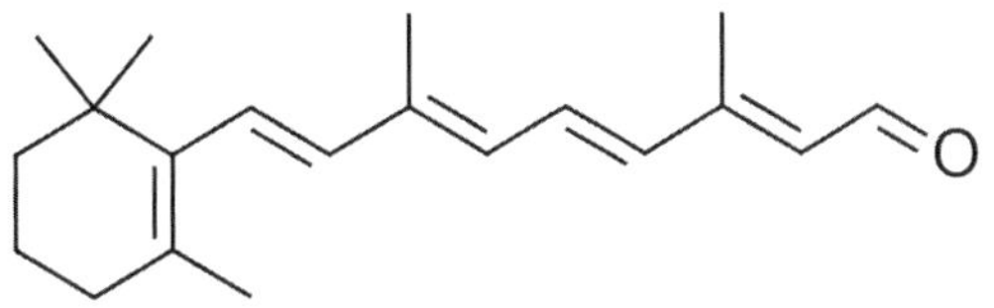

Figure 5. Molecule with a conjugated system (retinal)

Conjugated systems have a lower energy than those with isolated multiple bonds because of resonance stabilization. Consequently, they are generally detectable using UV-VIS spectroscopy, which utilizes lower electromagnetic energy.

Aromatic compounds are conjugated cyclic molecules with a planar structure that satisfies an additional criterion known as Hückel's rule, which means they have $4n + 2$ π-electrons, where n is 0 or any positive integer. The most important and well-known example of an aromatic compound is benzene; it has 6 π electrons, so $n = 1$. Aromatic rings containing atoms other than carbon are known as heterocycles. These include pyridine (present in the vitamin niacin), pyrimidine and purine (present in nucleic acids), imidazole (present in many important drugs), and pyrrole (which is a component of the porphyrins contained in heme). An aromatic compound known as borazine is a ring made up of alternating boron and nitrogen atoms. It also satisfies Hückel's rule where $n = 1$. Its chemical properties are strikingly similar to those of benzene, so as you can see, aromaticity is not limited only to benzene and its derivatives.

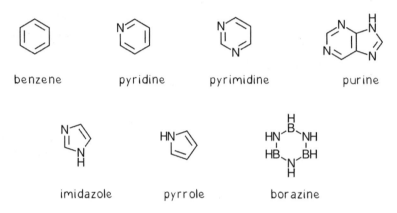

Figure 6. Aromatic compounds

One of the simplest but most striking examples of the chemical effects of resonance has to do with bond length. For example, the standard depiction of benzene has alternating C–C and C=C bonds. The bond length of C–C bonds is 154 pm, while C=C bonds have a length of 133 pm. The length of the carbon-carbon bonds in the benzene ring is 139 pm, which is intermediate between these two values. This is direct confirmation that electron delocalization exists in the benzene molecule.

More evidence is provided by the heat of hydrogenation of benzene compared to cyclohexene. The hydrogenation of cyclohexene, in which cyclohexene is converted to cyclohexane, is an exothermic process that releases 120 kJ/mol of energy. If the double bonds were localized in benzene, its hydrogenation would release $3 \times 120 = 360$ kJ/mol of energy. In actuality, the hydrogenation of benzene releases only 208 kJ/mol. The difference, 152 kJ/mol, reflects the resonance stabilization of benzene. It's worth pausing to ensure that you understand *why* this is the case. Hydrogenation of benzene releases less energy because benzene has lower internal energy due to resonance stabilization.

Resonance can also stabilize a charge on a molecule. For example, alcohols (with an –OH group) are generally very weakly acidic, but phenols, in which the –OH group is attached to a benzene ring, are more acidic. Loss of a proton from the –OH group on phenol produces a negative charge that is resonance stabilized, so phenol has a greater tendency to donate a proton, forming the phenoxide ion. Alternatively, resonance can stabilize the additional positive charge in a carbocation, which affects various reaction mechanisms. We will return to these topics in Chapter 11.

2. Isomers and Stereochemistry

This section will discuss molecules that share the same molecular formula but differ in their structure. Such molecules are called **isomers**. How molecules are arranged in space is known as **stereochemistry**. Stereochemistry is one of the highest-yield domains in organic chemistry for the MCAT. This is because stereochemistry is key to understanding why molecules behave the way they do.

The first category of isomers is known as **structural**, or **constitutional**, **isomers**. These are molecules with the same molecular formula but that differ in the way in which their constituent atoms are connected to each other. For example, C_5H_{12}, shown in Figure 7, can be pentane, isopentane (also known as 2-methylbutane), or neopentane (also known as 2,2-dimethylpropane). As suggested by the IUPAC nomenclature of these compounds, despite having the same molecular formula, they have completely different structures.

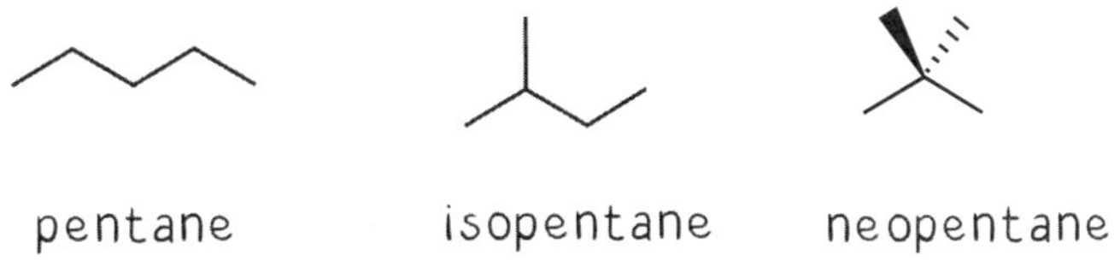

Figure 7. Structural isomers of pentane

Another example is provided by compounds with the molecular formula $C_5H_{12}O$. This could be 1-pentanol, 2-pentanol, or 3-pentanol. Moreover, as shown in Figure 8, the molecular formula corresponds to other compounds, as well not all of which are alcohols!

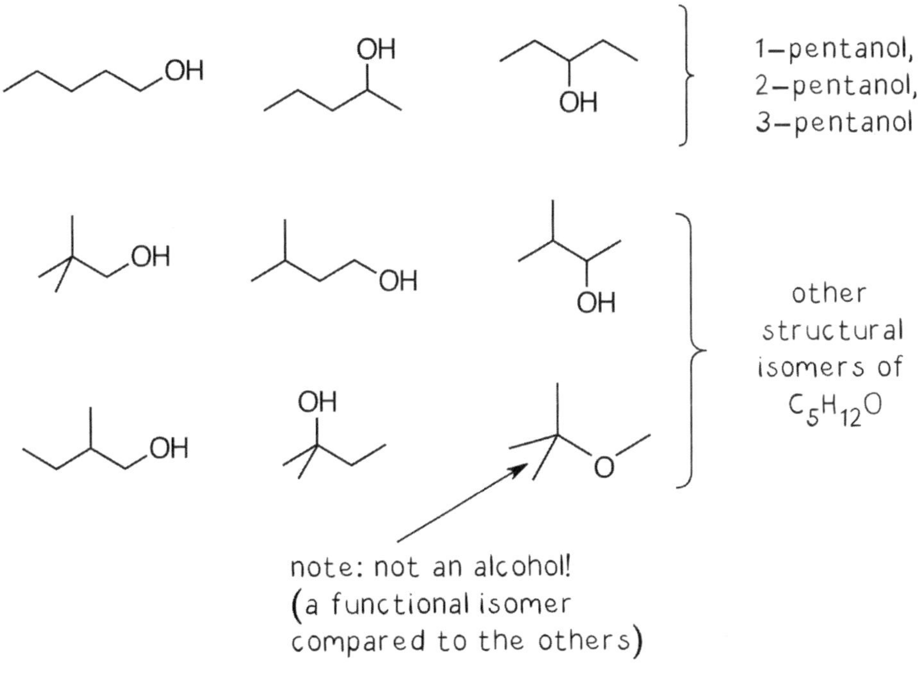

Figure 8. Structural isomers of $C_5H_{12}O$

As you see from the above example, structural isomers may have fundamentally different chemical properties. An ether has very different chemical and physical properties from those of an alcohol. Structural isomers with different functional groups are known as **functional isomers**. Figure 9 shows further examples of structural isomers.

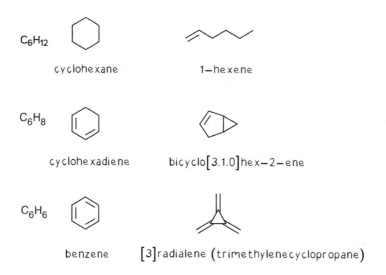

C_6H_{12}

cyclohexane   1-hexene

C_6H_8

cyclohexadiene   bicyclo[3.1.0]hex-2-ene

C_6H_6

benzene   [3]radialene (trimethylenecyclopropane)

Figure 9. Structural isomers

Tautomers are structural isomers that interconvert with each other and are in equilibrium. The most commonly encountered is **keto-enol isomerism** (also called **keto-enol tautomerism**), which is illustrated in Figure 10. At room temperature, the keto form is favored, but the enol form contributes significantly to some reaction mechanisms, and the deprotonated intermediate (known as an enolate ion) is also important for some reactions, as discussed further in Chapters 10 and 11.

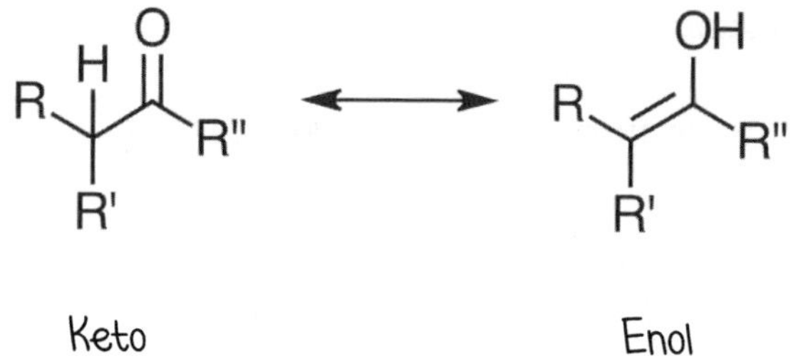

Keto   Enol

Figure 10. Keto-enol tautomerism

Although keto-enol tautomerism is the most important example of tautomerism for the MCAT, it is not the only one. As shown in Figure 11, tautomerization also occurs between enamines and imines (the second most important example), lactams and lactims, and amides and imidic acids. It is important to understand that tautomers and resonance structures are not the same thing. Resonance is a phenomenon in which electrons are delocalized. In contrast, tautomers are two *different* structures that interconvert via the breaking and reforming of bonds (see Chapter 11 for more details).

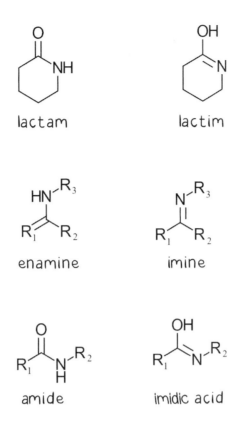

Figure 11. Other examples of tautomerism

Next we discuss **stereoisomers**. This broad category describes how molecules with a single pattern of connectivity among their constituent atoms can have different spatial configurations. There are multiple ways this can occur:

1. Arrangements of single bonds. Single bonds can freely rotate without being broken, but some of the resulting configurations—known as conformational isomers—are more favorable than others.

2. Orientation across a double bond. Double bonds do not freely rotate, so a substituent can be located on one side or another of the double bond. The designations *cis* or *trans*, as well as *E* or *Z*, are used to describe the orientations.

3. Orientation at a chiral center. A chiral center is formed by a carbon that has four different substituents. There are multiple ways to describe the differences in connectivity, most notably the *R/S* system and the *d/l* system.

Let's start with rotation around a single bond, which generates **conformational isomers**. One common example of a conformational isomer involves butane, which is visualized using **Newman projections**. In a Newman projection a carbon-carbon bond extends directly into the page, with the front carbon represented by a central dot and the back carbon represented by a circle. The carbon substituents are represented spatially by three lines radiating from each carbon in either staggered or eclipsed (overlapping) conformations.

Some of these conformations are more stable and predominate in solution. Conformations with **eclipsed, bulky substituents** experience torsional strain and are higher in potential energy, which makes them much more unstable than **staggered conformations** that maximize the separation between bulky substituents.

Staggered conformations can be 'anti' or 'gauche.' The anti conformation is the most stable because the bulky substituents are maximally separated at an angle of 180°. In the gauche conformation, the substituents are staggered, with a separation of 60° between bulky substituents. Eclipsed conformations contain overlapping substituents. Totally eclipsed conformations with bulky substituents that directly overlap are more unstable. Figure 12 illustrates the structures and potential energies of butane conformational isomers.

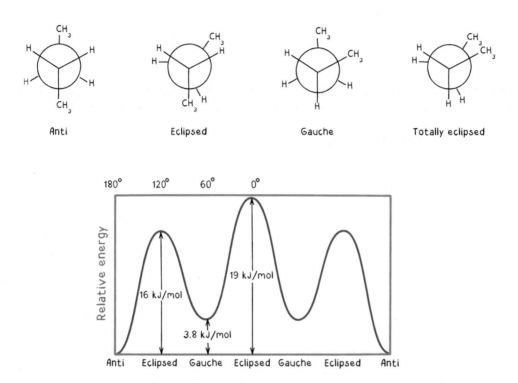

Figure 12. Structures and potential energies of butane conformational isomers

Other conformational isomerism occurs in cycloalkanes due to angle, torsional, and steric strain. **Angle strain** occurs when the angle between single-bonded carbon atoms deviates from the ideal tetrahedral bond angle of 109.5° for sp^3-hybridized carbons, whereas **torsional strain** is created by eclipsing substituents on neighboring atoms. **Steric strain** results when substituents (even hydrogen substituents!) are too close in space. In order to resolve these forms of strain, cyclohexane alternates between chair, twist-boat, and boat conformations. The chair conformation is the most stable and is preferred by cyclohexane.

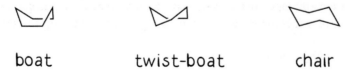

Figure 13. Conformational isomers of cyclohexane

The substituents of cyclohexane can either be in an **axial orientation** (vertical to the ring) or in an **equatorial orientation** (extending in the approximate plane of the ring). Each carbon in a cyclohexane ring has one axial and one equatorial substituent, as shown for the hydrogens in cyclohexane in Figure 14.

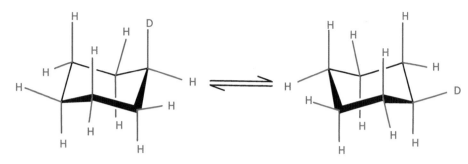

Figure 14. Axial and equatorial flipping in cyclohexane

Figure 14 also illustrates an important point: at equilibrium, two different chair conformers interconvert via bond rotation, which allows a given substituent to alternate between equatorial and axial positions. For cyclohexane, the bulkier substituents prefer equatorial positions where repulsions are minimized, so the equatorial conformation will predominate at equilibrium.

Free rotation about the C-C bond cannot occur in a cycloalkane. If a cyclohexane ring, for example, has two substituents that both point up or down, it is referred to as *cis*. Otherwise, the configuration is *trans*.

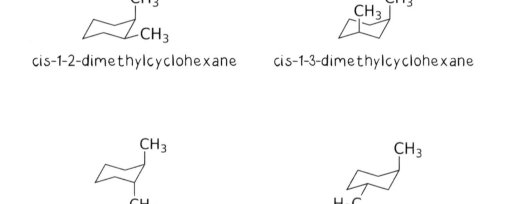

Figure 15. *Cis* and *trans* substituted cyclohexanes

Notice that a *cis* isomer cannot be converted to a *trans* isomer without breaking and reforming a bond. However, the chair conformations of each of these isomers *can* interconvert to minimize steric hindrance. This is shown in Figure 16.

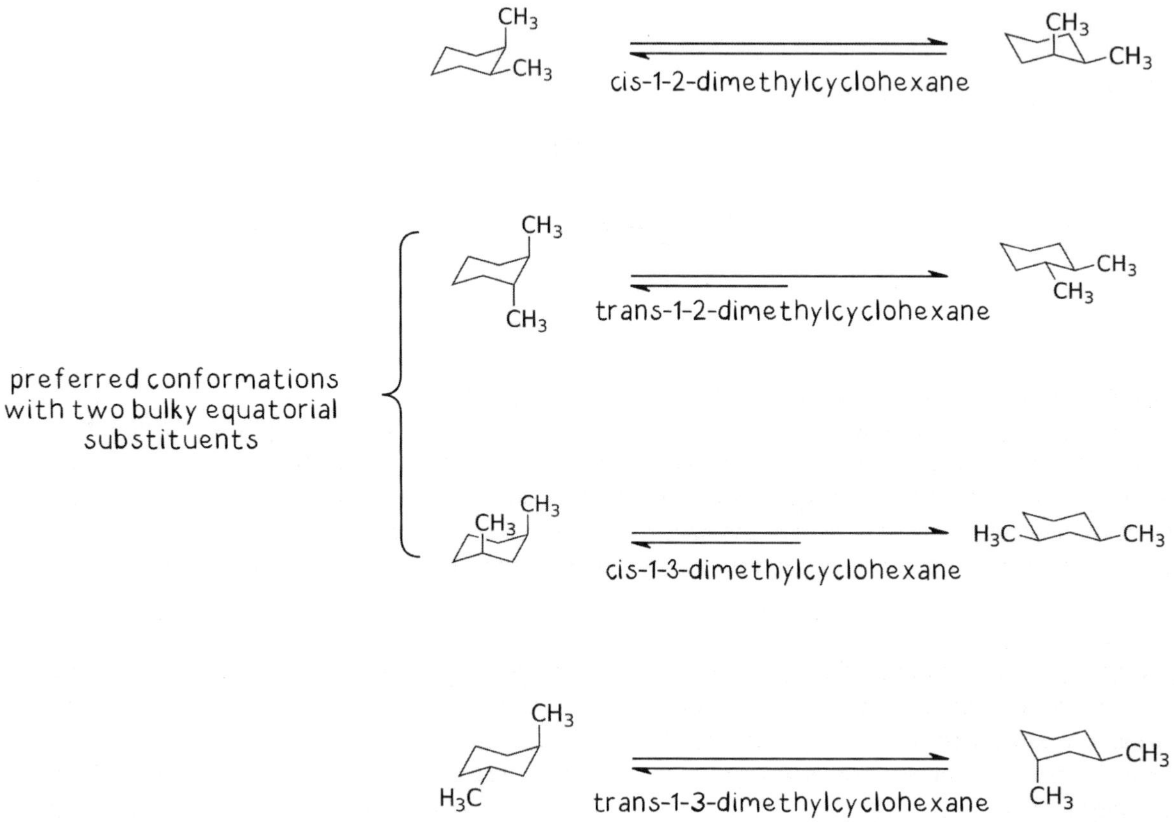

CH₃

cis-1-2-dimethylcyclohexane

CH₃
CH₃

CH₃
CH₃

preferred conformations
with two bulky equatorial
substituents
{

CH₃

CH₃

trans-1-2-dimethylcyclohexane

CH₃
CH₃

CH₃
CH₃

cis-1-3-dimethylcyclohexane

H₃C
CH₃

CH₃

H₃C

trans-1-3-dimethylcyclohexane

CH₃
CH₃

Figure 16. Interconversion of disubstituted cyclohexanes

In the above example, the two substituents are the same, but if there is a situation where one substituent is bulkier than the other (for example, if you have one methyl group and one *tert*-butyl group), the conformation with the bulkier substituent in an equatorial position will be preferred.

Geometric isomerism describes the spatial orientation of atoms around a double bond. Recall that while linear C–C bonds can rotate freely, that is not true for C=C bonds, which are in a fixed plane. ***Cis-trans*** refers to the positioning of two identical substituents across a double bond. When both substituents are on the same side of the double bond, a *cis* double bond is formed. When two identical substituents are diagonal across a double bond, a *trans* double bond is formed. This is shown in Figure 17.

trans

cis

Figure 17. *Cis* and *trans* isomers of butene

The terms *cis* and *trans* are frequently used to describe the orientation of bonds in fatty acid chains. Unsaturated fatty acids contain double bonds, whereas saturated fatty acids have only single bonds. Figure 18 compares *cis* and *trans* unsaturated fatty acids. Unsaturated fatty acids produced in nature almost always have the *cis* orientation, preventing them from evenly stacking. In contrast, *trans* fats are produced in industrial processes, stack easily, and have been shown to have detrimental effects on human health.

>> CONNECTIONS <<

Chapter 9 of Biochemistry

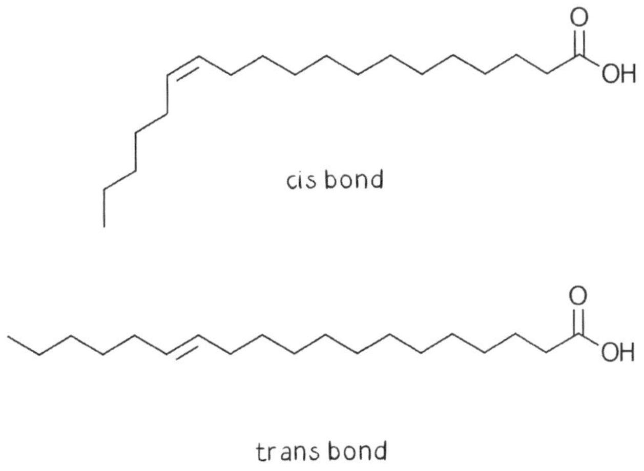

Figure 18. *Cis* and *trans* fatty acids

A more generic system for classifying geometric isomers is the **E-Z classification scheme**. The distinction from *cis-trans* isomerism is that E-Z isomerism specifies the orientation of the two highest-priority substituents, which are not necessarily identical to one another. In this system, the two highest priority substituents are on the same side of the double bond in (Z)-isomers and on the opposite side in (E)-isomers. According to the **Cahn-Ingold-Prelog priority rules**, the priority of substituent groups is determined by the atomic weights of the atoms attached to the central atom, with heavier atoms taking higher priority. If two bonded atoms are identical, the atomic weights of the atoms attached to each of those atoms are compared, and so forth. Multiple bonds are higher priority than single bonds when their atomic weights are the same.

A common point of confusion is that all *cis* isomers are (Z)-isomers and all *trans* isomers are (E)-isomers. Examine 2-bromo-2-butene in Figure 19. Notice that the two methyl groups on either side of the double bond make this molecule a *trans* isomer. First, look at the left carbon attached to the double bond. It is connected to a carbon and hydrogen. Carbon takes priority, and we know that it is pointing down (don't forget the hydrogen, which is pointing up!). Next, look at the right carbon attached to the double bond. It is attached to bromine and carbon. Bromine takes priority and is pointing down. Since both are on the same side, it is a (Z)-isomer.

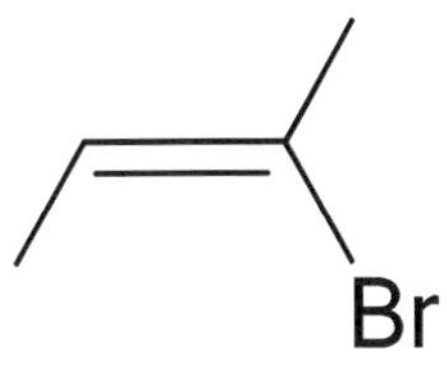

Figure 19. Structure of (Z)-2-bromo-2-butene

The E-Z classification scheme comes from German because much of the foundational research in organic chemistry in the 19ᵗʰ century was conducted in Germany. E stands for *entgegen* 'opposite,' and Z stands for *zusammen* 'together.' If you don't happen to know German, commit to memory that (Z)-isomers are on the "zame" side and (E)-isomers are on the "epposite" side!

Last but not least, we need to explore the spatial orientation of substituents at **chiral centers** (also called stereocenters), which are atoms that are connected to an sp^3-hybridized carbon with four unique groups. For example, the central carbon in the structure shown in Figure 20 is a stereocenter because it is attached to four unique substituents. This molecule is therefore chiral because it is not superimposable upon its own mirror image.

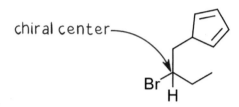

Figure 20. A chiral molecule

A helpful visual analogy is to consider handedness: your right and left hands are mirror images, but cannot be superimposed on one another. This principle is further exemplified in Figure 21, which illustrates the chirality of amino acids. Molecules that are non-superimposable mirror images are called enantiomers. In contrast, achiral molecules possess a plane of symmetry and are superimposable.

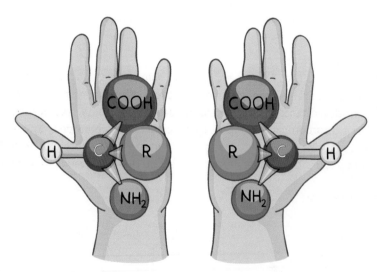

Figure 21. Amino acid chirality

The maximum number of stereoisomers possible for a given structure is equal to 2^n, where *n* is the number of stereocenters. Consider the structure of testosterone shown below. It has six chiral centers, so a maximum of $2^6 = 64$ stereoisomers.

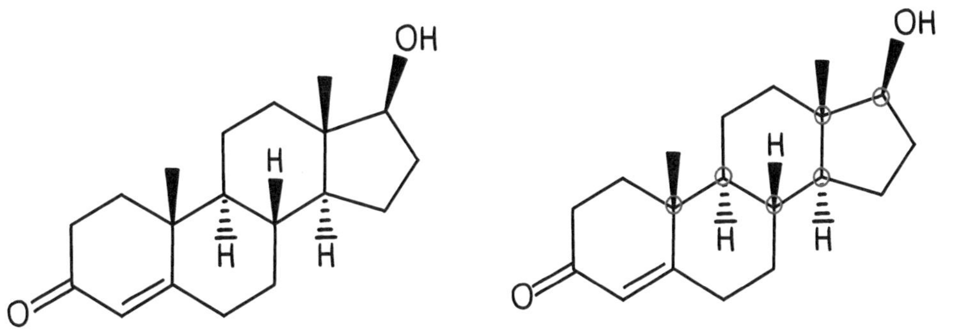

Figure 22. Chiral centers in testosterone

In Figure 22, each chiral center has a substituent denoted with a bold line or a dashed line. Bold lines represent atoms pointing out from the plane of the page (towards the reader), and dashed lines represent atoms pointing into the page (away from the reader). This is a common feature of how chiral centers are represented, and as such can be a valuable shortcut if you encounter a question on test day asking you to identify how many stereocenters there are in a given molecule. However, you should be careful to double-check that there are indeed four *distinct* substituents at every site. As shown in Figure 23, it is possible for bold/dashed lines to denote substituents of a non-chiral carbon and for a chiral carbon not to have bold/dashed lines.

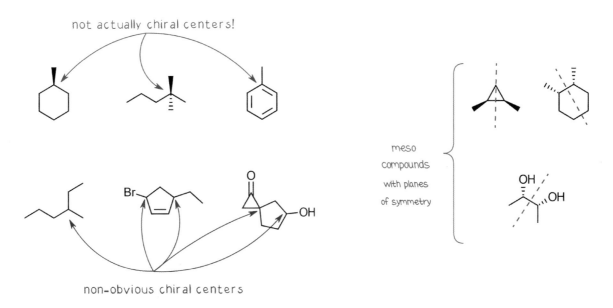

Figure 23. Misleading achiral and chiral compounds

Meso compounds are molecules that have multiple stereocenters (usually two in most examples you'll see on the MCAT) but are not chiral because they have a plane of symmetry that results in two superimposable mirror images. Suppose you identify a compound that has two stereocenters and an internal plane of symmetry. In that case, it is highly likely to be a meso compound if the substituents at both stereocenters are pointed either into or out of the plane of the page. Examples of meso compounds are shown in Figure 23.

An interesting manifestation of chemical 'handedness' (chirality) is that solutions of chiral compounds rotate planes of polarized light at angles unique to each stereoisomer. This is defined as the **specific rotation [α]** of the molecule. Compounds that produce clockwise (+) rotation of plane-polarized light are dextrorotatory (*d*), and compounds that produce counterclockwise (–) rotation are levorotatory (*l*). The specific rotation of a chiral compound in solution can be calculated according to the equation:

Equation 1.

$$[\alpha] = \frac{\alpha}{c\ell}$$

In Equation 1, α is the observed rotation in degrees, c is the concentration in g/mL, and ℓ is the length of the polarimeter tube in decimeters (dm).

A mixture with a 50:50 composition of two enantiomers of a given compound is known as a **racemic mixture**. Such mixtures do not rotate plane-polarized light at all because the optical activity of each enantiomer cancels out that of the other. If one enantiomer has a specific rotation of [+ α], its opposite enantiomer will have a rotation of [–α].

We can work backward from the observed rotation of a mixture—if we know [α]—to calculate the distribution of enantiomers in a solution. The formula we can use for this is given below:

Equation 2.

$$\text{enantiomeric excess (\%)} = \frac{[\alpha]_{observed}}{[\alpha]_{pure}} \times 100$$

Equation 2 gives us a quantity known as **enantiomeric excess**, which gives the percentage difference between two enantiomers in a sample. If we know, for example, that the optical activity ($[\alpha]_{pure}$) of the (*d*) enantiomer of a compound is + 20°, and we observe a rotation ($[\alpha]_{observed}$) of + 10°, substituting these values into Equation 2 will yield 50%. This does *not* mean that the (*d*) enantiomer comprises 50% of the sample; after all, that would be a racemic mixture, with an optical activity of 0°. Instead, it means that the percentage of the (*d*) enantiomer must exceed that of the (*l*) enantiomer by 50 percent, which means that the (*d*) enantiomer makes up 75% of the solution, while the (*l*) enantiomer makes up only 25%.

Optical activity is one way to refer to the different enantiomers of a compound. This was done historically and is still used in some contexts, but it has limitations as a form of chemical nomenclature because it describes nothing about the structure of a compound. We cannot predict which way a compound will rotate plane polarized light. Moreover, the problem gets worse when we have to account for molecules with multiple chiral centers (remember our example of testosterone with 64 possible stereoisomers!). Consequently, chemists developed a system of absolute configuration (known as the **R/S system**) that utilizes the Cahn-Ingold-Prelog priority rules discussed above for *E/Z* isomerism. To determine whether a given stereocenter has an *R* or *S* notation, use the following steps:

1. Assign priorities to each substituent. Atoms with greater atomic weights receive higher priority.

2. If the lowest priority substituent is in the back, move on to step 3. If not, draw the molecule so that it is in the back.

3. Determine the order of the remaining substituents from highest to lowest priority. If moving from highest to lowest gives a clockwise rotation, the configuration is R. If the rotation is counterclockwise, it is S.

4. If the orientation of the lowest priority group is in the front rather than the back, the true absolute configuration will be the opposite of that found in step 3.

Let's see how this works in practice with an example. What is the absolute configuration of the two stereocenters in 2,3-butanediol?

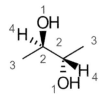

1. The compound has two stereocenters. First, we assign priorities to each substituent.

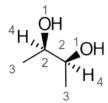

2. Next, we place the lowest priority substituent in the back at each stereocenter.

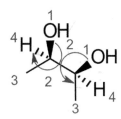

3. Then, we draw an arrow from the highest to lowest priority to determine the absolute configuration.

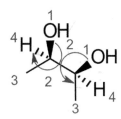

4. The orientation of the lowest priority substituent at position 3 of the right carbon is out of the plane of the paper as originally depicted, so the absolute configuration at that position must be reversed if you skip step 2 (R→S). Therefore, the name of this compound is (2R,3S)-2,3-butanediol.

When working with molecules that have multiple chiral centers, a distinction is made between **enantiomers** and **diastereomers**. As we have discussed, enantiomers are non-superimposable mirror images. For this to be true in a compound with multiple stereocenters, *all* the stereocenters in its stereoisomer must be oppositely oriented. In contrast, diastereomers are compounds that do not satisfy this criteria. In diastereomers, not all stereocenters in the stereoisomer are opposites. Figure 24 provides a simple illustration of how this works for compounds with two chiral centers.

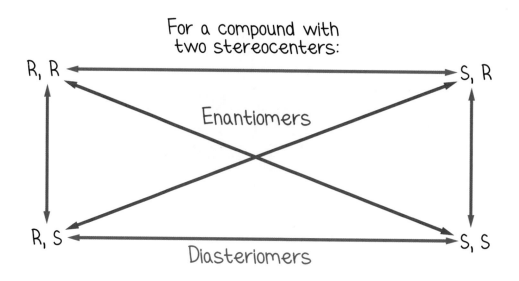

Figure 24. Enantiomers versus diastereomers

Now that we've reviewed the various types of isomers you may encounter on the MCAT, it is useful to look back at the bigger picture. Figure 25 presents a flowchart of the various types of isomerism.

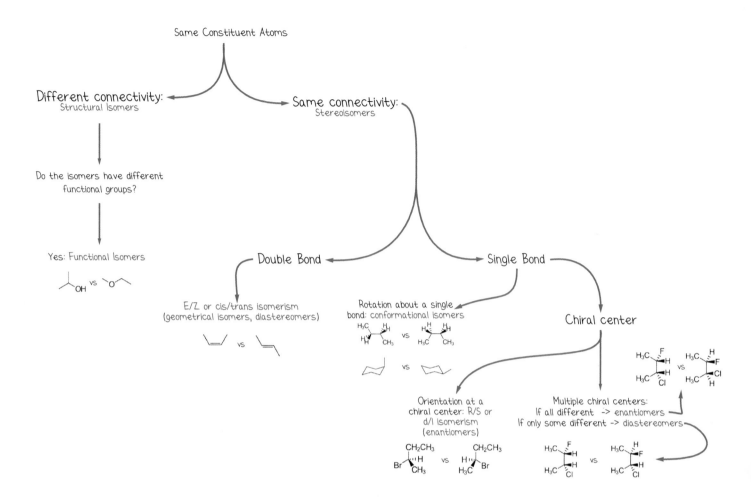

Figure 25. Isomerism flowchart

3. Must-Knows

> IUPAC nomenclature for alkanes:
  — (1) identify and name longest carbon chain (1C = methane, 2C = ethane, 3C = propane, 4C = butane, 5C = pentane, etc.).
  — (2) label carbons such that substituents have lowest possible #'s; (3) identify all substituents (methyl, ethyl, etc.).
  — (4) place substituents in alphabetical order.
  — Other functional groups have a suffix (when they are the highest-priority group): –COOH (-oic acid) is highest priority, followed by carboxylic acid derivatives, aldehydes/ketones (suffix: -al/-one, prefix: oxo-), alcohols (suffix: -ol, prefix: hydroxy-), amines (suffix: -amine, prefix: amino-), thiols (suffix: -thiol, prefix: mercapto-), and hydrocarbons.

> Resonance:
  — When more than one equivalent Lewis structure can be drawn for a compound. Multiple structures indicate electron delocalization.

> Aromatic compounds: conjugated cyclic molecules with planar structure + satisfy Hückel's rule: having $4n + 2$ π-electrons, where n is 0 or an integer.
  — Common example: benzene.

> Cahn-Ingold-Prelog rules for assigning priority to substituents:
  — (1) look at atoms directly connected to the stereocenter; heavier atoms have higher priority.
  — (2) if two atoms are the same, move one atom further down the substituents and re-rank by substituents.
  — (3) continue until a difference is encountered; multiple bonds are higher-priority than single bonds.
  — E/Z system for double bonds: E if higher-priority substituents are on opposite sides of double bond, Z if higher-priority substituents are on the same side.
  — R/S system for chiral centers: orient molecule such that lowest-priority substituent faces into the page and connect substituents from high to low priority; if doing so traces a clockwise pattern.
  — Molecule is R; if counterclockwise, S.

> Chirality: non-superimposable mirror images (enantiomers):
  — C must have 4 different substituents. When there is more than one chiral center, enantiomers have opposite orientation at *all* chiral centers, while diastereomers only differ at some.
  — For n chiral centers, there is a maximum of 2^n stereoisomers.

End of Chapter Practice

The best MCAT practice is realistic, with a focus on identifying steps for further improvement. For those reasons, we recommend completing practice questions in an online setting that simulates the real MCAT interface, and taking advantage of advanced analytic features to help you determine how best to move forward in your MCAT study journey.

With that in mind, online end-of-chapter questions for Biology, Biochemistry, Chemistry + Organic Chemistry, Physics, and Psychology/Sociology are available through your Blueprint MCAT account.

As a further supplement, given the importance of active learning for effective studying, we also suggest that you consult the Must-Knows as a basis for creating a study sheet, in which you list out key terms and test your ability to briefly summarize them.

This page left intentionally blank.

Key Functional Groups and Their Reactions

0. Introduction

Functional groups can be used to predict the behavior of molecules, both in terms of physical properties and in terms of reactivity.

For each functional group, the MCAT expects you to be aware of: (1) nomenclature; (2) physical properties; (3) important reactions; and (4) general principles affecting reactivity. This chapter discusses the functional groups necessary for the MCAT, with the goal of providing a systematic overview of the above four points.

The nomenclature is previously discussed in Chapter 9, but is presented here as well. In this chapter, important reactions are presented schematically, in terms of reactants and products. Use this chapter as such:

> Use this chapter for a comprehensive overview of the nomenclature, physical properties, and important reactions associated with each functional group.

> Consult Chapter 9 if you need to review the principles of IUPAC nomenclature.

> Use Chapter 11 to study organic reaction mechanisms in more detail.

Most MCAT questions on functional groups can be divided into the following three categories: (1) recognition; (2) basic properties; and (3) reactions. In order to reliably succeed on recognition questions, you must review *all* functional groups and their nomenclature. Questions about physical and chemical properties will often deal with topics such as acidity/basicity and electrophilicity/nucleophilicity, so be sure to understand how the structure of each functional group contributes to those properties. For reactions, be sure to review common reactions in terms of their reactants and products, and understand that you may be required to apply those principles to reactions involving unfamiliar molecules.

1. Alkanes, Alkenes, and Alkynes

Alkanes, **alkenes**, and **alkynes** are **hydrocarbons**—the simplest examples of organic molecules, are made up only of carbon and hydrogen atoms. Alkanes have only single bonds between carbons, and end with the suffix –ane. Alkenes have at least one double carbon-carbon bond (C=C), and end with the suffix –ene. An alkene with two double bonds is a diene, and an alkene with three double bonds is a triene. Alkynes have at least one triple carbon-carbon bond (C≡C), and have the characteristic suffix –yne. Hydrocarbons are not, in and of themselves, an especially high-yield class of molecules for the MCAT because they are not particularly relevant biologically, but they are worth reviewing because their nomenclature is the foundation for naming other molecule types and because some of their derivatives are involved in important reactions.

In addition to the basic nomenclature for hydrocarbons (–ane, –ene, and –yne), you should be aware of how alkane substituents on other molecules are named. The general rule is to use –yl as the suffix (leading to the term "alkyl" to refer to alkane substituents in general). Methyl, ethyl, propyl, and butyl (also known as *n*-butyl) are used relatively intuitively, but be sure that you can also recognize isopropyl, *sec*-butyl, and *tert*-butyl or *t*-butyl, as shown below in Table 1.

Methyl	H_3C-R	Isopropyl	
Ethyl		*sec*-Butyl	
Propyl		*t*-Butyl	
Butyl			

Table 1. Alkyl substituents

Hydrocarbons tend to have relatively low melting points and boiling points because the only intermolecular forces they experience are London dispersion forces, which are relatively weak. For the purposes of the MCAT, alkanes and alkenes can be treated as basically equivalent in this regard. The melting points and boiling points of alkanes and alkenes are primarily influenced by molecular weight (higher molecular weight → higher melting/boiling points) and, to a lesser extent, by branching, with more highly branched molecules exhibiting lower melting/boiling points because they stack less efficiently. This is shown in Table 2, in which the boiling points are compared for straight-chain versus branched isomers for various alkanes.

NUMBER OF CARBONS	STRAIGHT-CHAIN ISOMER			BRANCHED ISOMER		
	Name (formula)	Structure	Boiling point	Name (formula)	Structure	Boiling point
1	Methane (CH_4)	H–C–H with H above and H below	−161°C	None		
2	Ethane (C_2H_6)	H_3C-CH_3	−89°C			
3	Propane (C_3H_8)		−42°C			
4	Butane (C_4H_{10})		−1°C	2-Methylpropane (C_4H_{10})		−12°C
5	Pentane (C_5H_{12})		36°C	2,2-Dimethylpropane (C_5H_{12})		9°C
6	Hexane (C_6H_{14})		68°C	2,3-Dimethylbutane (C_6H_{14})		58°C

Table 2. Boiling points of alkanes according to molecular weight and branchedness

Hydrocarbons have no acid-base chemistry to speak of. They are very stable and not particularly reactive molecules, and show no meaningful tendency to become protonated or deprotonated. For example, the pK_a of pentane is approximately 45, which means that in an entire mole of pentane, comprising 6.02×10^{23} molecules (an almost unfathomably large number, corresponding to roughly 81 *trillion* times the current population of earth), you could expect to find literally about 20 protons at a given time. This means that spontaneous dissociation of pentane into H+ and its conjugate base is extraordinarily rare.

Haloalkanes, or **alkyl halides**, are alkanes with halogen substituents (F, Cl, Br, or I). They can be made from alkanes through a free-radical mechanism, from alkenes through hydrohalogenation, or from alcohols through substitution with hydrogen halides, as shown in Figure 1.

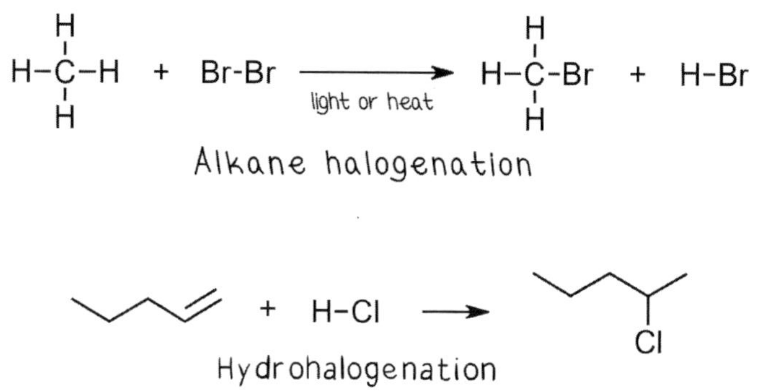

Figure 1. Formation of haloalkanes

Haloalkanes are mostly of note for the MCAT because they are quite reactive and readily undergo substitution and elimination reactions due to halogens being excellent leaving groups. Since halogens are highly electronegative, the carbon attached to the halogen substituent becomes electron-deficient, making it an electrophile. Figure 2 shows examples of substitution and elimination reactions in which haloalkanes are used to generate alcohols and alkenes, respectively. The mechanisms of these reactions are discussed in more detail in Chapter 11.

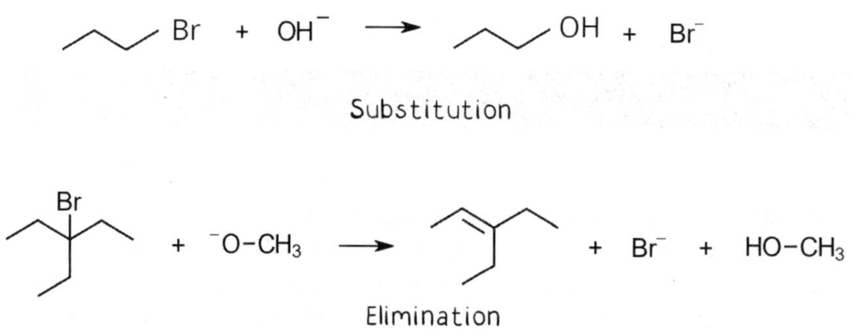

Figure 2. Substitution and elimination reactions of haloalkanes

Alkenes are largely important for MCAT organic chemistry for two main reasons that have little to nothing to do with their reactivity. First, alkenes and alkene derivatives are the prototypical examples used to illustrate E/Z (cis/trans) isomerism, as discussed in Chapter 9. Second, molecules with alternating C=C double bonds form conjugated systems of bonds, which involve connected p-orbitals with delocalized electrons. Conjugated systems are often visualized well in ultraviolet (UV) spectroscopy, as discussed in greater detail in Chapter 12.

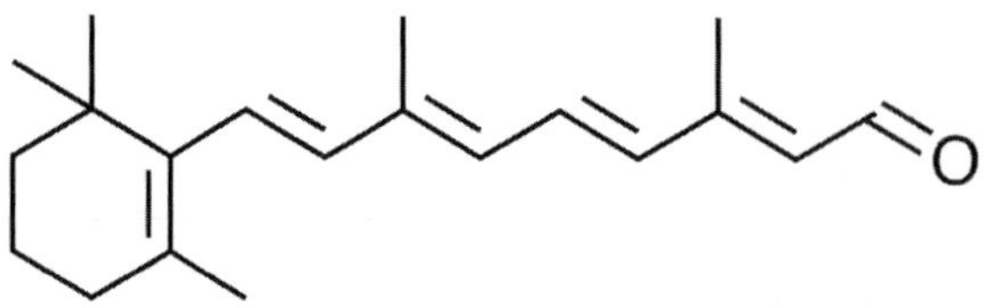

Figure 3. Molecule with a conjugated system (retinal)

Similarly to alkanes, alkenes are involved in some reactions that are relevant for the MCAT not primarily because of their products but because they provide a simple case of useful principles that can be applied to other, more complicated reactions. In particular, alkenes provide a useful example illustrating how to think about **reduction** and **oxidation** in organic chemistry. For example, alkenes can be reduced in a process known as **hydrogenation**, in which an alkene reacts with H_2 in the presence of a catalyst (usually Ni, Pd, or Pt) to form an alkane. Alkenes can also be oxidized in a variety of ways. One example is the reaction of alkenes with cold, dilute $KMnO_4$ to form a 1,2-diol. These reactions are shown in Figure 4.

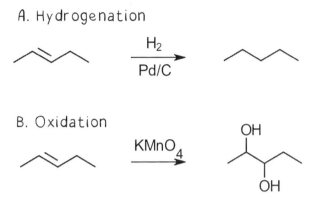

Figure 4. (A) Hydrogenation of an alkene. (B) Oxidation of an alkene with cold, dilute $KMnO_4$

The results of these reactions are not particularly important for the MCAT. The more important question is why the reaction in Figure 4A is reduction, while the reaction in Figure 4B is oxidation. In Figure 4A, each carbon breaks a C–C bond and forms a C–H bond, meaning its oxidation state decreases (reduction). In Figure 4B, a C–C bond is broken and a C–O bond is formed, meaning that the oxidation state of carbon increases (oxidation). Working through oxidation state changes for each reaction can be time-consuming, so it may be helpful to learn the following equivalent definitions for reduction and oxidation in the context of organic chemistry.

REDUCTION	OXIDATION
Gain of an electron	Loss of an electron
Decreased oxidation state	Increased oxidation state
Formation of a C–H bond (e.g., alkene → alkane)	Loss of a C–H bond (e.g., alkane → alkene)
Loss of a C–O or C–N bond (or any bond between carbon and an electronegative atom)	Gain of a C–O or C–N bond (or any bond between carbon and an electronegative atom)

Table 2. Reduction and oxidation in organic chemistry

2. Alcohols

Alcohols have the functional group –OH, also known as a hydroxyl group. In IUPAC nomenclature, alcohols are denoted using the suffix –ol, while hydroxyl substituents in molecules with other, higher-priority functional groups are named using the prefix hydroxy-. In common nomenclature, the alcohol group can be denoted using an –yl suffix, followed by "alcohol," such that "ethyl alcohol" is the common name for ethanol.

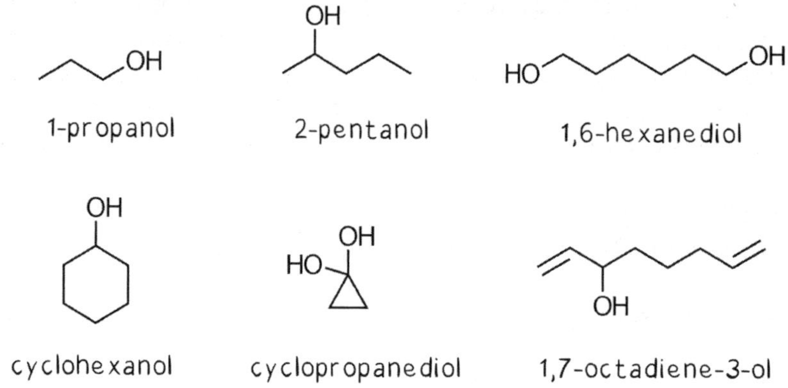

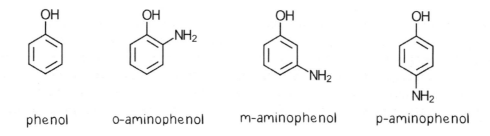

Figure 5. Examples of alcohols

Throughout this chapter, we will want to pay attention to a special set of alcohols, in which a hydroxyl group is bonded to an aromatic benzene ring. These compounds are known as **phenols**, and have special nomenclature, as well as distinct chemical and physical properties due to the ability of resonance to stabilize the conjugate base forms of these molecules (known as phenoxides). The terms *ortho* (*o*), *meta* (*m*), and *para* (*p*) are used to describe the orientation of two substituents on a benzene ring with regard to each other. Let's consider examples of phenols with an additional substituent. If the additional substituent is adjacent to the hydroxyl group, then the molecule is described as *ortho* (*o*). If the additional substituent and the hydroxyl group are separated by a single carbon, the molecule can be described as *meta* (*m*), while *para* (*p*) is used to describe substituents on the opposite sides of the benzene ring, separated by two carbons. Examples of this are given in Figure 6.

Figure 6. Examples of phenols

Alcohols have high melting and boiling points because they readily undergo hydrogen bonding. This effect increases with additional hydroxyl groups, as shown in Table 3.

STRUCTURE	NUMBER OF HYDROXYL GROUPS	BOILING POINT
Pentane	0	36.1°C
2-Pentanol	1	119.3°C
1,5-Pentanediol	2	242°C
1,3,5-Pentanetriol	3	320.2°C

Table 3. Melting points of alcohols

In general, alcohols are weakly acidic, and their conjugate bases (alkoxides) are weak bases. Alcohols tend to have pK_a values in the range of 15-17, making them weaker acids than water ($pK_a = 14$). However, phenols are notably more acidic due to resonance stabilization of the conjugate base. For example, phenol itself has a pK_a of approximately 10, which makes it a weak acid, but one that is strong enough to be relevant for acid-base chemistry. The acidity of alcohols and phenols can be increased by adding electron-withdrawing substituents that help stabilize the negative charge on the conjugate base, or decreased by adding electron-donating substituents. This is technically true of all acids and bases, but phenols are an especially good example because of the very wide range of pK_a values that can be generated this way. For example, 2,4-dinitrophenol (which contains two electron-withdrawing groups) has a pK_a of 4.11. This pK_a value is still weakly acidic, technically speaking, but is more than low enough for 2,4-dinitrophenol to be meaningfully acidic in biological contexts. For comparison, the pK_a values of the side chains of aspartic acid and glutamic acid are 3.9 and 4.07, respectively, and that of acetic acid is 4.76.

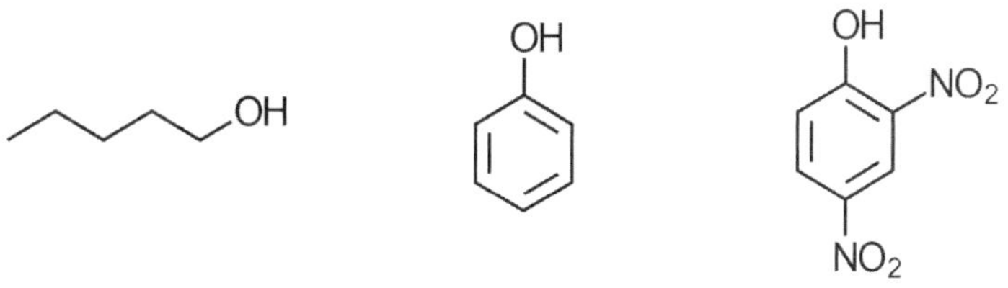

pentanol
$pK_a = 16.8$

phenol
$pK_a = 10.0$

2,4-dinitrophenol
$pK_a = 4.11$

Figure 7. Alcohols and phenols with various pK_a values

To summarize, there are two basic things to understand about the physical and chemical properties of alcohols and phenols: (1) hydrogen bonding, (2) weak but modifiable acidity.

The largest set of MCAT-relevant reactions involving alcohols is **oxidation**. In this context, oxidation means the conversion of a hydroxyl group bound to a carbon to a carbonyl group (C=O, corresponding to either an aldehyde or ketone depending on its location within the molecule) or a carboxylic acid (COOH). Oxidation of an alcohol can be thought of as proceeding in two steps: first, oxidation to a carbonyl group, and then further oxidation to a carboxylic acid. The outcome of the oxidation of alcohols depends on whether the alcohol is primary or secondary, and on the oxidizing agent that is used.

Pyridium chlorochromate (PCC) is a **weak oxidizing agent** that turns C–OH groups into carbonyl (C=O) groups. When applied to a primary alcohol, this results in an aldehyde, whereas a ketone results when a secondary alcohol is treated with PCC.

MCAT STRATEGY >>>

If you see a primary alcohol oxidized to an aldehyde (terminal C=O) on the MCAT, the oxidizing agent must have been PCC.

Stronger oxidizing agents, such as $NaCr_2O_7$, $K_2Cr_2O_7$, and CrO_3, oxidize primary alcohols to carboxylic acids. When applied to secondary alcohols, they result in ketones, because the oxidation process can go no further in that location.

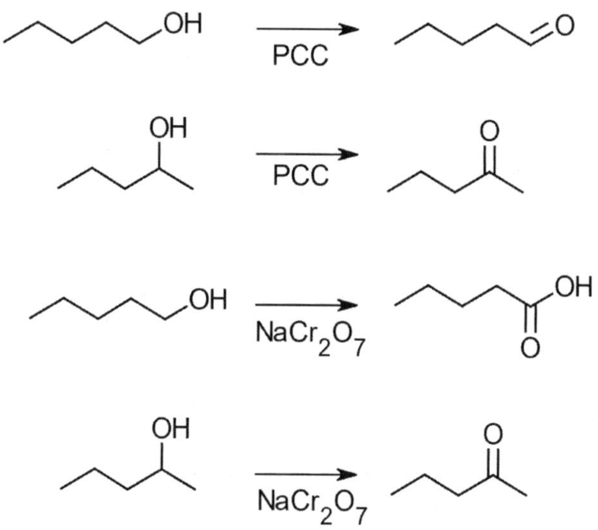

Figure 8. Oxidation of alcohols

The oxidation of certain phenols is biologically relevant, although the actual chemistry is not meaningfully different than how other alcohols are oxidized. The molecule *p*-benzenediol, also known as hydroquinone, becomes quinone (2,5-cyclohexadiene-1,4-dione) when oxidized. Note that quinone itself is *not* an aromatic molecule, although it is entirely possible for derivatives of quinone to contain aromatic rings bonded to the parent quinone structure. Derivatives of quinone are known as **quinones**, and form a class of biologically important molecules that generally serve as electron acceptors.

An especially important example of a biologically important quinone is **ubiquinone**, also known as coenzyme Q. Ubiquinone is an electron carrier involved in complexes I, II, and III of the electron transport chain. Its amphipathic structure (polar head and long alkyl tail) allows it to be both lipid-soluble and a functional electron carrier. When carrying one electron, one of its carbonyl (C=O) groups is reduced to an alcohol, resulting in a molecule known as ubisemiquinone, and when carrying two electrons—as is commonly the case—both carbonyl (C=O) groups are reduced, and the molecule is known as ubiquinol. Similar reactions underpin the function of other biological electron carriers, such as NAD^+/NADH and FAD/FADH/$FADH_2$.

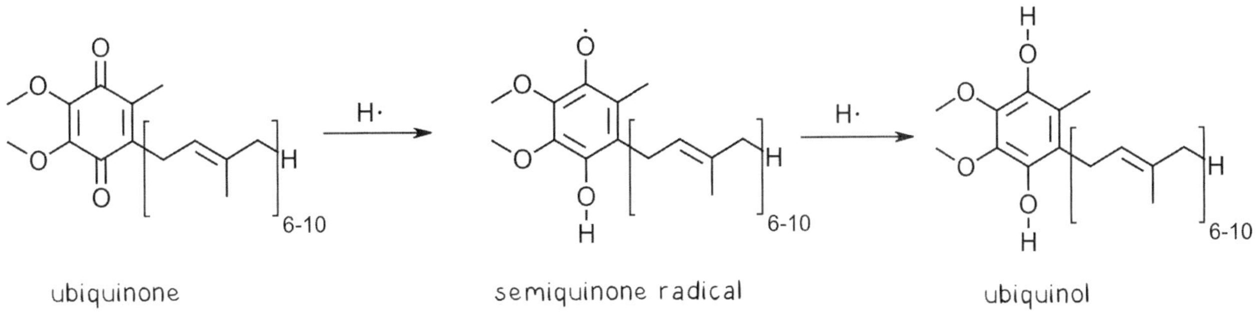

Figure 9. Ubiquinone, semiquinone, and ubiquinol

Alcohols are generally fairly reactive molecules, and in organic synthesis it may become necessary to "protect" an alcohol group to ensure that another functional group on a molecule undergoes a reaction without altering the alcohol group. Consider the example shown in Figure 10, where we have a molecule with an alkene and a hydroxyl group, and we want to use HBr to carry out hydrohalogenation of the alkene group. How do we prevent HBr from engaging in a substitution reaction to replace the –OH group with –Br, potentially resulting in a complex mixture of products?

The answer to this dilemma is to protect the –OH group by reversibly treating it with another compound that makes the –OH group non-reactive. Once the desired reaction is completed, the protecting group can be removed. Many types of **protecting groups** have been developed, but there are three major classes that you should be aware of for the MCAT: silyl ethers, mesylates, and tosylates. Silyl ethers involve a Si–O bond that can be broken with fluoride after the desired reaction is completed. Mesylates and tosylates are formed by reacting the alcohol with methylsulfonyl chloride and toluenesulfonyl chloride, respectively. Mesylates and tosylates are also good leaving groups, so the effect of treating alcohols with methylsulfonyl chloride or toluenesulfonyl chloride may be either to protect them or to facilitate a substitution reaction in which the hydroxyl group is replaced by an incoming nucleophile. The specific outcome depends on details of the reaction setup that are beyond the scope of the MCAT.

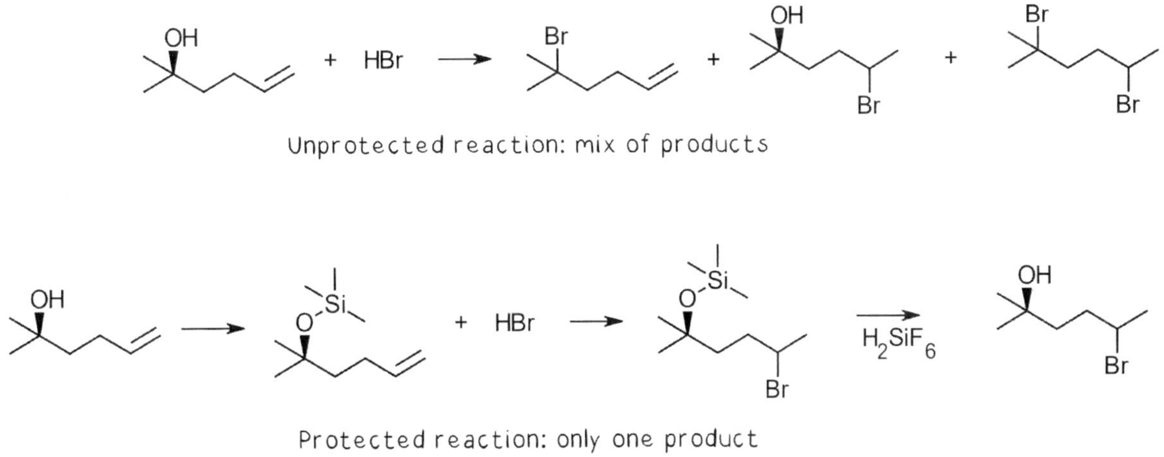

Unprotected reaction: mix of products

Protected reaction: only one product

Figure 10. Unprotected and protected hydrohalogenation reactions

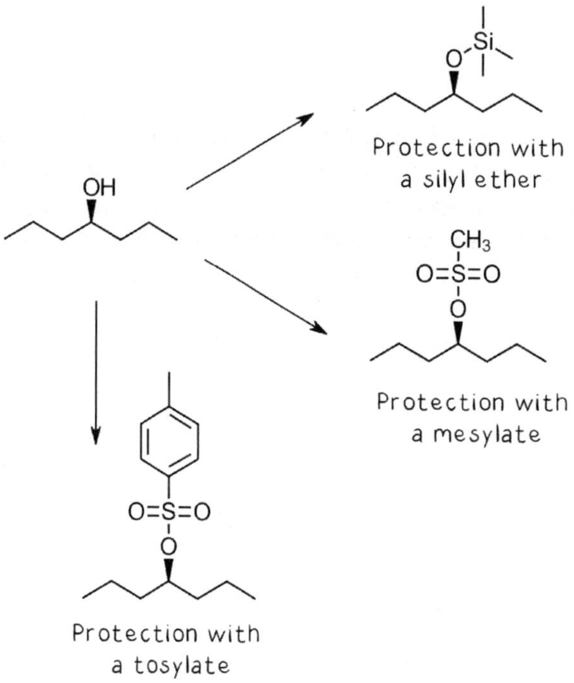

Figure 11. Alcohols protected with silyl ethers, mesylates, and tosylates

In addition to being protected, alcohols can also be used to protect other functional groups. Consider the compound in Figure 12. Imagine that we want to reduce the carboxylic acid functional group (–COOH) to an alcohol using $LiAlH_4$, while not affecting the carbonyl group (C=O). The challenge here is that $LiAlH_4$ is capable of reducing both groups. Treatment of the carbonyl carbon with two equivalents of an alcohol (often accomplished by using a single equivalent of a diol) results in the formation of an **acetal** group, which is not affected by $LiAlH_4$, and can easily be removed under acidic conditions after the carboxylic acid functional group is reduced.

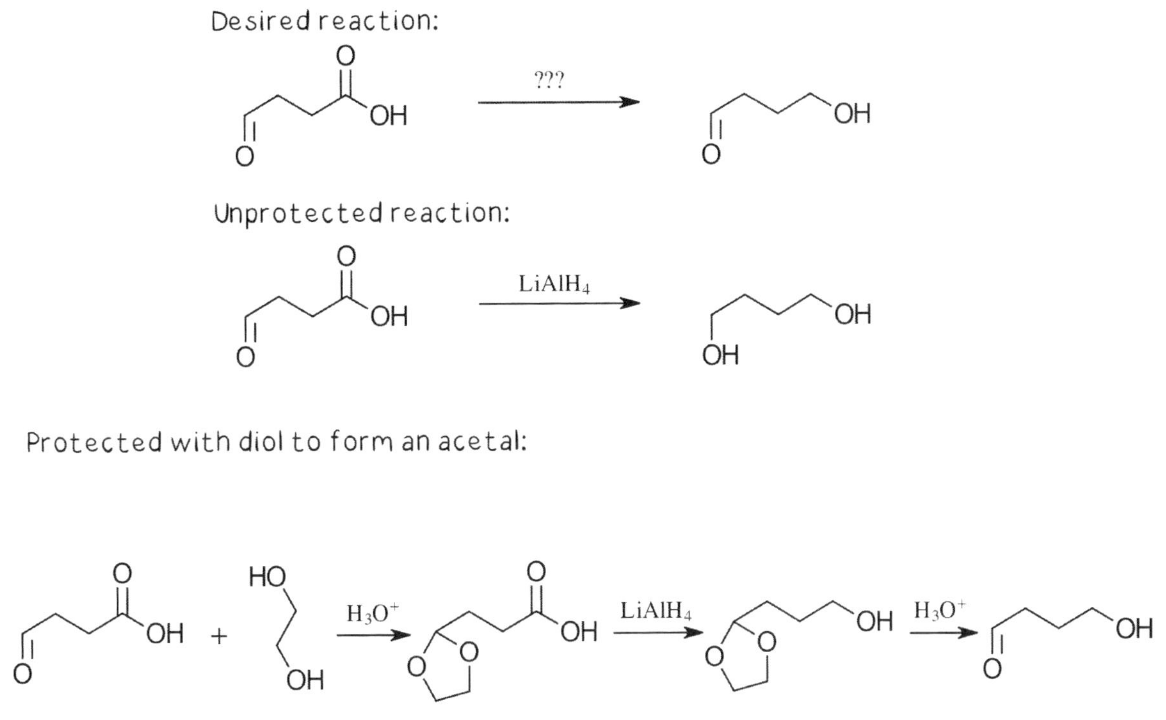

Desired reaction:

Unprotected reaction:

Protected with diol to form an acetal:

Figure 12. Protection using acetal formation

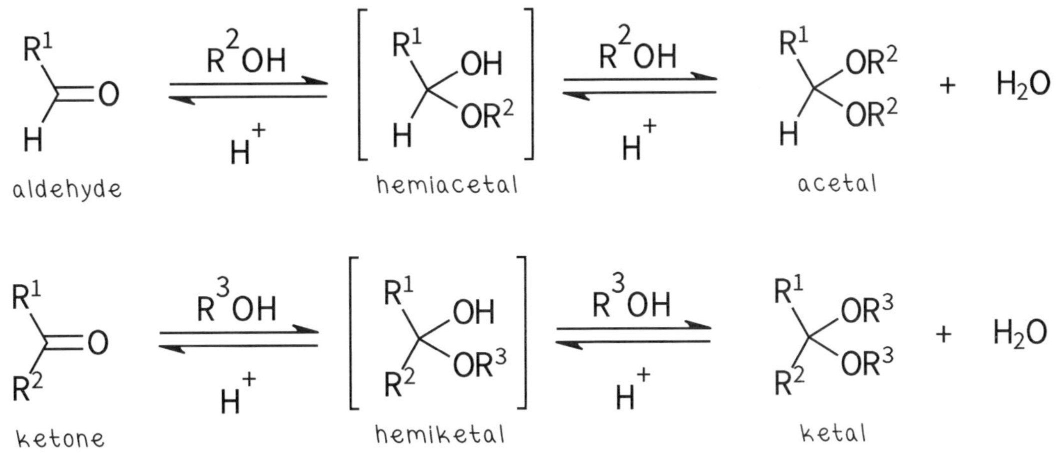

Figure 13. Acetals, hemiacetals, ketals, and hemiketals

As shown in Figure 13, the central C atom in acetals is connected to one H, one R1 group, and two OR2 groups. Hemiacetals are an intermediate step in the formation of acetals and include one –OH group in place of one of the two OR2 groups found in acetals. Ketals and hemiketals are the corresponding structures for ketones. In laboratory conditions, hemiacetals are often very unstable, and quickly proceed to acetals. However, cyclic hemiacetals and hemiketals are common in sugar chemistry, corresponding to the cyclic forms of glucose and fructose, respectively.

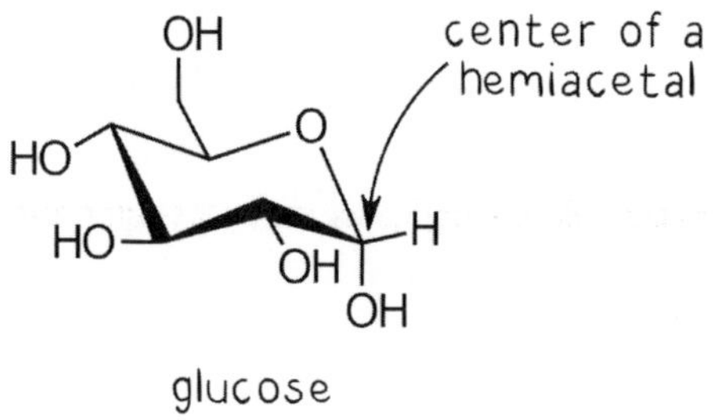

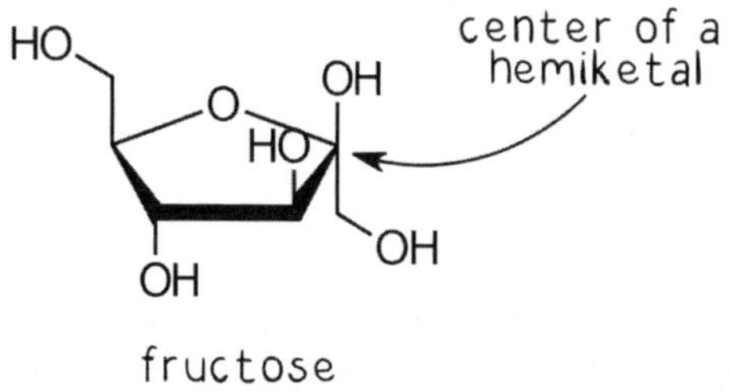

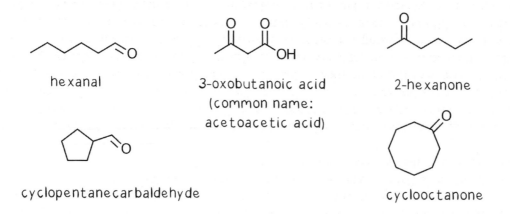

Figure 14. Cyclic forms of glucose and fructose as hemiacetals and hemiketals

glucose

center of a
hemiacetal

center of a
hemiketal

fructose

>> CONNECTIONS <<

Chapter 6 of Biochemistry

3. Aldehydes and Ketones

Aldehydes and ketones are defined by the presence of a **carbonyl (C=O) group**. In **aldehydes**, the carbonyl group is terminal (at the end of the molecule), while in **ketones** it occurs within the molecule proper. Aldehydes end in the suffix –al, and ketones end in the suffix –one. If an aldehyde is attached to a ring, the suffix –carbaldehyde may be used instead. The prefix –oxo is used if another, higher-priority functional group is present, although –keto may be used in some biological contexts. For some ketones, the traditional name is still generally used, and the most common example of this is acetone, the simplest ketone.

hexanal

3-oxobutanoic acid
(common name:
acetoacetic acid)

2-hexanone

cyclopentanecarbaldehyde

cyclooctanone

Figure 15. Nomenclature and structures of aldehydes and ketones

The physical and chemical properties of aldehydes and ketones are determined by the **carbonyl group**. The carbonyl group contains a strong dipole, meaning that aldehydes and ketones experience **dipole-dipole interactions**. This raises their melting and boiling points compared to alkanes, but these interactions are not as strong as the hydrogen bonding that is characteristic of alcohols. Therefore, the melting/boiling points of aldehydes and ketones are between those of alkanes and alcohols. For example, the boiling point of pentanal is 102°C, which is much higher than that of pentane (31.6°C), but also markedly lower than that of 1-pentanol (137°C).

In terms of acidity and basicity, the action for aldehydes and ketones takes place at the **α-hydrogen**—that is, hydrogens attached to carbons adjacent to the carbonyl carbon. (Recall that the α-carbon is adjacent to a functional group, the β-carbon is one carbon removed from a functional group, and so on for γ and δ if needed). At first this may seem puzzling, because hydrogens on alkyl chains are not generally acidic. What makes the α-hydrogen on aldehydes and ketones special? The answer is **resonance stabilization**. Removal of the α-hydrogen generates a negative charge on the carbon, resulting in a carbanion. However, in aldehydes and ketones, resonance can stabilize this negative charge by shifting it onto the carbonyl oxygen in some of the major resonance contributors to the deprotonated molecule. This structure is known as an **enolate**, because these major resonance contributors can be thought of as having a double C=C bond and a deprotonated hydroxyl group (with the negative charge on the oxygen).

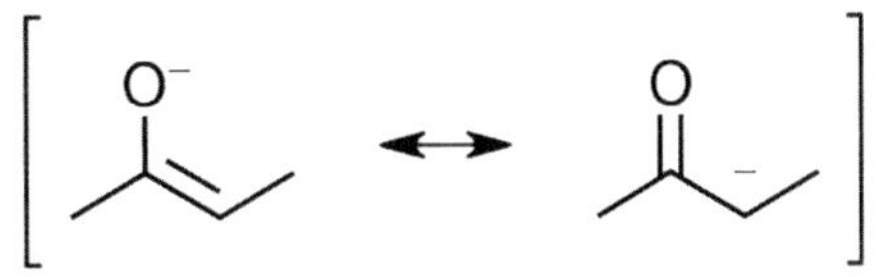

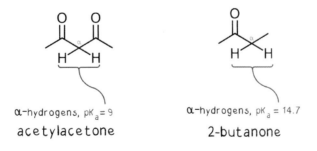

Figure 16. Resonance stabilization of an enolate

These α-hydrogens are still only weakly acidic; their pK_a values tend to be in the range of 17-19, which is still less acidic than water. The α-hydrogens of ketones tend to be less acidic than those of aldehydes due to the electron-donating effects of the additional alkyl substituent in ketones. However, these hydrogens are just acidic enough to be removed by an extremely strong base (such as NaH), which is the initial step in many reactions involving carbanions. Additionally, in β-dicarbonyl compounds (that is, compounds with two carbonyl groups separated by a carbon), the pK_a value of the α-hydrogen between the two carbonyl groups can be as low as 9, which is reasonably acidic for a weak organic acid and certainly acidic enough to be deprotonated by a strong base, such as NaOH. The reason for this is that the presence of two adjacent carbonyl groups increases the extent of resonance stabilization, and the electron-withdrawing effects of the carbonyl oxygen also help to stabilize the additional negative charge.

α-hydrogens, pK_a = 9
acetylacetone

α-hydrogens, pK_a = 14.7
2-butanone

Figure 17. Structures and pK_a values of selected α-hydrogens (acetylacetone and 2-butanone)

Trends in the acidity of α-hydrogens are useful because they illustrate two general trends that you can apply when reasoning about molecules you've never seen before. First, electron-donating groups, such as alkyl substituents, stabilize positive charges (e.g., carbocations), but destabilize negative charges (e.g., carbanions). Second, resonance plays a role in delocalizing and stabilizing charges, and the more contributing resonance structures present, the greater the effect.

Aldehydes and ketones are involved in a broad range of reactions that you are expected to be familiar with on Test Day. A special feature of aldehydes and ketones is that they can act as **nucleophiles** and **electrophiles**, depending on the reaction. This statement may seem surprising at first, but it contains nothing paradoxical. Because the α-hydrogens of aldehydes and ketones are acidic, reactions can take place in three locations: (1) the carbonyl carbon, which has a δ+ charge, making it electrophilic; (2) the carbonyl oxygen, which carries a δ- charge and can act as a nucleophile; and (3) an α-carbon carbanion formed in the presence of strong base, which has a negative charge and therefore also acts as a nucleophile. These mechanisms are explained in more detail in Chapter 11, however, it is worth noting that in reactions involving the carbonyl carbon, aldehydes tend to be somewhat more reactive than ketones due to the steric hindrance imposed by the additional R group in ketones compared to the –H in aldehydes.

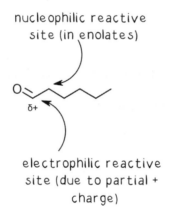

nucleophilic reactive site (in enolates)

δ+

electrophilic reactive site (due to partial + charge)

Figure 18. Nucleophilic and electrophilic sites in aldehydes and ketones

Aldehydes and ketones can be thought of as occupying an intermediate place on the spectrum of oxidation and reduction between alcohols (most reduced) and carboxylic acids (most oxidized). Aldehydes can be further oxidized to carboxylic acids by any oxidizing agent stronger than PCC, with common examples including $Na_2Cr_2O_7$, $K_2Cr_2O_7$, CrO_3, $KMnO_4$, Ag_2O, and H_2O_2. One important oxidation of aldehydes is use of a compound known as Tollens' reagent to selectively oxidize aldehydes to carboxylic acids – and that's the only reaction for Tollens' reagent as far as the MCAT is concerned! This historically made Tollens' reagent extremely useful as an experimental test for sugars, so don't be surprised to see it mentioned in a passage about carbohydrates. Ketones cannot be further oxidized by anything but the strongest oxidizing agents because it is impossible to do so without breaking a C–C bond. Aldehydes and ketones can be reduced to alcohols both by $NaBH_4$, a milder reducing agent, and $LiAlH_4$, a stronger reducing agent.

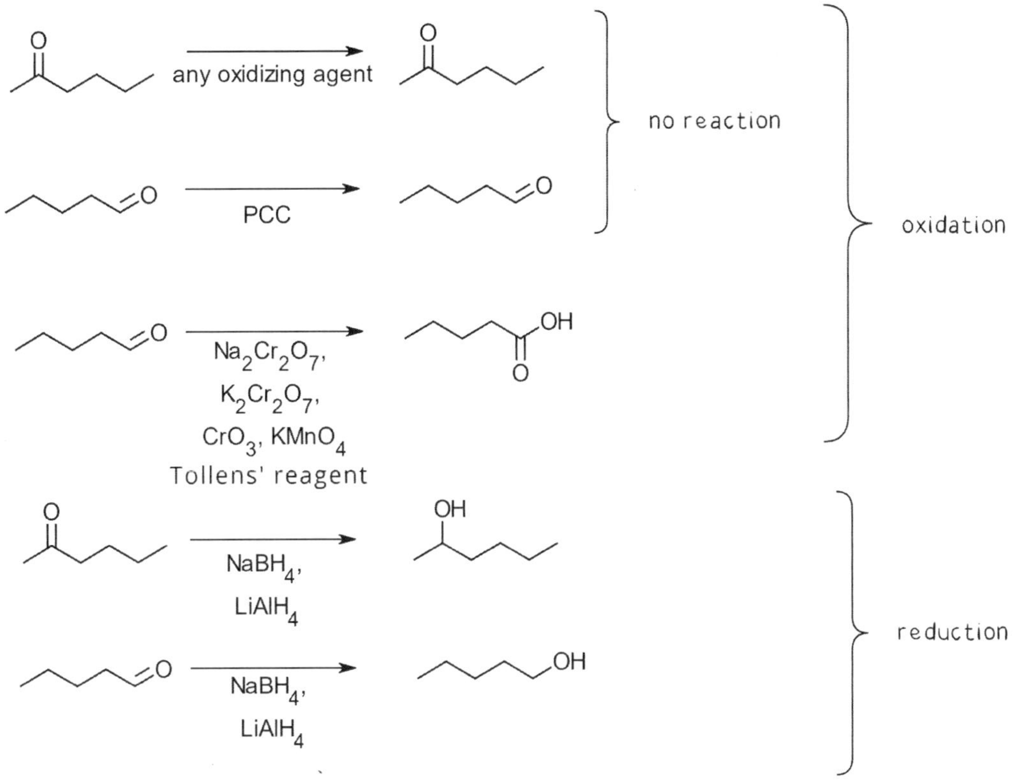

Figure 19. Oxidation and reduction of aldehydes and ketones

Aldehydes and ketones undergo several reactions in which a nucleophile attacks the carbonyl carbon and either adds a substituent or replaces the carbonyl oxygen. These reactions are summarized below in Table 4, and illustrated in Figure 20.

NUCLEOPHILE	WHAT HAPPENS?	PRODUCT	NOTES
Water (H_2O)	–OH adds to the carbonyl C.	Geminal diol (two –OH groups on the carbonyl C).	This process is referred to as hydration.
Alcohol (ROH)	–OR adds to the carbonyl C; in acidic conditions, second –OR addition occurs and original carbonyl O is protonated and leaves.	Hemiacetal/hemiketal (one equivalent of ROH), acetal/ketal (two equivalents of ROH).	In laboratory conditions, reaction usually goes to completion and acetals/ketals are formed.
Hydride reagents ($NaBH_4$, $LiAlH_4$)	Hydrogen is added to the carbonyl group.	Alcohol.	This is how aldehydes and ketones are reduced.
Amine (NH_3, etc.)	The nitrogen from the amine "replaces" the carbonyl oxygen; a C = N double bond is formed.	Imine.	Imines undergo tautomerization and form an equilibrium with enamines, as discussed in section 5.
Hydrogen cyanide (HCN)	The carbon in the deprotonated CN^- (cyanide) ion adds to the carbonyl carbon.	Cyanohydrin (former carbonyl carbon now has an –OH group and a –C≡N group).	

Table 4. Nucleophilic addition reactions to the carbonyl carbon

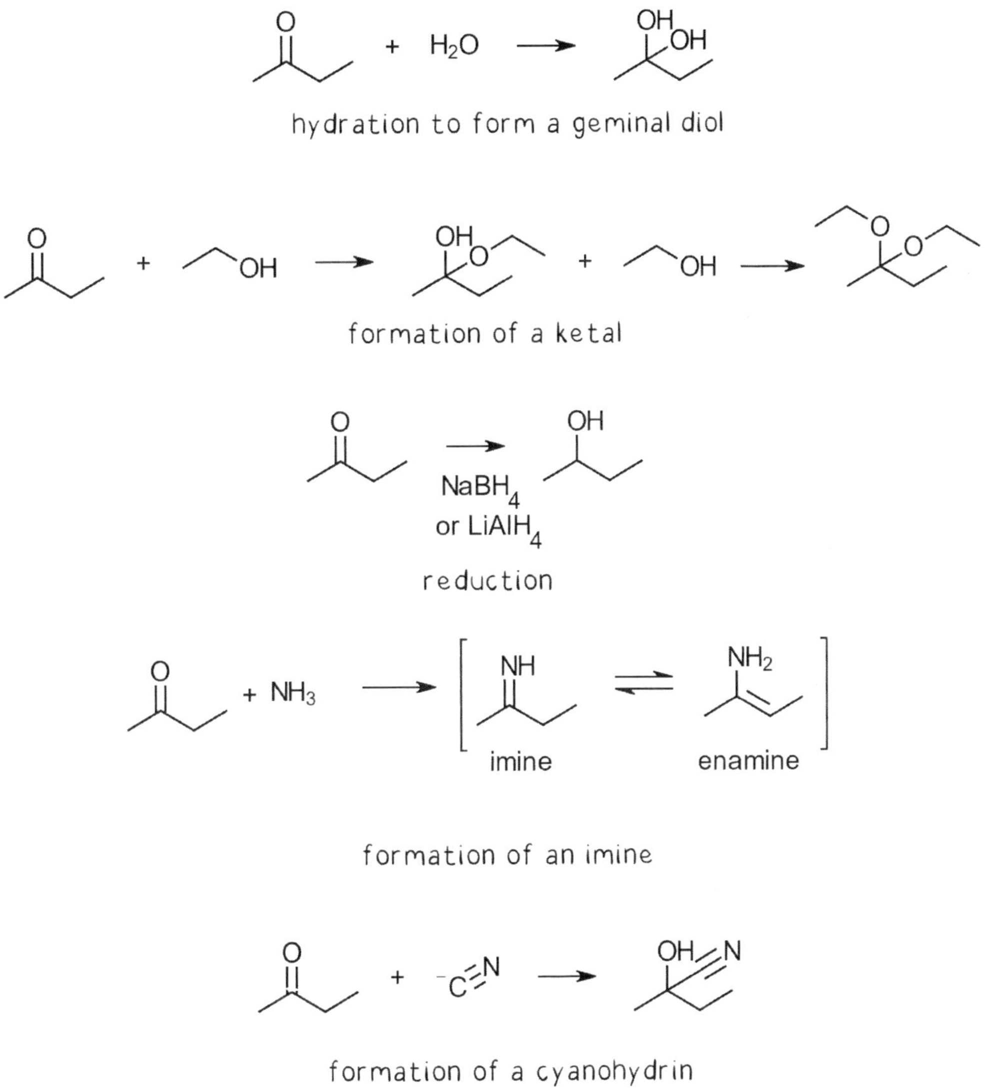

hydration to form a geminal diol

formation of a ketal

reduction

formation of an imine

formation of a cyanohydrin

Figure 20. Nucleophilic addition reactions to the carbonyl carbon

Aldehydes and ketones also undergo a set of important reactions involving the α-carbon. Before exploring these reactions, it is necessary to cover some prerequisites. The acidity of the α-hydrogens enables ketones to undergo **keto-enol tautomerization**, that is, an equilibrium process in which ketones convert between keto forms (the standard structural representation of a ketone) and enol forms, which have a C=C double bond (hence the "en" part of the name, like "alkene") and a –OH group attached to the carbonyl carbon (like an alcohol, hence the "ol" part of "enol"). In most cases, the keto tautomer is predominant under standard conditions, with the notable exceptions of phenols, in which the enol form is stabilized by the aromatic ring. This process means that any aldehyde or ketone with a chiral α-carbon will be converted into a racemic mixture due to the interconversion between the aldehyde and ketone forms. This process is known as α-racemization.

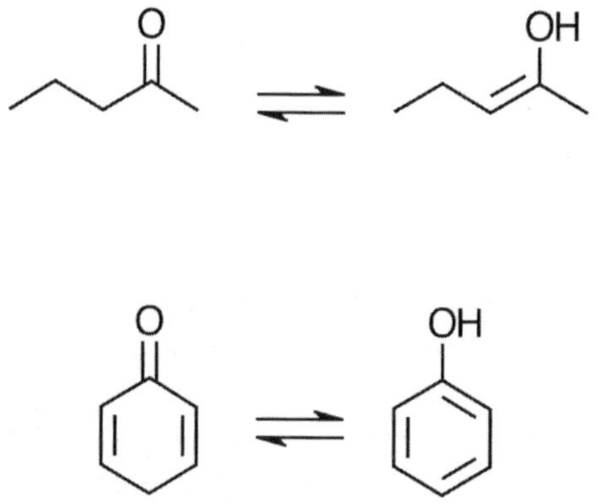

Figure 21. Keto-enol tautomerization

MCAT STRATEGY >>>

Keto-enol tautomerization is a relatively higher-yield topic within this subject area, because it involves a relatively limited amount of knowledge that can either be tested directly, resulting in straightforward discrete or pseudodiscrete questions, or applied to solve passage-based questions.

So far, we have not discussed where the double bond is formed in an enol isomer or an enolate (it is often more useful to discuss this process in terms of enolates, which can be thought of as both the deprotonated version of an enol and the major resonance contributor to the carbanion generated by removing the α-hydrogen). For symmetric compounds like acetone, this is irrelevant—although we could imagine drawing the double bond on either the left or the right side of the oxygen, that would not correspond to any actual chemical difference. However, for asymmetric ketones, this does correspond to a real difference between two enolate compounds.

It turns out that different enolates are favored in different reaction conditions, with corresponding implications for the eventual products of the reaction. A distinction is made between **kinetically favored** and **thermodynamically favored enolates**. By definition, the kinetically favored enolate is formed more quickly, but is less stable over the long term. In kinetically favored enolates, the double bond tends to involve the less substituted carbon because less steric hindrance is present. Therefore, **kinetic control** tends to exist in reactions that are rapid and irreversible, are conducted at low temperatures, and use strong and sterically hindered bases to deprotonate the α-hydrogen (because those bases will tend to favor the less sterically hindered α-carbon). In contrast, thermodynamically favored enolates form less quickly, but are more stable over the long term. **Thermodynamic control** generally leads to the double bond being present between the carbonyl carbon and the more substituted α-carbon, and is favored with the opposite set of conditions: high temperatures, weaker and less sterically hindered bases, and slower and more reversible reaction conditions that allow the formation of the product that is ultimately more stable.

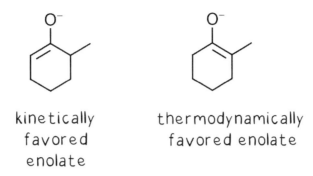

kinetically
favored
enolate

thermodynamically
favored enolate

Figure 22. Kinetic versus thermodynamic control of enolate formation

Aldehydes and ketones can react with each other in an important reaction known as **aldol condensation.** The basic mechanism involves the nucleophilic enolate ion of one aldehyde/ketone attacking the electrophilic carbonyl carbon of the other. The molecules join together, and the immediate result is an aldol—that is, a molecule that combines the features of an aldehyde (or ketone) and an alcohol—and is technically known as a β-hydroxyaldehyde or β-hydroxyketone. This simply refers to the fact that there is a single carbon separating the carbonyl and hydroxyl functional groups.

That accounts for the "aldol" part of "aldol condensation," but what about the "condensation" part? Condensation refers to the next step in the reaction, in which the –OH is removed through an elimination reaction catalyzed by a strong base, resulting in a compound known as an α,β-unsaturated aldehyde or ketone (where "unsaturated" refers to the presence of a double bond, similarly to the terminology used to discuss fatty acids, and "α,β" specifies the location of the double bond relative to the carbonyl group), or, as a conjugated enone (where "conjugated" describes the alternating double bonds present in the molecule, and "enone" describes the alk*ene* and ket*one* functionalities of the molecule).

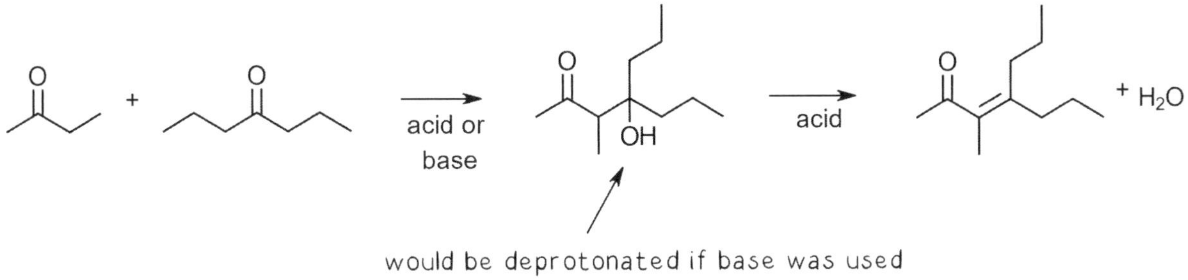

acid or
base

OH

acid

+ H₂O

would be deprotonated if base was used

Figure 23. Aldol condensation

The aldol condensation process is reversible, and the reverse reaction is known as the **retro-aldol reaction.** It breaks the bonds between the α and β-carbons of an aldehyde or ketone. In laboratory conditions, it is favored by high temperatures and basic conditions, and under physiological conditions, it can be catalyzed. It actually takes place in the fourth step of glycolysis, in which fructose-1,6-bisphosphate is cleaved by fructose-bisphosphate aldolase to form glyceraldehyde-3-phosphate and dihydroxyacetone phosphate, which are both ultimately converted to pyruvate in later steps of the pathway.

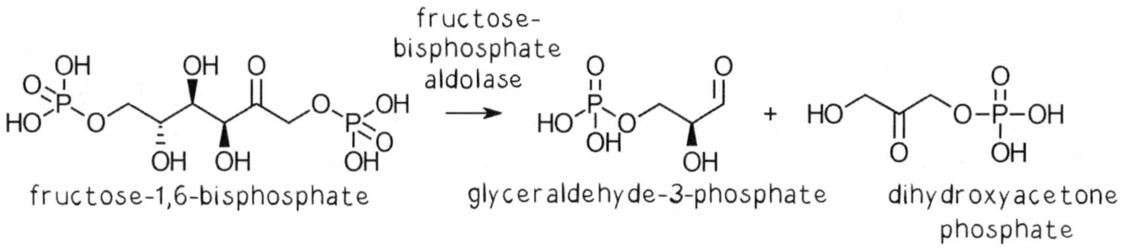

Figure 24. Retro-aldol reaction in glycolysis

4. Carboxylic Acids and Derivatives

Along with aldehydes and ketones, carboxylic acids and their derivatives are among the most important functional groups for the MCAT. They are especially relevant for the biochemistry of amino acids and proteins, two perennial high-yield biochemistry topics.

MCAT STRATEGY >>>

The key to deciphering aldol condensation/retro-aldol problems is to stay calm and work through the geometry of the molecules carefully. Remember the basics, use your scratch paper, and don't panic!

>> CONNECTIONS <<

Chapter 2 of Biochemistry

The nomenclature of carboxylic acids and their derivatives is important to master, because doing so can allow you to answer relatively straightforward questions simply and effectively: Test Day is not the time to get confused about the difference between an amide and an amine, or an ester and an ether!

Carboxylic acids are characterized by a –COOH functional group, while in **carboxylic acid derivatives**, the –OH is replaced by something else. That is, all carboxylic acid derivatives essentially have a carbonyl group plus *something*, although that something can vary. The carboxylic acid derivatives you must know for the MCAT are amides, esters, anhydrides, and acyl halides.

Carboxylic acids are characterized by the suffix "-oic acid" in IUPAC nomenclature. Many carboxylic acids fall under the biochemical category of fatty acids, and many such carboxylic acids have common names ending in –ic acid; for example, pentanoic acid is also known as valeric acid. The most frequently encountered example of this is likely acetic acid (ethanoic acid), although you should also be prepared to encounter formic acid (methanoic acid) and proprionic acid (propanoic acid). Carboxylic acids have the highest priority of all functional groups in the IUPAC nomenclature system, although the prefix "carboxy-" can be used if needed. Cyclic carboxylic acids are named using the name of the cyclic compound followed by "-carboxylic acid," such as "cyclohexanecarboxylic acid." However, many cyclic carboxylic acids are commonly referred to using common names that you do not have to be aware of for the MCAT. Carboxylic acids with two –COOH groups are referred to with the suffix "-dioic acid."

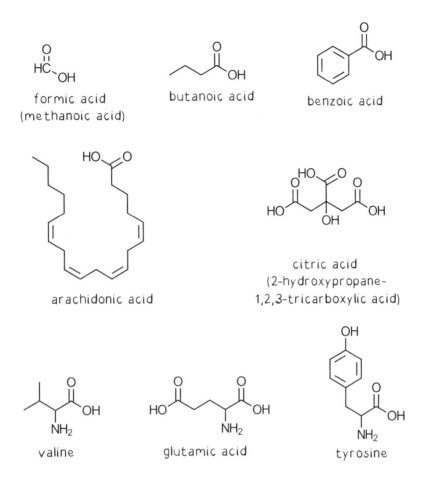

Figure 25. Selected carboxylic acids

Similarly to alcohols, the physical properties of carboxylic acids are fundamentally defined by their ability to hydrogen-bond. The intermolecular interactions present within carboxylic acids are even stronger than those that take place among alcohols, due to the strong molecular dipole in the carbonyl carbon that is bound to two electronegative oxygen atoms. For instance, the boiling point of 1-pentanol is 137°C, while that of pentanoic acid is 186°C.

Carboxylic acids are quite acidic for organic weak acids, with typical pK_a values in the range of 4-5, with lower values possible in the presence of other structural factors that stabilize the carboxylate ion corresponding to an acid's conjugate base. Additionally, similar to aldehydes and ketones, the α-hydrogens on the carbon chain can be acidic in certain structures known as β-dicarboxylic acids—that is, molecules with two carboxylic acid functional groups separated by a single carbon. In such molecules, resonance can stabilize the negative charge generated by removing this proton to the point that it is weakly acidic, with pKa values on the order of 9 to 14.

A special case of acid-base chemistry involving carboxylic acids is known as **saponification** (Latin *sapo* means "soap," so this literally means something like "soapification"). Under basic conditions (e.g., when mixed with NaOH or KOH), carboxylic acids are deprotonated and their conjugate bases form salts, according to the following template: $RCOOH + Na^+ + OH^- \rightarrow RCOO^-Na^+ + H_2O$. The acid-base chemistry of this process is straightforward; saponification is mostly of note for historical interest and because its wide range of applications opens the door for it to be introduced as a way of testing organic chemistry and general chemistry principles in a passage on Test Day.

Amides are carboxylic acid derivatives with an amine (–NH$_2$, –NHR, or -NR^{1}R^2) attached to the carbonyl carbon instead of the –OH group. Instead of the suffix "-oic acid," they have the suffix "-amide," and substituents attaching to the nitrogen of the amide group are named with *N*. A completely different name exists for cyclic amides; such molecules are known as **lactams**. Classes of lactams are named using Greek letters to refer to which non-carbonyl carbon binds to the nitrogen atom to form a cyclic structure: lactams where the β-carbon plays this role are known as β-lactams, with other classes of lactams including γ-lactams and δ-lactams. One of the major reasons that the MCAT expects you to be aware of lactams is the fact that β-lactams form a very large class of broad-spectrum antibiotics, including penicillin and its derivatives as well as many other medically important drugs.

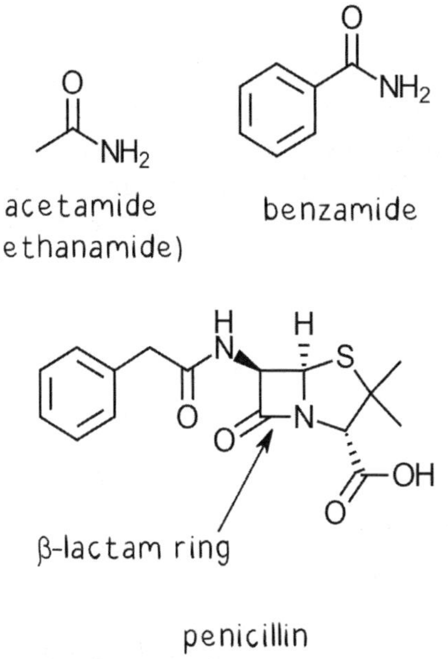

acetamide
(ethanamide)

benzamide

β-lactam ring

penicillin

Figure 26. Selected amides

The physical properties and acid-base chemistry of amides are strongly dependent on whether the nitrogen atom in the amide has alkyl substituents. In particular, the more hydrogens present on this atom, the greater the degree to which amides can participate in hydrogen bonding. Nonetheless, the intermolecular forces present in amides tend to be weaker than those in carboxylic acid. Thus, pentanamide has a boiling point of approximately 101°C, which is markedly lower than the corresponding values for pentanol (137°C) or pentanoic acid (186°C). If the molecular weight is held constant, the presence of alkyl substituents will tend to reduce the melting/boiling points by reducing the ability of the amide to undergo hydrogen bonding.

Amides are extremely weak bases, to the point that for the purposes of the MCAT you can consider them as essentially not involved in acid-base chemistry. The reason for this is the adjacent carbonyl group and its oxygen, which has two consequences: first, the electronegativity of the oxygen attracts the lone pair of electrons on the amide nitrogen; and second, the lone pair of electrons on the nitrogen is involved in a resonance system with the carbonyl group, delocalizing the electrons. The latter fact about amides is relevant for some of the structural properties of peptide bonds.

> > CONNECTIONS < <

Chapter 2 of Biochemistry

In **esters**, the –OH group is replaced by an –OR group. The nomenclature of esters is a bit tricky because esters contain two alkyl groups that must be included and differentiated in the nomenclature. The suffix

"-oate" is applied to the main alkyl chain that contains the carbonyl group, and the esterifying group is named as a prefix ending in "-yl." Be sure to practice with this until it becomes familiar, because this is a relatively rare opportunity for the MCAT to ask about nomenclature in a tricky way. Like amides, special nomenclature exists for cyclic esters. Cyclic esters are known as lactones. Similarly to lactams, lactones are named as β-lactones, γ-lactones, and δ-lactones depending on which carbon from the main alkyl chain bonds with the oxygen to form the ester.

> **MCAT STRATEGY >>>**
>
> Keep lactams and lactones straight by remembering that lact*ams* are *am*ides, while lact*ones* have oxygen like ket*ones*. Additionally, make sure you don't confuse esters with ethers!

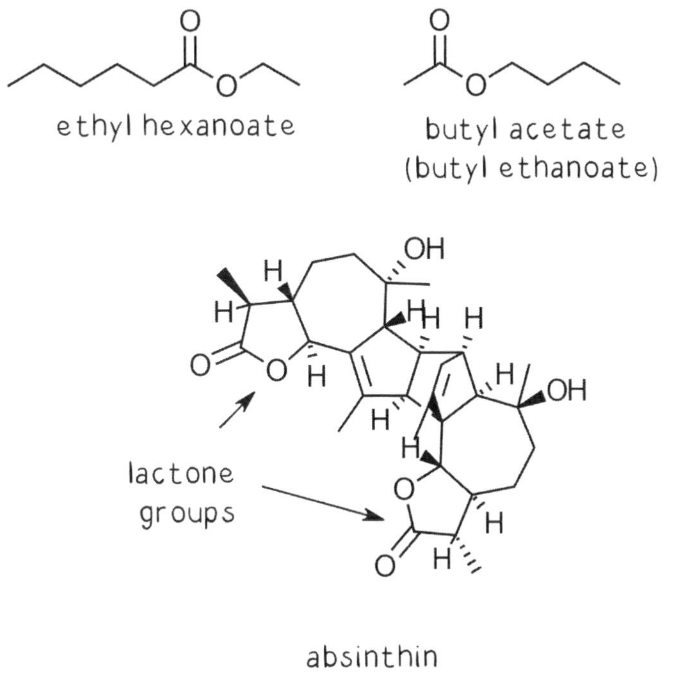

ethyl hexanoate

butyl acetate
(butyl ethanoate)

lactone groups

absinthin

Figure 27. Selected esters

The physical and chemical properties of esters are generally unremarkable. Their melting and boiling points are relatively low due to their inability to engage in hydrogen bonding; for instance, the boiling point of methyl butanoate is 102°C, which is close to that of pentamide and much less than those of pentanol and pentanoic acid. Esters do not engage in acid-base chemistry to any appreciable extent. However, esters are quite relevant for biochemistry, because triglycerides—which, along with their derivatives, form a major class of lipids—are esters formed between fatty acids and glycerol.

Acid anhydrides are formed by the condensation of two carboxylic acids; that is, the substituent that replaces the –OH of one carboxylic acid is actually another carboxylic acid. Symmetric anhydrides are named by replacing the word "acid" with "anhydride," and asymmetric anhydrides are named by listing the names of the acid chains in alphabetical order with the suffix "-oic," such as butanoic ethanoic anhydride. Cyclic anhydrides do exist, but no special nomenclature exists for them except

> **>> CONNECTIONS <<**
>
> Chapter 9 of Biochemistry

for a tendency to use common names instead of IUPAC nomenclature, such as phthalic acid (corresponding to the IUPAC name of 2-benzofuran-1,3-dione).

Acid halides are one final derivative of note, wherein a halogen atom replaces the –OH group of a carboxylic acid. You can spot them by their name because they'll end in something like "-oyl chloride" instead of "oic acid," butanoyl chloride for example. These are super useful starting materials for the other derivatives, because halide ions are much better leaving groups than –OH. The most common halogen used in acid halides is chlorine, because a nice, quick synthesis involves simply treating the corresponding carboxylic acid with a reagent called thionyl chloride ($SOCl_2$). If you want to make a carbonyl group that will get rapidly attacked by just about any nucleophile, it doesn't get much easier than that! If you see an acid chloride in a chemistry passage, expect it to act as a strong electrophile, getting attacked at the carbonyl carbon.

A strong reducing agent is needed to **reduce** carboxylic acids to alcohols. For the purposes of the MCAT, this means $LiAlH_4$, *not* $NaBH_4$. It is difficult to reduce carboxylic acids to aldehydes, because this essentially means stopping halfway through the process; $NaBH_4$ is too weak to do any reduction at all, and $LiAlH_4$ is so strong that the reaction will proceed all the way to alcohol formation. A reducing agent known as diisobutylaluminium hydride (DIBAL or DIBALH) can do this, however, but only if care is taken with the stoichiometry to include only one unit of DIBAL for each unit of carboxylic acid.

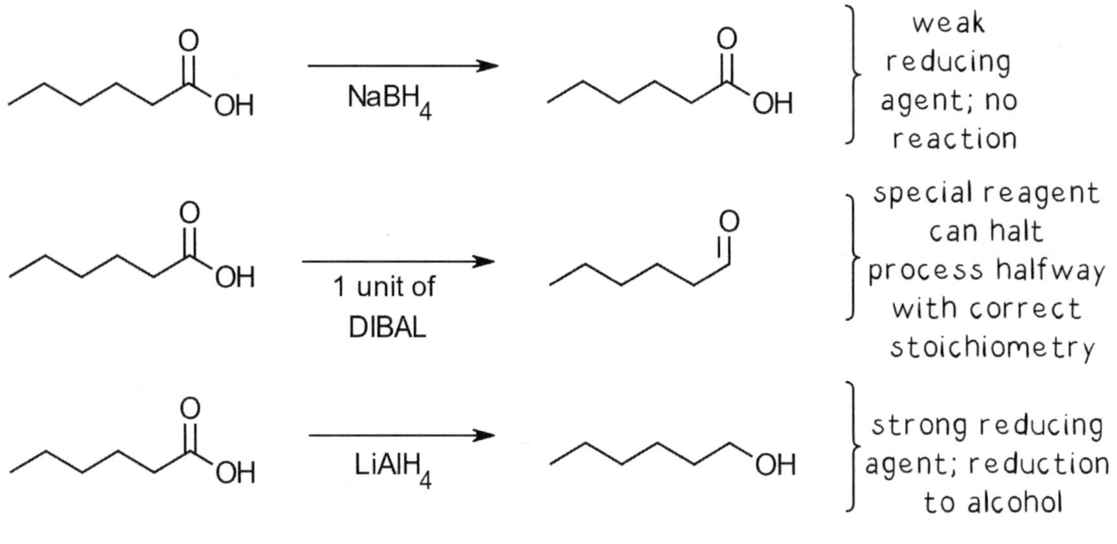

Figure 28. Reduction of carboxylic acids

Carboxylic acids with another carbonyl group separated by a single carbon (that is, 1,3-dicarboxylic acids and β-ketoacids) can also lose a –COOH group in a process known as **decarboxylation**, in which the –COOH group is lost as CO_2. This process is favored by high temperatures and can also be significantly upregulated by enzymatic activity. It is a fundamentally important type of reaction in many biochemical pathways, perhaps most notably because it occurs in the conversion of pyruvate to acetyl-CoA and at two points in the Krebs cycle, corresponding to changes in the number of carbons in the substrate. It is also important from a pharmacological perspective. The non-psychoactive compound Δ9-tetrahydrocannabinolic acid found in cannabis undergoes decarboxylation when heated to form the derivative Δ9-tetrahydrocannabinol, which is responsible for the psychoactive effects of cannabis. This is why raw cannabis leaves are non-psychoactive.

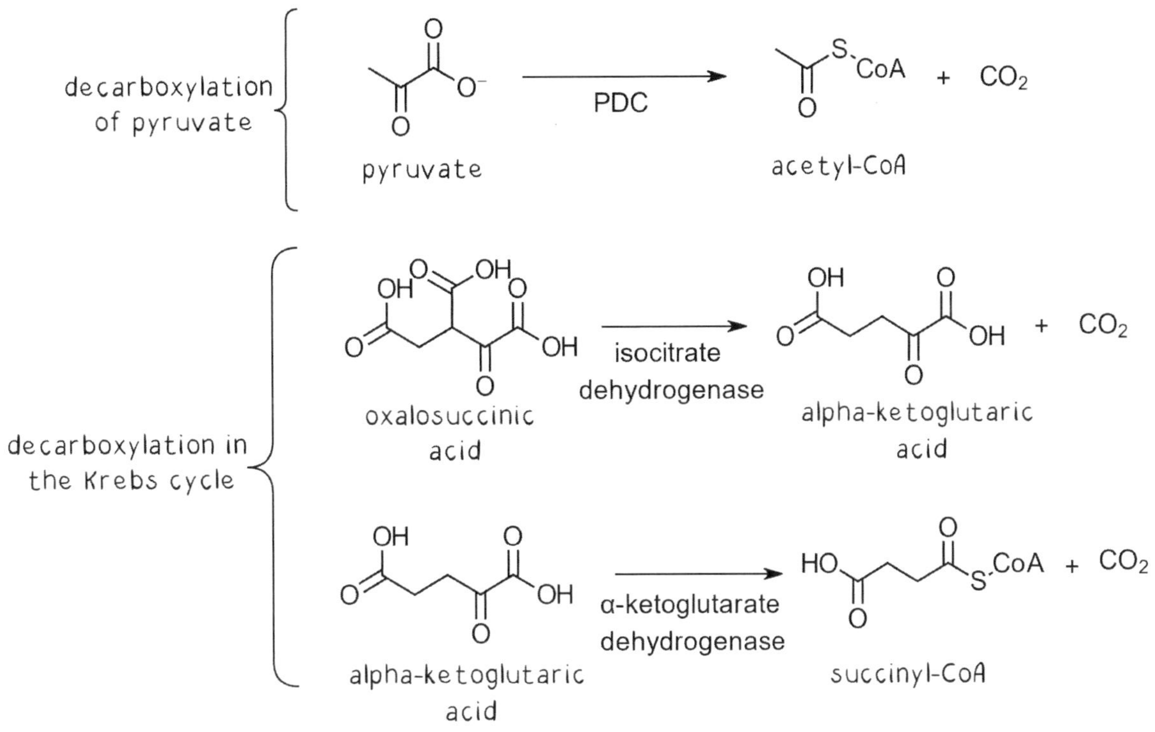

Figure 29. Decarboxylation of pyruvate and Krebs cycle intermediates

Carboxylic acids undergo many reactions involving **nucleophilic substitution** at the carbonyl carbon. Unlike aldehydes and ketones, carboxylic acids have an excellent leaving group (–OH)—or, more accurately, a functional group that can be *converted* to an excellent leaving group by protonation—so essentially an appropriate nucleophile can replace the –OH group. This is how the major carboxylic acid derivatives are formed: amides are formed when ammonia or an amine acts as the nucleophile, esters are formed when an alcohol acts as a nucleophile (in a process known as Fischer esterification), and acid anhydrides are formed when a carboxylic acid acts as the nucleophile. These are considered condensation reactions, because in each of these reactions, two larger molecules are joined together with the loss of water. This mechanism is discussed at greater length in Chapter 11, but the schematic results are presented below in Figure 30.

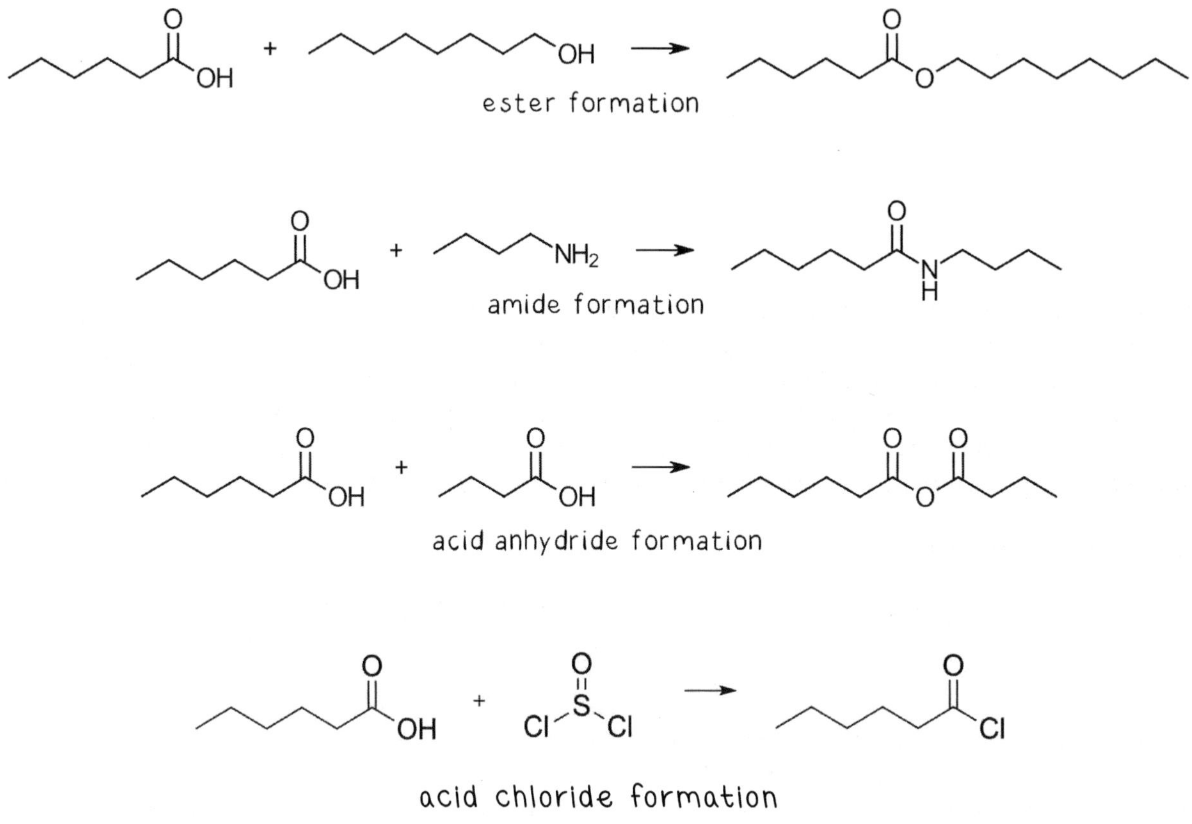

Figure 30. Formation of major carboxylic acid derivatives

A final reaction involving carboxylic acids to be aware of is **Hell-Volhard-Zelinsky halogenation**, in which carboxylic acids are halogenated at the α-carbon due to the slight acidity of the α-hydrogen, as discussed above. Using bromination as an example, this reaction occurs by the addition of a catalytic amount of PBr_3 followed by Br_2. First, an acyl halide is formed, in which a –Br substituent replaces the –OH. At this point, keto-enol tautomerism generates an enol form, and the Br_2 can react with the alkene bond of the enol to brominate the α-carbon. The first bromine (the one that replaced the –OH group of the carboxylic acid) is then spontaneously lost.

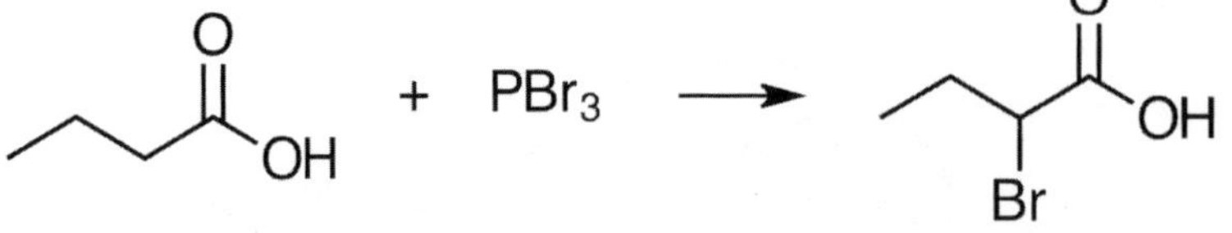

Figure 31. Hell-Volhard-Zelinsky halogenation

Since carboxylic acid derivatives are closely interrelated molecules, it is not surprising that they can be interconverted among each other. This process follows a scale of **reactivity**; more reactive carboxylic acid derivatives can be converted to less reactive carboxylic derivatives through nucleophilic substitution, but not vice versa. To "climb" the reactivity scale would be to convert a carboxylic acid derivative back to a carboxylic acid and then generate a new carboxylic acid derivative according to the processes described above. This flow chart is illustrated in Figure 32.

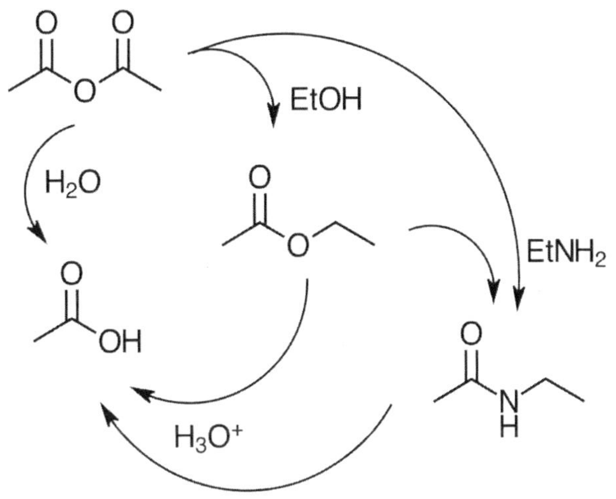

Figure 32. Interconversion of carboxylic acid derivatives

The relative reactivity of carboxylic acid derivatives can be thought of in terms of how electrophilic the carbonyl carbon is, which in turn reflects the partial positive charge created by adjacent or nearby electron-withdrawing groups. Anhydrides have three nearby electronegative oxygens, while esters have two, and amides have a less strongly electronegative nitrogen atom in place of an oxygen. This consideration affects the general reactivity of these classes of molecules, but when considering the reactivity patterns of a *specific* reaction, it is important to consider steric hindrance as well. Steric hindrance will cause carboxylic acid derivatives (and molecules in general) to be less likely to undergo nucleophilic attack.

There are also some special reactions involving carboxylic acid derivatives that you should be aware of for the MCAT. One of these is **transesterification**, which occurs when an ester is reacted with an alcohol distinct from the original alcohol that makes up the ester (the esterifying group). The result is that these alcohol molecules replace each other, resulting in a different alcohol and a different ester. For example, if ethyl hexanoate reacted with propanol, transesterification would result in propyl hexanoate and ethanol.

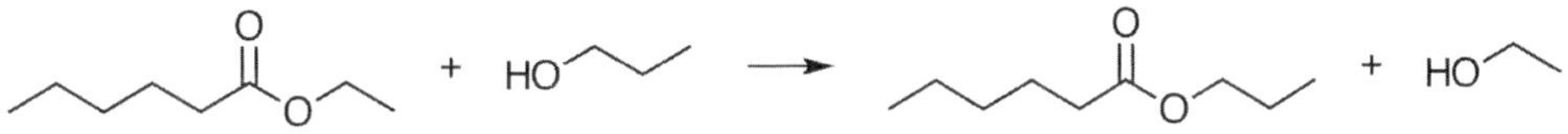

Figure 33. Transesterification

Another reaction to be aware of is the **hydrolysis of amides** to the parent carboxylic acid and an amine. Hydrolysis is a very common reaction type, and this reaction is not especially remarkable from a strictly mechanistic point of view. However, it is important to be familiar with for two main reasons. First, it is the only interconversion reaction that amides undergo, since amides are the least reactive of carboxylic acid derivatives. Second, and most notably, the hydrolysis of amides is the mechanism involved in breaking peptide bonds in amino acid sequences. Enzymes (peptidases) exist that can catalyze this process with considerable specificity.

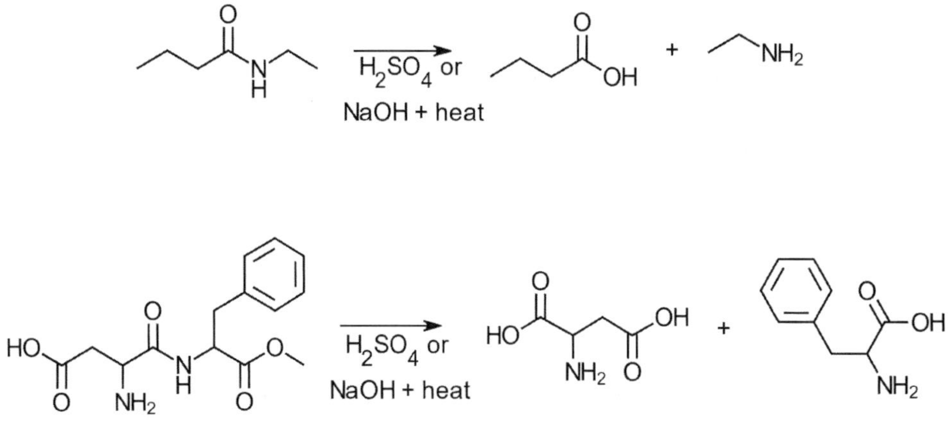

Figure 34. Hydrolysis of an amide

When attempting to predict the outcome of a reaction involving carboxylic acid derivatives, you should keep the following principles in mind:

1. <u>Relative reactivity.</u> As discussed above, acyl halides > anhydrides > esters > amides. Simple nucleophilic substitution can move you down that scale, but not up.

2. <u>Steric hindrance.</u> Molecules with greater steric hindrance are less likely to undergo nucleophilic substitution reactions.

3. <u>Electronic effects.</u> Electron-withdrawing groups, such as oxygen, tend to make the carbonyl carbon more reactive. Resonance can stabilize negative charges, increasing (for example) the acidity of carboxylic acids both at the –OH group and at the α-hydrogen.

4. <u>Strain.</u> In cyclic molecules, ring strain increases reactivity. An example of this is provided by β-lactam antibiotics. As shown in Figure 26, β-lactam molecules have a strained 4-member ring, which is an important reactive site both for how they interact with penicillin-binding proteins to inhibit peptidoglycan sequences and for how they are cleaved by β-lactamase enzymes that provide bacteria with resistance to these drugs.

5. Amines, Imines, and Enamines

Amines, imines, and enamines are nitrogen-containing compounds. Amines are actually not included on the list of key functional groups that you are expected to know as part of the organic chemistry content of the MCAT, but they are nonetheless important for two reasons. First, they occur as precursors of several structures that you are responsible for, such as amides. Second, they are very important in biochemistry, because a knowledge of the properties of amines is essential for understanding the structure and function of amino acids.

Amines are derivatives of ammonia (NH_3), in which one or more of the hydrogens are replaced by a *single bond* to an organic substituent. They are named with the suffix "-amine" or the prefix "amino-" if a higher-priority functional group is present. Amines undergo hydrogen bonding unless all three hydrogen atoms are replaced by organic substituents, and they therefore generally have moderately high melting and boiling points. For instance, the boiling point of pentylamine is approximately 94-110°C, which is in the range of that of pentanal (102°C), much higher than that of pentane (31.6°C), but also much lower than that of 1-pentanol (137°C).

Amines are weak bases, as they contain a lone pair of electrons. However, alkyl amines, in which the organic substituents are alkyl groups, are distinguished from aryl amines, which have an aromatic substituent. This is similar to the distinction between alcohols and phenols. Aromatic amines, such as aniline (shown in Figure 35) are less basic than typical alkyl amines. The reason for this is that the lone pair of electrons is delocalized throughout the resonance structure of the aromatic ring. Essentially, the aromatic ring provides support for that lone pair, such that the nitrogen doesn't "want" to use it to pick up an extra hydrogen in an acid-base reaction.

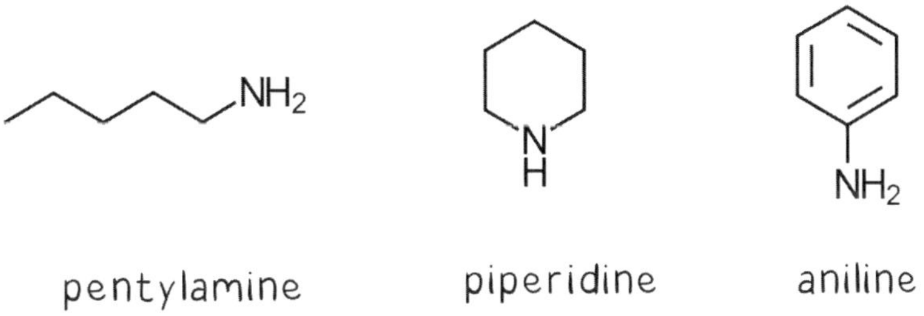

Figure 35. Amines

Amines are defined by single bonds between nitrogen and carbon. In contrast, **imines** are characterized by a C=N double bond. You should think of them as being analogous to carbonyl groups. Like oxygen, nitrogen has at least one available lone pair in many organic contexts and is more electronegative than carbon. As discussed in section 3, imines are formed from carbonyl groups. The analogy with oxygen-containing compounds can be extended. Just as enols have a C=C bond and a C–O bond, **enamines** (named using the same principle: *en* for alk*ene* plus *amine*) have a C=C bond and a C–N bond. Moreover, imines and enamines are tautomers that interconvert in a process very similar to keto-enol tautomerism. Imines in which an organic R group replaces the remaining hydrogen are known as **Schiff bases**. This term may be familiar from your organic chemistry coursework, but the chemistry of Schiff bases is beyond the scope of the MCAT.

As discussed in section 4, **amides** are carboxylic acid derivatives with an amine group instead of a hydroxyl group.

A very common and entirely preventable source of error regarding nitrogen-containing functional groups on the MCAT is becoming confused about which structures are referred to by the similar-sounding terms "amine," "amide," "imine," and "enamine." Be sure to review Figure 36 below until they are familiar.

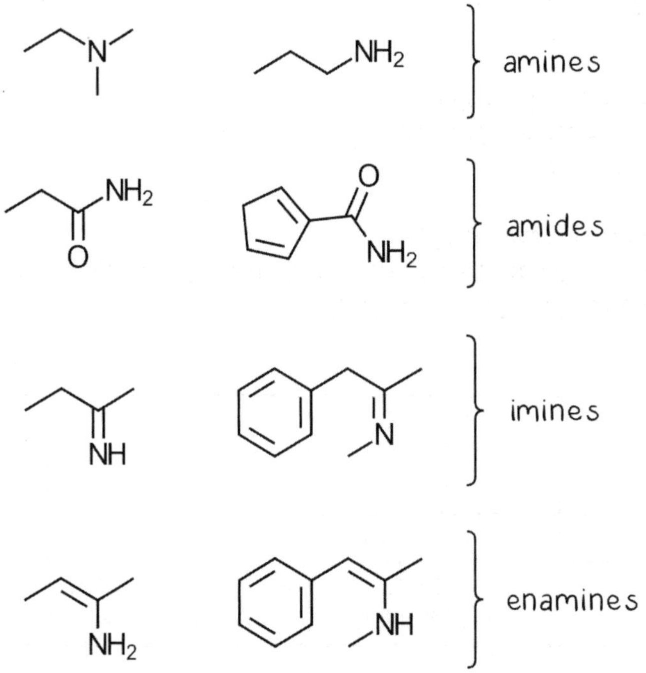

Figure 36. Nitrogen-containing compounds

>> CONNECTIONS <<

Chapters 2 and 12 of Biochemistry

MCAT STRATEGY >>>

When you see "thio-," think of sulfur! Usually this will point you in the direction of the correct structure, as long as you replace oxygen with sulfur.

6. Sulfur-Containing Groups

Sulfur-containing functional groups are not a major area tested by the MCAT, but you should be aware of them in general terms. There are three sulfur-containing groups you should know as structures similar to major oxygen-containing functional groups: **thiols** (-RSH, analogous to alcohols), **sulfides** or **thioethers** (R-S-R', analogous to ethers), and **thioesters** (R-CO-S-R', analogous to esters). Thioesters are highly reactive and play a notable role in several biochemical pathways, most notably in the form of acetyl-CoA. Additionally, you should be aware of **disulfides** (R-S-S-R'; this is analogous to a peroxide [R-O-O-R'], but peroxides are not critical for the MCAT). Disulfides are an important structure because disulfide bonds between cysteine amino acid residues are a crucial aspect of the tertiary structure of proteins.

7. Must-Knows

> Nomenclature and major chemical/physical properties:

NAME	NOMENCLATURE	STRUCTURE	RELEVANT NTERMOLECULAR FORCES	MELTING/ BOILING POINT	ACID-BASE PROPERTIES
Alkanes	-ane	C_nH_{2n+2}	London dispersion forces	Low	Negligible
Alkenes	-ene -en-	C_nH_{2n}	London dispersion forces	Low	
Alcohol	-ol hydroxy-	RC–OH	Dipole-dipole, H-bonding	High	Very weak acids (phenols stronger)
Aldehyde	-al oxo-	RC(O)H	Dipole-dipole	Medium	Negligible
Ketone	-one oxo-, keto-	R(C=O)R'			
Carboxylic acid	-oic acid	R(C=O)OH	Dipole-dipole, H-bonding	High	Weak acids
Amide	-amide	$R(C=O)NH_2$, R(C=O)NHR', R(C=O)NR'R''	Dipole-dipole, H-bonding (maybe)	Medium	Very weak bases
Ester	X-yl Y-ate (X = esterifying group)	R(C=O)OR'	Dipole-dipole	Medium	Negligible
Acid anhydride	X-oic Y-oic anhydride	R(C=O)O(C=O)R'	Dipole-dipole	Medium	Negligible
Amine	-amine amino-	$R–NH_2$, R–NHR', R–NR'R''	Dipole-dipole, H-bonding (maybe)	Medium	Weak bases
Imine	-imine	R=NH, R=NR'			
Enamine	enamine	RC=CNH, C=CNHR', C=CNR'R''			

> Major reactions:
  — Reduction/oxidation on scale OH > C=O > COOH.
    • Mild oxidizing agent: PCC; strong oxidizing agents: $NaCr_2O_7$, $K_2Cr_2O_7$, and CrO_3; mild reducing agent: $NaBH_4$, strong reducing agent: $LiAlH_4$.
  — Keto-enol tautomerism.
  — Acetal/hemiacetal formation.
  — Aldol condensation and retro-aldol reaction.
  — Formation of carboxylic acid derivatives.
  — Transesterification.
> General principles:
  — Factors affecting acidity, most notably resonance.
  — Factors affecting reactivity: electron-withdrawing groups, resonance, steric effects, strain.

End of Chapter Practice

The best MCAT practice is realistic, with a focus on identifying steps for further improvement. For those reasons, we recommend completing practice questions in an online setting that simulates the real MCAT interface, and taking advantage of advanced analytic features to help you determine how best to move forward in your MCAT study journey.

With that in mind, online end-of-chapter questions for Biology, Biochemistry, Chemistry + Organic Chemistry, Physics, and Psychology/Sociology are available through your Blueprint MCAT account.

As a further supplement, given the importance of active learning for effective studying, we also suggest that you consult the Must-Knows as a basis for creating a study sheet, in which you list out key terms and test your ability to briefly summarize them.

This page left intentionally blank.

This page left intentionally blank.

Organic Reaction Mechanisms

0. Introduction

In this chapter, we discuss *how* organic reactions happen. Reaction mechanisms can be an intimidating topic, but for the MCAT, focus on the essential principles. The best strategy for the MCAT is to focus on the key reaction types and then extend that knowledge to less common reactions.

Two basic parameters govern reaction mechanisms: sterics (that is, whether the reactants can physically interact with each other in the way needed to push the reaction forward) and charge-based interactions. On a very simple level, the attractive forces between positive and negative charges drive reactions forward, but we also need to account for factors that stabilize or destabilize charge in certain structures.

Reactions occur when a bond forms between an electrophile and a nucleophile. **Electrophiles** are species that 'want' more electrons. Often, electrophiles are positively charged or partially-positively charged. In contrast, nucleophiles are species with an excess of electrons and therefore 'want' to use those electrons to bond with an electrophile. **Nucleophiles** are defined by the presence of at least one free pair of valence electrons.

In common practice, the formation of an organic bond is indicated by drawing arrows in so-called 'electron-pushing' notation. This means that the arrows focus on the movement of electrons, which can correspond either to breaking a bond or forming a bond, depending on the context. Though sometimes confusing, but it's essential that you become familiar with this notation.

The first topic discussed in this chapter is S_N1, S_N2, and elimination chemistry, which is the single most important topic to master in the organic chemistry mechanisms for the MCAT. We'll then proceed to cover some important examples of nucleophilic addition and substitution, followed by a review of some other representative mechanisms and concluding with a presentation of the mechanisms involved in enolate chemistry.

In order to get the most out of this chapter, be sure to study each mechanism carefully, and focus on which atom acts as a nucleophile and which as an electrophile in each reaction. It is possible that on test day, you will see a reaction *mechanism* that you have studied in the context of *molecules* that you haven't seen before, so your real task in this chapter is to push beyond studying reactions as input-output pairings of functional groups (as presented in Chapter 10) towards understanding the principles of reactivity that can be applied in seemingly novel contexts.

1. S~N~1, S~N~2, and elimination

Nucleophilic substitution is probably the single most-tested reaction mechanism on the MCAT, so let's step back and think about what that term implies. The term 'nucleophilic' tells us that the reaction mechanism will involve a nucleophile (that is, an electron-rich atom) attacking an electrophile. 'Substitution' means that the attacking nucleophile replaces a substituent on the target molecule, which is known as the **leaving group**. For nucleophilic substitution reactions, you ultimately want to identify three things:

1. <u>What is the nucleophile? What makes it nucleophilic?</u> In other words, you want to find the compound with one or more free lone pairs of electrons that will be shared with the target molecule.

2. <u>What is the electrophile? What creates an electrophilic region on the target molecule?</u> In this step, your goal is to pinpoint where the electrons on the attacking nucleophile will go. This generally means finding an area of positive or partial positive charge on the target molecule.

3. <u>What is the leaving group?</u> Nucleophilic *substitution* (compared to nucleophilic addition, which we will discuss more below) is characterized by a substituent being 'kicked out' or 'leaving.' You'll want to identify which substituent is likely to be the leaving group, although context may make it obvious. In general, a good leaving group will be a species that has a positive formal charge or is characterized as a halogen. You may also need to think about possible steps that make the leaving group better. As we will see, protonation is a frequent option.

Figure 1 shows the general scheme of a nucleophilic substitution reaction, where *Nu* indicates the nucleophile, *El* the electrophile, *LG* the leaving group, and *R* indicates whatever other substituents the electrophile may have.

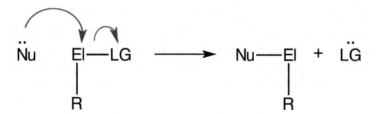

Figure 1. General nucleophilic substitution reaction

The general scheme in Figure 1 is fairly simple, but we have to account for some complications in real-world reaction scenarios. First, let's note that Figure 1 contains two steps: (1) the nucleophilic attack and (2) the transfer of electrons to the leaving group as the bond between it and the electrophile is broken. It turns out that these steps can occur in either order, which is at the heart of the difference between the S~N~1 and S~N~2 mechanisms we will discuss below. Additionally, as mentioned above, some reaction mechanisms include steps—most commonly, protonation—that make the leaving group more likely to leave.

For the MCAT, you will have to distinguish between two types of nucleophilic substitution mechanisms: **S~N~1** and **S~N~2**. The 'S' stands for 'substitution' and the subscript 'N' stands for 'nucleophilic,' while the numbers '1' and '2' describe the rate laws associated with the reaction. In S~N~1 reactions, the rate law depends only on the concentration of the substrate, while in S~N~2 reactions, the rate law depends on the concentrations of both the substrate and the nucleophile. Both the S~N~1 and S~N~2 mechanisms are generally illustrated with alkyl halides, although S~N~2 mechanisms in particular can occur with other substrates.

Let's first look at the **S~N~1 mechanism**. The key idea with the S~N~1 mechanism is that the leaving group leaves *first*, generating a **carbocation** (that is, a positively charged, electron-deficient carbon). This step is slow because even a good leaving group will be relatively stable in its default state and because carbocations are inherently unstable, highly reactive species. The next step is nucleophilic attack, followed by deprotonation of the nucleophile once it is attached to the target molecule. The S_N1 mechanism is shown in Figure 2.

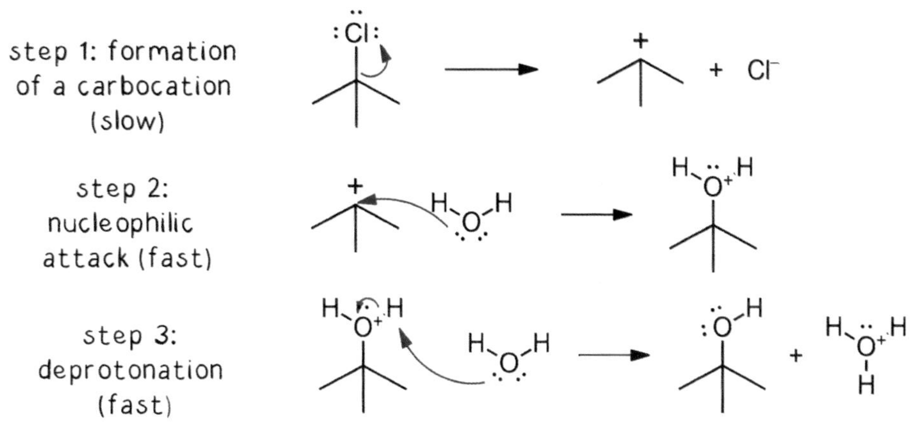

Figure 2. S_N1 mechanism.

There are a few things we should note about the S_N1 mechanism. First, step 1 (the formation of a carbocation) is slow, while the other steps are fast, and thus the carbocation formation step is the rate-limiting step of the reaction. This is why the rate law of an S_N1 reaction depends only on the concentration of the substrate. Another consequence here is that anything that promotes the stability of the carbocation increases the reaction rate. As mentioned above, carbocations are generally unstable, highly reactive species, so anything that increases the stability of the carbocation will increase the rate of an S_N1 reaction. Carbocation stability is enhanced by the degree to which the carbon is substituted. Tertiary carbocations (a carbon with three other non-hydrogen substituents, as in Figure 1) are more stable than secondary carbocations, which are more stable than primary carbocations, which are more stable than methyl carbocations. As a rule of thumb, a carbocation must be on a tertiary or secondary carbon for the reaction to proceed to any significant extent. A third important consequence is that this reaction proceeds through an extremely active carbocation intermediate. Thus, the nucleophile doesn't have to be especially strong for the reaction to go forward. To summarize, *S_N1 reactions are all about forming the carbocation!*

A final point to note about S_N1 reactions is that the mechanism is not stereochemically sensitive. An S_N1 reaction can certainly occur at a carbon with four different substituents and is, therefore, a chiral center, but the chirality is lost as soon as the carbocation is formed. Therefore, when an enantiomerically pure substrate undergoes an S_N1 reaction, the product will exhibit racemization. The outcome may not be a perfect 50:50 racemic mixture because nothing in chemistry is that simple, but the original chiral orientation will certainly not be preserved.

In **S_N2 reactions**, in contrast, the nucleophilic attack pushes the reaction forward. The carbon that is attacked is a relatively weak electrophile, with a partial positive charge due to the inductive electron-withdrawing effect of the halide. The nucleophile attacks the electrophilic carbon on the opposite side of the halide substituent in what is known as a **backside attack**. The electron-rich nucleophile "tries" to approach at an angle maximally distant from the electron-rich halide leaving group. This leads to the formation of a complex transition state in which a new bond is being formed between the nucleophile and electrophile while a bond is being broken between the electrophile and the leaving group. As the leaving group leaves, the stereochemical orientation of the target molecule is inverted. A common analogy is how an umbrella can be turned inside out by the wind. Figure 3 shows the S_N2 mechanism.

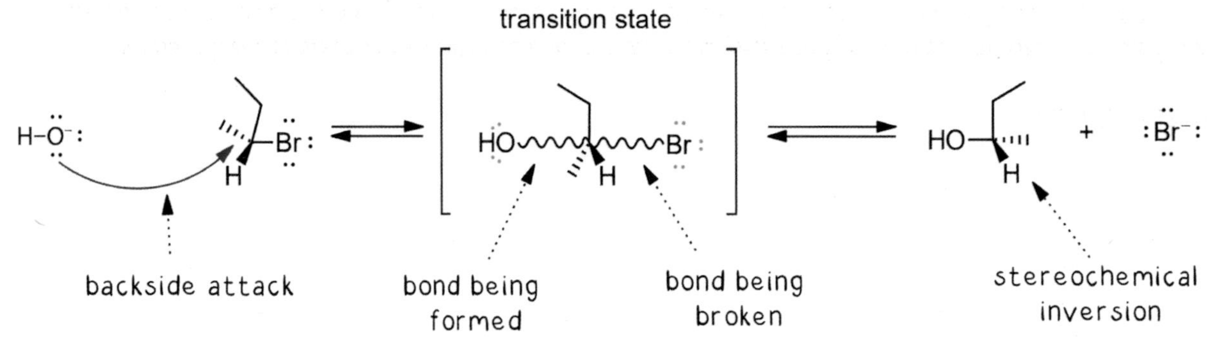

transition state

backside attack · bond being formed · bond being broken · stereochemical inversion

Figure 3. S_N2 mechanism

S_N2 reactions are initiated by a nucleophilic attack, so one prerequisite is having a strong nucleophile. Figure 2 showed an S_N1 reaction using H_2O, which is only a weak nucleophile, whereas in Figure 3, the S_N2 reaction uses OH^-, which is a strong nucleophile. However, it's not enough just for the nucleophile to be strong. It also has to encounter the electrophilic carbon. This is where steric considerations come in. First, we want to make sure that the nucleophile is both strong and *small*; a big bulky base like *tert*-butoxide will not work effectively here. Second, we need to think about the sterics of the reaction substrate. The less substituted the electrophilic carbon is, the easier it will be for the nucleophile to contact the electrophile. Therefore, S_N2 reactions are favorable at methyl carbons and primary carbons, but less so at secondary carbons, and will essentially not occur at any meaningful rate at tertiary carbons (Note that the example shown in Figure 3 is not favorable because it takes place at a secondary carbon! This choice illustrates the stereochemical inversion more clearly).

Also, the solvent can also be a factor favoring one reaction mechanism over another. The relevant distinction is between polar protic and polar aprotic solvents. Nonpolar solvents are not generally useful for these reactions. **Polar protic solvents** are those with the ability to donate a hydrogen bond, most typically involving an O–H or N–H bond. Typical examples include water, methanol, and ethanol. Polar protic solvents engage in hydrogen bonding to the leaving group, which stabilizes the carbocation. These solvents favor the S_N1 reaction because even a weak nucleophile can attack the carbocation without interference from the leaving group. **Polar aprotic solvents** contain a permanent dipole due to a polar bond (typically C=O), but cannot act as hydrogen bond donors. Acetone is a typical example, as is dimethyl sulfoxide (DMSO). As is suggested by the definition of polar protic versus aprotic solvents, the difference in their properties has to do with the presence or absence of hydrogen bonding. These solvents favor S_N2 reactions since there are no hydrogen bonds from the solvent. This results in less steric hindrance blocking the nucleophile, so the nucleophile can initiate a backside attack more easily.

With all of this in mind, we can summarize the characteristic features of S_N1 or S_N2 mechanisms. On test day, you may have to predict which reaction mechanism will occur in a given situation, but you may be given a Sn_1 or Sn_2 mechanism and then must predict something about the reaction. Either way, you should be familiar with the key features of these mechanisms presented in Table 1.

	S_N1	S_N2
'Key' to the mechanism	Carbocation stability.	Steric hindrance.
Rate law dependence	Unimolecular (substrate concentration only).	Bimolecular (substrate and nucleophile concentrations).
Number of steps	2.	1.
Substituents on carbon	3° > 2°.	0° (methyl) > 1° > 2°.
Strength of nucleophile	Doesn't really matter.	Strong (and non-bulky).
Solvent	Polar protic.	Polar aprotic.
Stereochemistry	Not preserved (racemization).	Inverted (backside attack).

Table 1. S_N1 and S_N2 reaction descriptions and important factors

In a reaction environment with a nucleophile present, alkyl halides can also undergo a type of reaction in which the halide is kicked out, but the nucleophile doesn't add itself as a substituent. Instead, a double C=C bond is formed. This type of reaction is known as **elimination**, and just as there are S_N1 and S_N2 mechanisms, there are E1 and E2 mechanisms.

Most organic chemistry courses emphasize the E1 and E2 mechanisms to the same extent that they do S_N1 and S_N2 reactions. This is *not* the case for the MCAT. S_N1 and S_N2 mechanisms are important mechanisms to study for the MCAT, however, elimination is helpful background information, but is unlikely to be directly tested. For this reason, we will only briefly review the two elimination mechanisms.

The E1 mechanism is similar to the S_N1 mechanism in that it has a unimolecular rate law and is driven by carbocation formation. However, it differs by instead of attacking the carbocation once it is formed, the nucleophile pulls off a proton from an adjacent carbon, which allows a double bond to form on the target molecule. This is illustrated below in Figure 4.

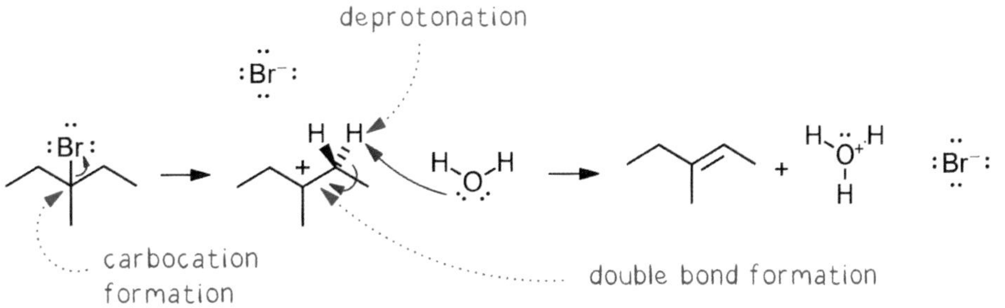

Figure 4. E1 mechanism

The E2 mechanism is also similar to its S_N2 counterpart in that it has a bimolecular rate law and is driven by nucleophilic attack. The difference is that in an E2 reaction, a strong base attacks a proton adjacent to the carbon with a halide substituent. Once that proton is removed, a double C=C bond is formed, which causes the leaving group to be kicked off.

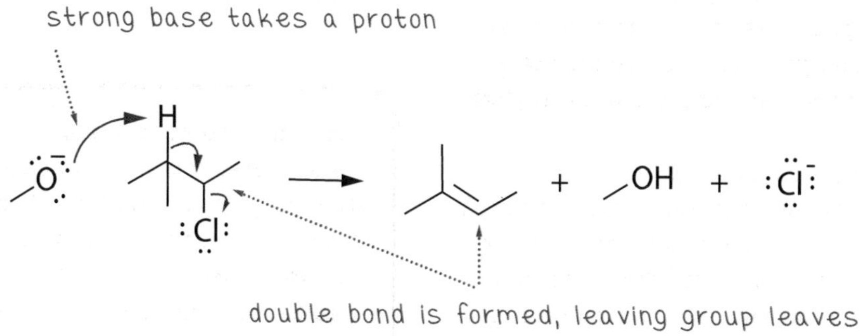

Figure 5. E2 mechanism

We use Zaitsev's rule to determine which C=C bond is most likely to be formed. Zaitsev's rule states that the alkene favored in an elimination reaction is the one that corresponds to the removal of a proton from the beta-carbon with the fewest associated hydrogens. The alkene formed from this reaction is more substituted and is, therefore, more stable.

It can be possible for elimination chemistry to occur at the same time as S_N1 or S_N2 chemistry. However, the details of this go beyond the scope of the MCAT. Instead, focus on being able to predict whether a mechanism will be S_N1 or S_N2 and know that elimination chemistry is another theoretical possibility that involves double bond formation.

2. Nucleophilic Substitution and Addition: Examples

Nucleophilic substitution—and its cousin, nucleophilic addition—are the mechanisms through which many biologically relevant reactions take place. In particular, they are common at carbonyl carbons because the carbonyl oxygen has a partial negative charge and the carbonyl carbon has a partial positive charge. This is also the case for the carbons in carboxylic acid functional groups, but even more so because of the additional –OH group. This means that the carbonyl carbon can act as an electrophile that is subject to nucleophilic attack.

A prototypical example of nucleophilic substitution at a carboxylic acid group is provided by a process known as Fischer esterification. Fischer esterification is an acid-catalyzed, highly practical technique for turning a carboxylic acid into an ester—replacing the –OH group of the carboxylic acid with the –OR functional group characteristic of an ester. To do this, a carboxylic acid is mixed with an alcohol under acidic conditions. The mechanism of Fischer esterification is shown below in Figure 6.

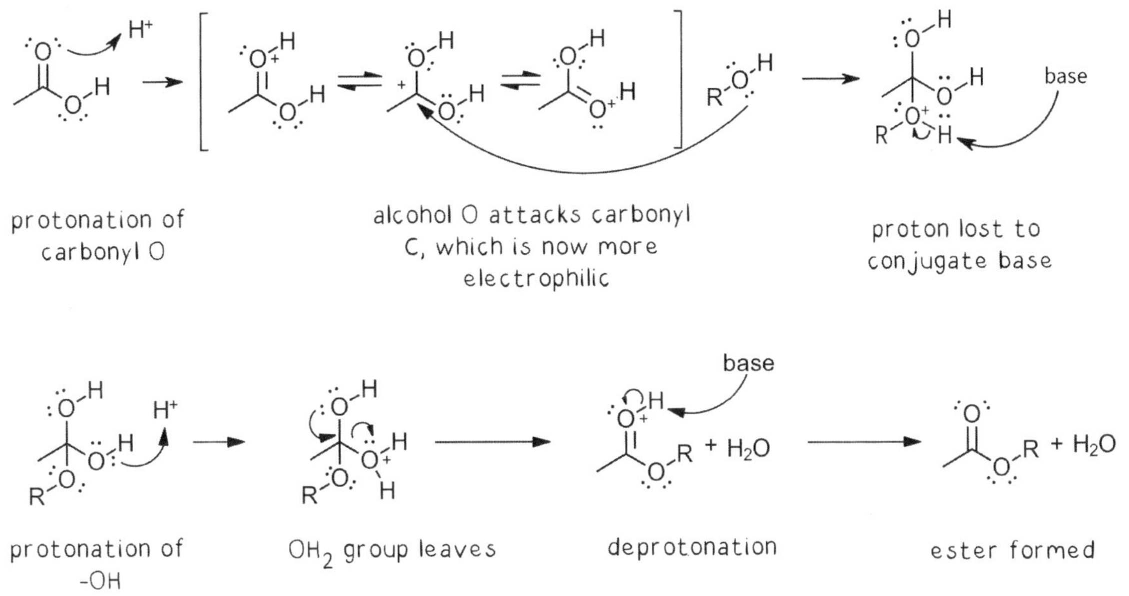

protonation of
carbonyl O

alcohol O attacks carbonyl
C, which is now more
electrophilic

proton lost to
conjugate base

protonation of
-OH

OH$_2$ group leaves

deprotonation

ester formed

Figure 6. Fischer esterification

The first step in Fischer esterification is protonation of the carbonyl oxygen. This is a typical first step in nucleophilic reactions involving carbonyl groups because it adds a positive charge that helps to make the carbonyl carbon even more electrophilic. After protonation, the positive charge is to some extent shared by the carbon through resonance. After this occurs, the carbonyl C is more electrophilic, so the oxygen in the alcohol can attack it. After this step, we have a complex four-membered structure known as a tetrahedral intermediate. Our goal is now to kick out the –OH group. In order to do that, proton shuffling, describes a which is facilitated by the acidic environment. A proton is eventually added to the –OH, making it a good leaving group. Then the oxygen that was originally the carbonyl oxygen executes a nucleophilic attack. This step forms a double bond, regenerating the carbonyl group, and kicks off the –OH$_2$ leaving group. The only remaining step is some additional proton shuffling to regenerate the ester.

As outlined in Section 1, there are three keys for understanding nucleophilic substitution reactions: (1) **find the nucleophile** (in this case, the oxygen in an alcohol), (2) **find the electrophile** (the carbonyl C, with protonation to activate it), and (3) **identify the leaving group** (–OH, protonated to H$_2$O). Protonation is important conceptually because, as shown in this mechanism, it can help activate the electrophile and prepare the leaving group. Luckily, you don't need to worry about protonation for the MCAT as much as you might have when drawing mechanisms by hand for organic chemistry coursework.

> **MCAT STRATEGY >>>**
>
> Fischer esterification is a classic example of how nucleophilic substitution works for carboxylic acids and their derivatives. Study this mechanism thoroughly, and you will be prepared for any variations you might encounter on your exam.

Fischer esterification can be reversed through **hydrolysis**, which describes a reaction in which a compound breaks down through the addition of water. The mechanism for the hydrolysis of an ester is essentially the same as ester formation, with the only difference is that water attacks and the –OR group is the leaving group. Hydrolysis is important physiologically because it is the main mechanism through which biological polymers, like proteins, are degraded. However, the specific mechanism of hydrolysis of biomolecules can vary. It is often the case that such reactions are technically favorable but would be very slow without a catalyst. The enzymes that catalyze these reactions can be very specific and involve individualized mechanisms and intermediate stabilizing steps. For the MCAT, you should be aware of the general idea of hydrolysis as a form of nucleophilic substitution, and you don't need to worry about the specific details.

Another important nucleophilic substitution reaction, **imine formation**, occurs at a carbonyl carbon (not a carboxylic acid group!). This reaction replaces the carbonyl carbon with a nitrogen, creating the C=N double bond that defines an imine (You may also hear the term 'Schiff base,' which refers to an imine with an additional carbon substituent [C=N–R]). The imine formation mechanism is shown in Figure 7.

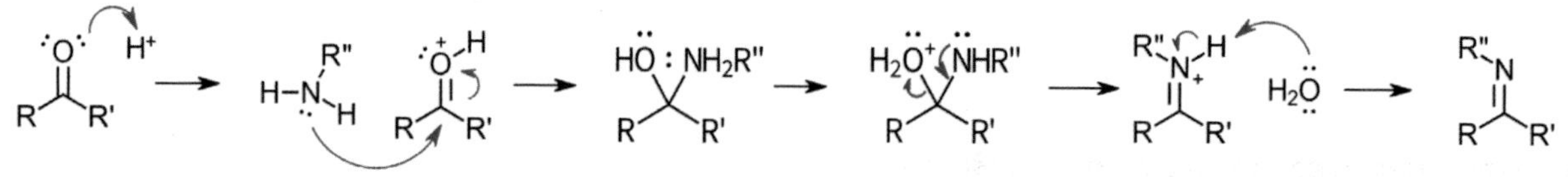

Figure 7. Imine formation

The first steps of imine formation follow a familiar pattern. The carbonyl oxygen is protonated, which activates the carbonyl carbon as an electrophile. This is followed by nucleophilic attack of the nitrogen atom in the reactant amine, which joins with the carbonyl carbon to form a tetrahedral intermediate. The nitrogen is initially positively charged, but acid-base interactions with the medium mediate proton transfer to the oxygen. Once that proton transfer happens, the nitrogen atom regains a nucleophilic lone pair of electrons. This lone pair forms a double bond with the carbon, kicking off the H_2O leaving group. The nitrogen now has a positive charge, which is then removed in a final deprotonation step, resulting in the imine.

To summarize imine formation using the rubric we used above, (1) the nucleophile is an amine; (2) the electrophile is a carbonyl carbon post-protonation; and (3) the leaving group is $-OH_2$, derived from the carbonyl oxygen. Note that the nitrogen atom executes *two* nucleophilic attacks, which is enabled by how proton transfer processes allow the nitrogen lone pair to be regenerated.

A similar, but distinct, mechanism is known as **nucleophilic addition**. As the name implies, nucleophilic addition is similar to nucleophilic substitution but without the leaving group. In a classic example, an alcohol can attack an aldehyde or a ketone (both characterized by a C=O bond and add to it. The resulting structure has a central—potentially chiral—carbon with an –OR group (derived from the alcohol) and an –OH group (derived from the carbonyl oxygen). If an aldehyde undergoes this reaction, the resulting structure is known as a hemiacetal, whereas a ketone that undergoes this reaction results in a hemiketal.

Figure 8 shows the mechanism of **hemiacetal formation**, comparing acidic and basic conditions. The mechanism shown in Figure 8 also works for **hemiketal formation** if the initial molecule is a ketone rather than an aldehyde, as in Figure 8. However, the difference between acid- and base-catalysis is worth exploring in some detail.

Acid-catalyzed hemiacetal formation

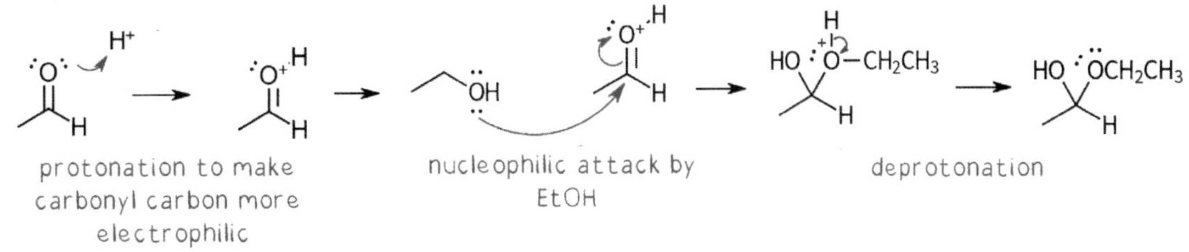

protonation to make
carbonyl carbon more
electrophilic

nucleophilic attack by
EtOH

deprotonation

Base-catalyzed hemiacetal formation

strong base deprotonates
EtOH, making it more
nucleophilic

nucleophilic attack by
EtO⁻

base gives up H to
reprotonate what was
originally the carbonyl O

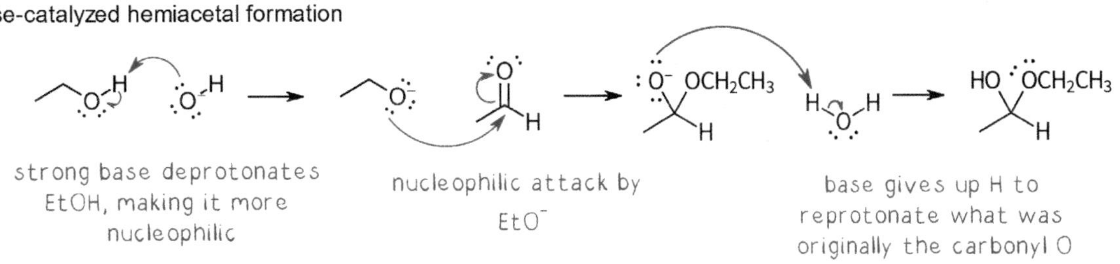

Figure 8. Hemiacetal formation

If you've thoroughly studied Fischer esterification, **acid-catalyzed hemiacetal formation** will be familiar. The oxygen is protonated to make the carbonyl carbon more electrophilic, the alcohol then executes a nucleophilic attack, and the result, after deprotonation, is a tetrahedral structure. **Base-catalyzed hemiacetal formation**, in contrast, follows a different logic. Whereas acid catalysis focuses on making the electrophile stronger via protonation, base catalysis works by making the nucleophile more intensely nucleophilic via deprotonation. The alcohol is deprotonated to form an alkoxide, which is a very strong nucleophile capable of directly attacking the carbonyl carbon. Once this happens, the hemiacetal is formed, and the only remaining step is reprotonation to generate the hemiacetal.

> > CONNECTIONS < <

Chapter 6 of Biochemistry

This mechanism is especially noteworthy in the biochemistry context because it is what takes place in sugars when they convert from linear forms to cyclic forms, which are predominant in aqueous solution in the body.

Interestingly, it turns out that you have to be very careful about stoichiometry to generate hemiacetals and hemiketals in laboratory conditions. If there is an excess of alcohol, the reaction can keep going, resulting in **acetals** and **ketals**, which have two –OR groups instead of one –OR and one –OH group, as seen in hemiacetals and hemiketals. These structures are shown in Figure 9.

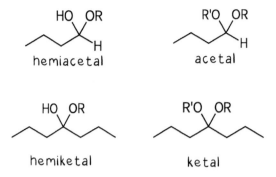

Figure 9. Hemiacetals, hemiketals, acetals, and ketals

For example, a **glycosidic bond** is formed between two monosaccharides (isolated sugar molecules) to form a disaccharide, a hemiacetal or hemiketal is converted into an acetal or ketal. This is shown and labeled in the diagram of sucrose, a disaccharide formed from glucose and fructose, Figure 10.

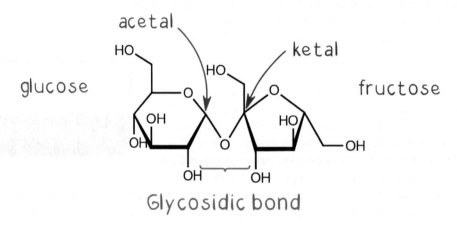

Figure 10. Glycosidic bond

To summarize, there are three major takeaways of the hemiacetal/hemiketal reaction mechanism:

1. It is an excellent example of acid catalysis (protonation makes the electrophile stronger) versus base catalysis (deprotonation makes the nucleophile stronger). Study this aspect of the mechanism carefully because these two types of logic can be applied to other reactions as well.

2. Nucleophilic addition can take place instead of substitution and stoichiometry can be necessary to obtain the desired reaction outcome.

3. Organic chemistry reactions can have close parallels in biological contexts that are not necessarily immediately obvious, because it can sometimes be challenging to visualize functional groups in cyclic conformations with large –R groups.

3. Keto-enol tautomerism

Tautomerism is a phenomenon in which a molecule has two structures that interconvert at equilibrium. The most common example is **keto-enol tautomerism**, although tautomerism is also found between enamines and imines (the second most important example), lactams and lactims, and amides and imidic acids. As noted before in Chapter

9, when tautomerism was introduced, tautomerism is not the same thing as resonance. In resonance, electrons are delocalized in the underlying structure of the molecule, and we use resonance structures as a relatively crude way of representing this fact. In contrast, tautomers are two *different* structures that interconvert via the breaking and reformation of bonds.

Keto-enol tautomerism describes the interconversion between ketone and enol forms. An enol is a functional group with a C=C double bond (hence the *en–* part of the name) and an –OH group (hence the *–ol* part of enol). The interconversion between these two forms is generated by proton transfer that can be accomplished in either acidic or basic conditions. The two mechanisms of keto-enol tautomerism are shown below in Figure 11.

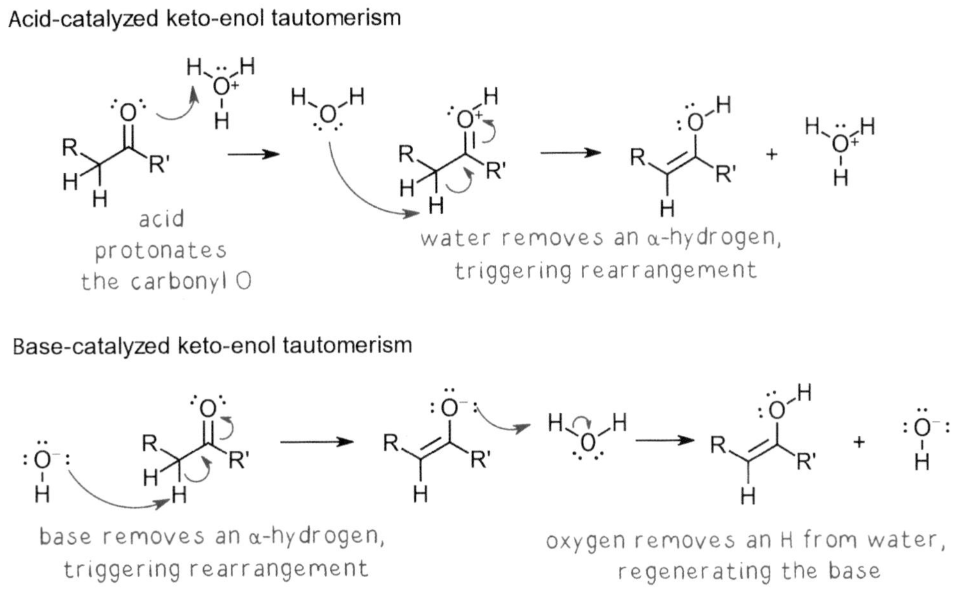

Acid-catalyzed keto-enol tautomerism

acid protonates the carbonyl O

water removes an α-hydrogen, triggering rearrangement

Base-catalyzed keto-enol tautomerism

base removes an α-hydrogen, triggering rearrangement

oxygen removes an H from water, regenerating the base

Figure 11. Mechanisms of keto-enol tautomerism

This mechanism provides another opportunity to compare the logic of acid catalysis with that of base catalysis. In **acid catalysis**, as usual, the first step is to protonate the carbonyl oxygen, after which the conjugate base of the acid (in this case, water) removes an α-hydrogen (that is, a hydrogen located on a carbon *next* to the carbonyl carbon), which triggers rearrangement into the enol form. In contrast, in the **base-catalyzed mechanism**, a base removes the α-hydrogen in the first step, which triggers the formation of a C=C double bond and the conversion of the C=O double bond to a C–O single bond. The negatively-charged oxygen then picks up a proton from the conjugate acid of the base catalyst, regenerating the base and resulting in the enol form.

In aqueous solution, the keto form generally predominates over the enol form. However, the enol form can predominate in some circumstances. Most importantly, if the enol form is resonance-stabilized, it will be preferred to a non-stabilized keto form. Additionally, hydrogen bonding can stabilize the enol form. Stabilization of a 1,3-diketone is a classic example. To some extent, the solvent can also affect the keto-enol equilibrium. Both resonance and internal hydrogen bonding stabilization of the enol forms are shown below in Figure 12.

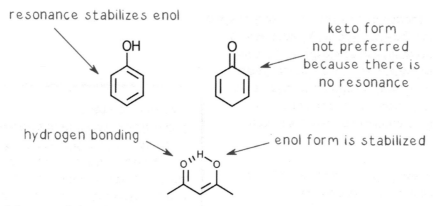

Figure 12. Enol stabilization of phenol and a 1,3-diketone

An important point about the keto-enol mechanism—in both its acid-catalyzed and base-catalyzed forms—is its dependence on α-hydrogens. If there is no α-hydrogen, tautomerization cannot take place. This means that if you're faced with a compound that might undergo keto-enol tautomerization on test day, be sure to double-check that there is at least one hydrogen on the adjacent alpha carbon(s).

4. Enolate chemistry and aldol condensation

Above, in Figure 11, we saw that base-catalyzed keto-enol tautomerism involves an intermediate with a negative charge. This structure is known as an **enolate**. Enolates are discussed in greater detail in Chapter 10, but the short version of why enolates are remarkable is that resonance allows that negative charge to be distributed onto the α-carbon to some extent, allowing it to act as a nucleophile.

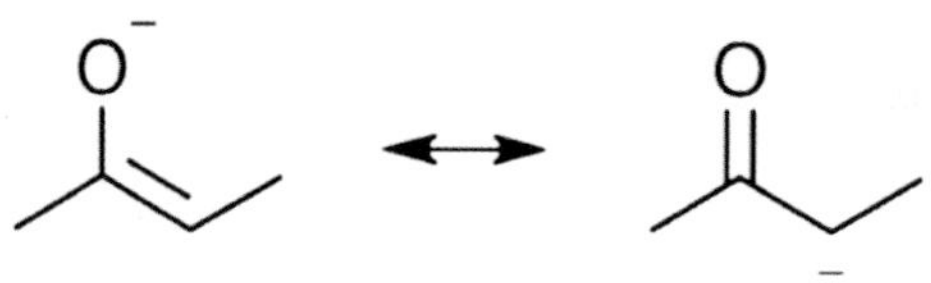

Figure 13. Resonance stabilization of an enolate

This property of enolates is exhibited in **base-catalyzed aldol condensation**. This is a two-step reaction between two molecules of an aldehyde (or ketone). The basic idea of an aldol condensation reaction is that the two aldehyde/ketone molecules combine via nucleophilic attack to form a product known as an **aldol**. Aldol refers to the product having one aldehyde (or ketone) and one alcohol functional group. Once the aldol is formed, it can undergo spontaneous reduction in which the alcohol group is kicked out and a C=C double bond is formed, creating an **α,β-unsaturated ketone or aldehyde**.

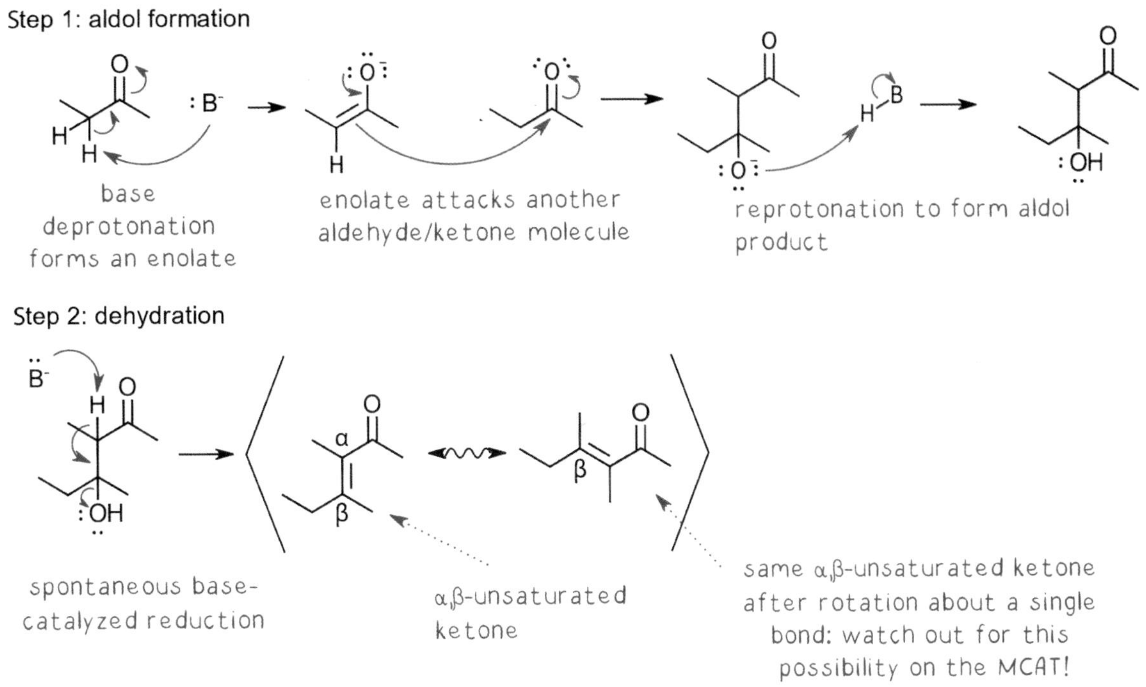

Step 1: aldol formation

Step 2: dehydration

Figure 14. Base-catalyzed aldol formation

As shown in Figure 14, in the first step of base-catalyzed aldol formation, a base removes an α-hydrogen, forming an enolate. This is the same first step that we saw in Figure 11 for base-catalyzed keto-enol tautomerization. In terms of similarities, you may note that the actual mechanism itself is virtually identical to the nucleophilic addition mechanism we saw for hemiacetal and hemiketal formation: a nucleophile attacks, is added, and then protonation/deprotonation occurs to get the final product. Important differences include the nature of the nucleophile, and in particular, the fact that the enolate ion is a structure that allows carbon to act as a nucleophile because of the resonance-distributed negative charge.

The second step is **spontaneous reduction/dehydration**. In this step, the base removes another α-hydrogen, which triggers the formation of a C=C double bond, at which point the –OH leaves. This generates a structure known as an α,β-unsaturated ketone/aldehyde. The terms 'saturated' and 'unsaturated' are used more often in biochemistry, but just to review, 'saturated' means a compound in which all the carbon-carbon bonds are single bonds—that is, a compound that is 'saturated' with as many hydrogens as possible.

The aldol condensation reaction can be catalyzed by an acid as well, although this mechanism is less important for the MCAT because it doesn't involve an enolate ion. In the **acid-catalyzed mechanism**, an enol molecule attacks with an activated (protonated) ketone/aldehyde molecule to form the condensation product. The dehydration step to an α,β-unsaturated compound can also occur via acid catalysis.

MCAT STRATEGY >>>

One way to cope with the potential difficulty of visualizing the outcomes of aldol condensation reactions is to implement simple safety checks like counting carbons and accounting for the location and orientation of double bonds. If nothing else, this will help you rule out answer choices that *cannot* be correct.

Although the aldol condensation reaction builds on mechanisms that should be familiar from simpler nucleophilic addition reactions, students often find it challenging. One reason for this is that the final product—especially after the dehydration step—is visually unlike the reactants. In general, the MCAT doesn't test you on retrosynthetic analysis, but aldol condensation is an exception. It's worth remembering that if you see an α,β-unsaturated carbonyl, aldol condensation is a possibility. Moreover, it can be important to remember that the possibility of rotation around single bonds means that the orientation of aldol products might not correspond to how you imagine the reaction happening in your head or how you would draw it out. This possibility is demonstrated at the end of the pathway in Figure 14.

Aldol condensation is an equilibrium process and can be reversed. The reverse reaction is known as the **retro-aldol reaction**. An important example of this is found in glycolysis, in which the six-carbon compound fructose-1,6-bisphosphate is cleaved to form the three-carbon compounds dihydroxyacetone phosphate and glyceraldehyde phosphate. Figure 15 shows this mechanism.

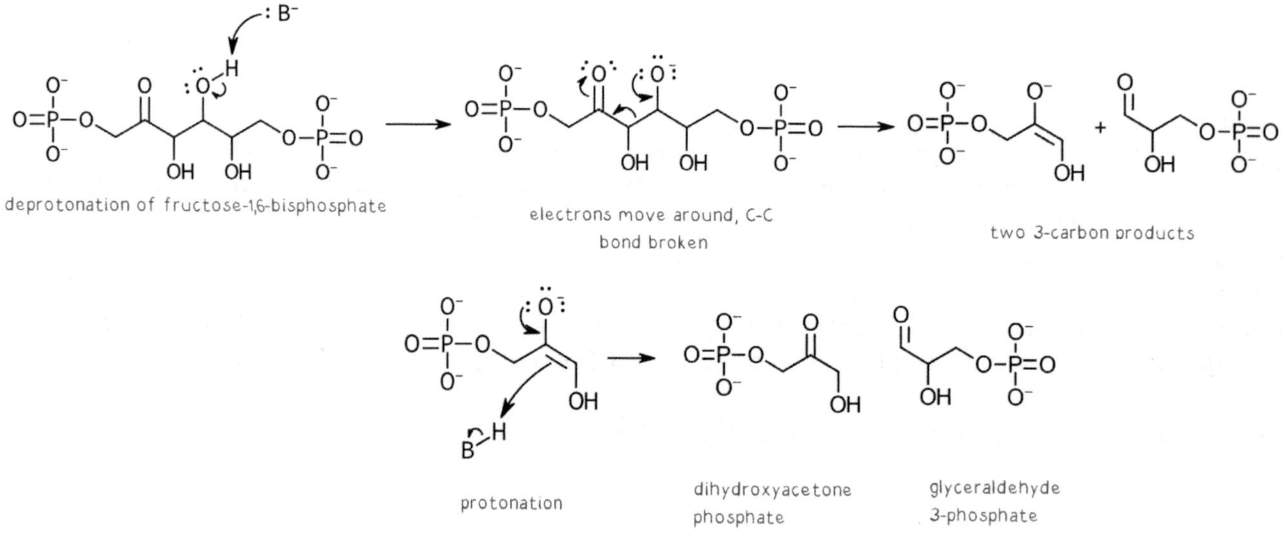

Figure 15. Cleavage of fructose-1,6-bisphosphate

It is unlikely that you will be directly tested on this mechanism, but you should know what retro-aldol reactions are generally, and it is useful to walk through this reaction as an example of how analyzing simple nucleophilic substitution reactions can be applied to systematically understand reaction mechanisms that might initially seem intimidating or unfamiliar.

The first step of this reaction is deprotonation of fructose-1,6-bisphosphate by a base. The surplus electrons on the deprotonated oxygen then attack the carbon, forming a C=O double bond. This break the C–C bond, and in a process of electron transfers, a C=C bond and a C–O⁻ are formed. This is followed by a protonation step that converts the C=C bond to a C–C bond and allows the C=O bond to reform, generating dihydroxyacetone phosphate. In physiological conditions, this reaction is catalyzed by an enzyme known as fructose-1,6-bisphosphate aldolase.

Be aware of two other applications of enolate chemistry: **Michael addition** and **Robinson annulation**. To understand these processes, our starting point is an α,β-unsaturated aldehyde or ketone, of the type that we can generate through aldol condensation. Let's take a closer look at this type of molecule, as shown in Figure 16.

Figure 16. An α,β-unsaturated aldehyde and an α,β-unsaturated ketone

A remarkable fact about α,β-unsaturated aldehydes and ketones is that they have two sites that nucleophiles can add to. The first is the carbonyl carbon, as is generally the case for carbonyl-containing compounds. The second is the β-carbon or the double-bonded carbon located farther from the carbonyl. Resonance explains this phenomenon. As shown in Figure 17, in one resonance structure, the double bond is placed between the α-carbon and the carbonyl carbon. Another resonance form places a negative charge on the oxygen atom and a positive charge on the β-carbon, which makes it electrophilic. Of course, this structure is not the *major* contributor to α,β-unsaturated aldehydes/ketones, but it makes enough of a contribution to matter for chemical reactions.

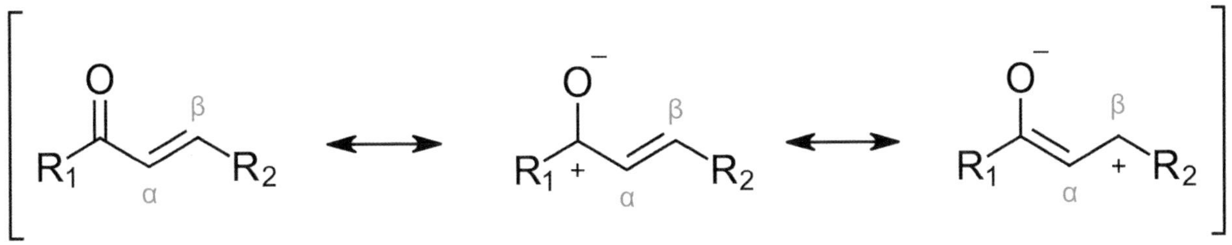

Figure 17. Resonance of α,β-unsaturated aldehyde and ketones

In a **Michael addition** reaction, as shown in Figure 18, an enolate attacks the β-carbon of an α,β-unsaturated aldehyde/ketone. In this mechanism, the double C=C bond is removed, initially resulting in a negative charge on the α-carbon. This negative charge is addressed by a quick protonation step, yielding a characteristic structure with two carbonyl groups that are separated by three carbon atoms—or, more technically, a 1,5-dicarbonyl structure. Note that alcohols, amines, cyanide, and even β-dicarbonyl compounds can function as the nucleophile instead of an enolate. That said, the reaction with an enolate nucleophile is by far the most likely version to appear on the MCAT. A key point underlying Michael addition is that the β-carbon in α,β-unsaturated aldehydes/ketones is another potential site for nucleophilic addition.

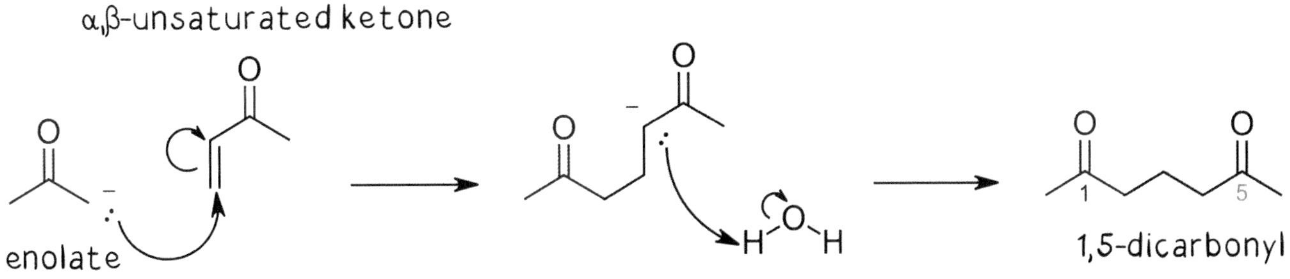

Figure 18. Michael addition between acetone enolate and methyl vinyl ketone (but-3-en-2-one)

Robinson annulation involves Michael addition followed by an aldol condensation. Therefore, let's take a closer look at the product of Michael addition, as shown in Figure 19.

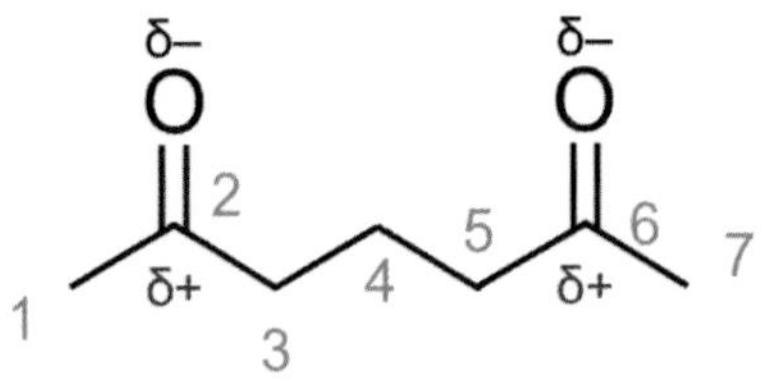

Figure 19. Structure of Michael addition product

Note how this structure has a linear seven-carbon stucture with two carbonyl groups at 2 and 6. So, what would an intramolecular aldol condensation look like for this molecule? In basic conditions, it forms an enolate. This is possible by using a strong base to remove a hydrogen from one of the α-carbons. More specifically, in order to form a stable ring structure without undue strain, we'll need to remove a hydrogen from an α-carbon at the end of the molecule, forming an enolate. We label that α-carbon as carbon 1. It acts as a nucleophile and attacks the carbonyl structure at the end of the molecule, which we label carbon 6. Protonation by water regenerates the hydroxide ion OH⁻, which then removes the hydrogen on carbon 1 and results in formation of a carbanion. The carbanion then forms a double bond within the ring while pushing off the –OH group. This results in an α,β-unsaturated *cyclic* ketone. The ring-forming mechanism is presented in Figure 20.

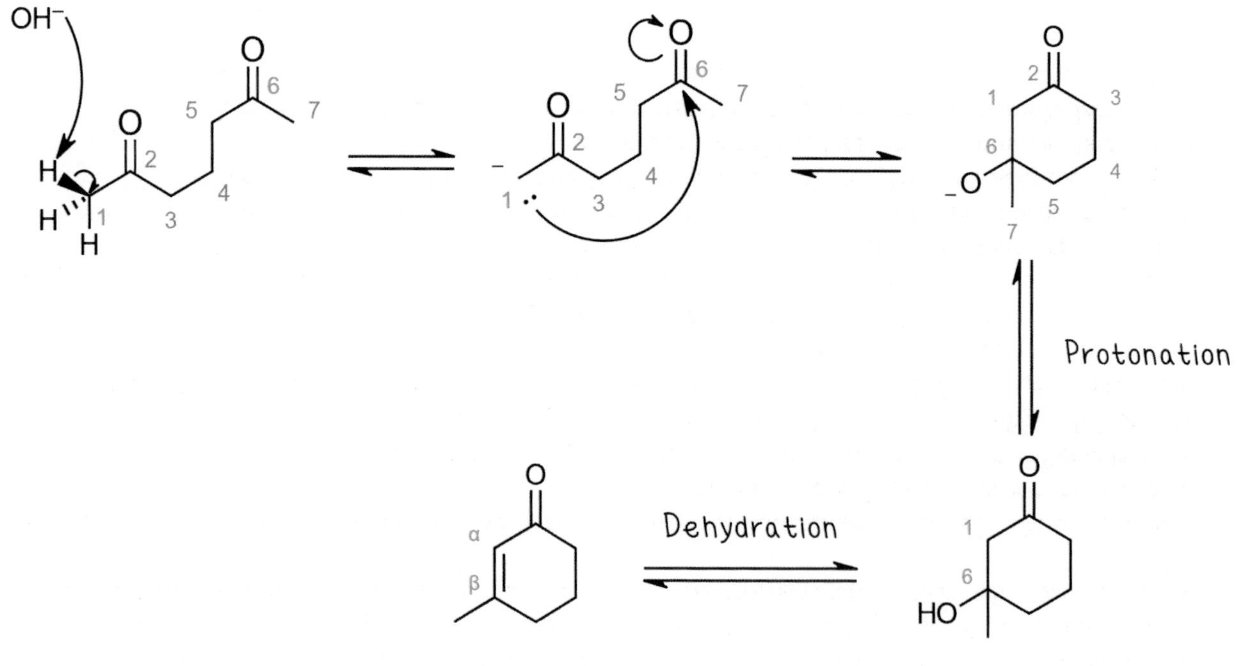

Figure 20. Robinson annulation, an intramolecular reaction

The Robinson annulation mechanism is interesting to organic chemists because it can form a six-membered ring, which has several important applications, such as the synthesis of steroid hormones and certain drugs. For our purposes, recognize that complex-seeming mechanisms are driven by a small set of principles—namely, enolates make good nucleophiles, and carbonyl-containing carbons can contain two distinct electrophilic sites.

5. Must-Knows

> Basic idea for reaction mechanisms: an electrophile and a nucleophile form a bond.
>   — Electrophile: an atom that 'needs' electrons (usually has positive or partial positive charge).
>   — Nucleophile: an atom that 'needs' to share its excess electrons (usually has negative or partial negative charge).
> S_N1: nucleophilic substitution with a first-order rate law (depends on substrate concentration only). Carbocation forms, then nucleophile attacks. Favorable factors: highly substituted carbons, polar protic solvent. Stereochemistry not preserved.
> S_N2: nucleophilic substitution with a second-order rate law (depends on substrate *and* nucleophile concentration). Nucleophile performs 'backside attack' and kicks out leaving group, inverting the stereochemistry. Favorable factors: methyl/primary carbons, strong and non-bulky nucleophile, polar aprotic solvent.
> Carboxylic acid: C has strong partial positive charge, is a good electrophile. Nucleophilic substitution is common, as in Fischer esterification and imine formation.
>   — Nucleophile attacks carboxylic acid C, then a leaving group is kicked off.
> Nucleophilic addition at carbonyl C (C=O): hemiacetals (–R, –H, –OH, –OR') formed from aldehydes, hemiketals (–R, –R', –OH, –OR'') from ketones. Reaction can repeat with excess alcohol to form acetals and ketals (another –OR group instead of –OH).
>   — Nucleophile attacks carbonyl C without a leaving group.
> Keto-enol tautomerism: can be catalyzed by acid or base, α-hydrogen removal is critical in both (first step in base-catalyzed mechanism, second step in acid catalysis).
> Enolate chemistry: resonance-stabilized negative charge on α-carbon allows carbon to be a nucleophile.
>   — Aldol condensation: nucleophilic α-carbon attacks electrophilic carbonyl C to form a new C–C bond.
>   — Retro-aldol: reverse of the aldol condensation process.
>   — Michael addition: an enolate attacks the β-carbon of an α,β-unsaturated aldehyde/ketone.
>   — Robinson annulation: Michael addition followed by aldol condensation.

End of Chapter Practice

The best MCAT practice is realistic, with a focus on identifying steps for further improvement. For those reasons, we recommend completing practice questions in an online setting that simulates the real MCAT interface, and taking advantage of advanced analytic features to help you determine how best to move forward in your MCAT study journey.

With that in mind, online end-of-chapter questions for Biology, Biochemistry, Chemistry + Organic Chemistry, Physics, and Psychology/Sociology are available through your Blueprint MCAT account.

As a further supplement, given the importance of active learning for effective studying, we also suggest that you consult the Must-Knows as a basis for creating a study sheet, in which you list out key terms and test your ability to briefly summarize them.

This page left intentionally blank.

This page left intentionally blank.

Spectroscopy and Separations

0. Introduction

You have now learned MCAT general chemistry, as well as some organic chemistry and reactions. This leads us to a new question: once a chemist has performed a reaction procedure, how can they be certain that the correct product was formed? And how can this desired product be separated from reactants or side products present in the same flask?

We answer these questions using separation and analytical techniques. **Separation techniques** separate a mixture into its pure components or, when this is not possible, to convert the original mixture into multiple mixtures that are each largely composed of a single component. The separation techniques discussed in this chapter are distillation, extraction, and chromatography. In contrast, **analytical techniques** identify a compound or determine its properties. In this chapter, the analytical techniques discussed are spectroscopy (infrared, nuclear magnetic resonance, and ultraviolet-visible) and mass spectrometry.

1. Infrared Spectroscopy and Nuclear Magnetic Resonance

Let's begin with analytic al techniques, which are largely spectroscopy methods. For the MCAT, familiarize yourself with spectroscopy (the analysis of organic compounds exposed to electromagnetic radiation). What exactly *is* electromagnetic radiation? It is light, but remember visible light forms only a small portion of the electromagnetic spectrum (Figure 1).

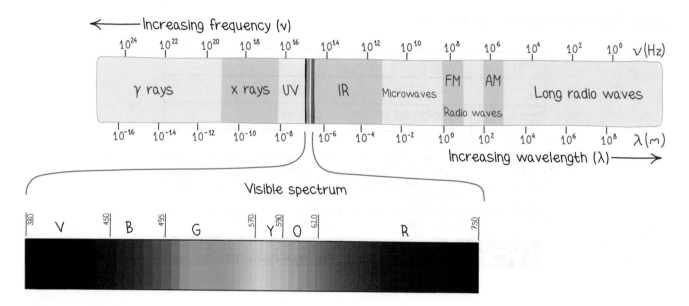

Figure 1. The electromagnetic spectrum

>> CONNECTIONS <<

Chapter 9 of Physics

MCAT STRATEGY >>>

The terms used to describe concepts can give away a great deal about their meanings. For example, "infra-" means "below," so "infrared" means "a frequency below that of red light." Conversely, "ultra" means "above," so "ultraviolet" light has a frequency higher than that of violet light.

This chapter discusses only two forms of electromagnetic radiation: **infrared radiation (IR)** and **ultraviolet radiation (UV)**. Infrared radiation is a form of electromagnetic radiation with a frequency just below that of visible light. **Infrared (IR) spectroscopy** uses infrared light to vibrate covalent bonds in molecules and measure the vibrations to collect information about functional groups.

Put simply, the bonds that appear on an IR spectrum must have a dipole moment, such as the polar O–H bond in water. In contrast, the Br–Br bond in Br_2 does not have a dipole and thus does not appear on an IR spectrum. The same is true for the N-N bond in N_2 and so on.

An example of an **IR spectrum** is shown in Figure 2. The y-axis displays percent transmittance (the proportion of IR light transmitted through the sample), which is the reciprocal of absorbance. Regions that have absorbed light will appear as peaks along the graph. The x-axis displays the frequency of light in a unit of measurement known as wavenumbers (cm^{-1}), with wavenumbers increasing from right to left along the x-axis.

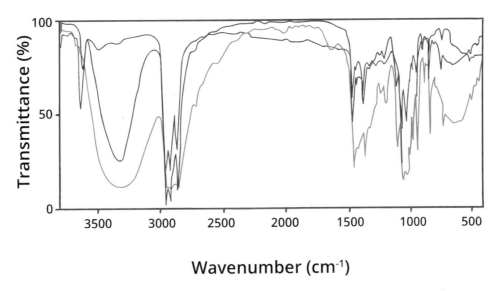

Figure 2. A sample IR spectrum showing multiple compounds, each corresponding to a separate line

Specific bonds are associated with characteristic absorption frequencies on an IR spectrum. Memorizing these frequencies may get you some quick, easy points on the MCAT! Most of these peaks appear within the 1500-4000 cm⁻¹ range. While it may initially appear that the region below 1500 cm⁻¹ contains a large number of notable peaks, this area, termed the fingerprint region, is specific to each compound. Since each molecule has a distinct fingerprint region, this range is generally not useful when identifying functional groups on an unknown molecule.

The IR frequencies of the most common covalent bonds are listed in Table 1. Among these frequencies, the most commonly tested are the carbonyl (C=O) functional group, which appears as a sharp peak near 1700 cm⁻¹, and the hydroxyl (–OH) functional group, marked by a broad peak in the range of 3100–3500 cm⁻¹. By "sharp," we mean that the peak is narrow and it slopes dramatically downward and back up. On the other hand, a broad peak is wider and takes up a larger area of the IR spectrum.

> **>> CONNECTIONS <<**
>
> **Chapter 10 of Chemistry**

Bond	Wavenumber (cm⁻¹)	Shape (if applicable)
C=N	1550-1650	–
C=C	1600-1680	–
C=O	1650-1780	Sharp
C≡C	2100-2260	–
C≡N	2220-2260	–
O-H	3200-3600	Broad
N-H	3300-3500	–

Table 1. IR spectrum frequencies of select bonds

Unlike IR, which identifies the *bonds* in a molecule, **nuclear magnetic resonance (NMR) spectroscopy** aims to characterize a molecule's *atoms*. Specifically, this technique places a sample in a magnetic field. If the sample has a nuclear spin due to an odd number of protons or neutrons, then it will be affected by the magnetic field. The atomic nuclei will align *with* the field (a lower-energy state) or *against* the field (a higher-energy state). The frequency of transition between these states, or resonance, is measured by NMR. The NMR type that you should understand for the MCAT is ^{1}H (proton) NMR. To be comprehensive, we will also briefly discuss ^{13}C (carbon) NMR, although it is far less likely to appear on the MCAT.

Before delving into these methods, we must discuss the general appearance of an NMR spectrum. **Resonance frequencies** are chemical shifts ranging from zero on the far right to positive values on the far left. A shift of zero is arbitrarily assigned to the peak corresponding to tetramethylsilane (TMS) as a reference point. Figure 3 depicts a sample NMR spectrum. Peaks that are shifted to the right are said to be located upfield, and peaks that are shifted to the left are said to be located downfield.

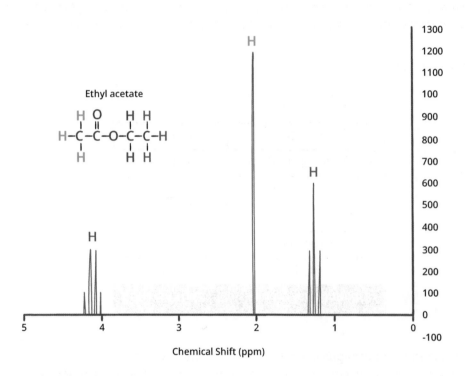

Figure 3. The ^{1}H NMR spectrum of ethyl acetate

Let's begin with ^{1}H NMR, as it is the more confusing and higher-yield of the two methods. In proton NMR, each hydrogen atom (or set of equivalent hydrogen atoms) produces a single peak on the spectrum. Equivalent hydrogen atoms are protons that exist in the same magnetic environment. For example, consider ethyl acetate ($CH_3COOCH_2CH_3$). The three H atoms on the CH_3 group adjacent to the carbonyl carbon rotate freely around the C–C bond and are essentially identical. Because these protons do not differ in any measurable way, they will correspond to only one peak on the spectrum, but the area under that peak will be *three times greater* than the area under a peak that corresponds to a single hydrogen atom. In other words, the **peak area** (or **integration**) directly correlates to the number of protons represented by that peak.

Peaks on a proton NMR spectrum can range from 0–12 ppm. The location depends on the extent of shielding or deshielding experienced by ^{1}H nuclei. Returning to Figure 3, let's consider the blue hydrogen atoms on ethyl acetate located on the terminal carbon of the ethyl group. These hydrogen atoms are surrounded by a relatively large amount of electron density, so they are considered to be **shielded** or blocked from experiencing the full extent of the magnetic field. As a result of shielding, the peak associated with these protons will shift upfield closer to 0 ppm.

In contrast, let's examine the two protons marked in red attached to the non-terminal carbon of the ethyl group. This carbon atom is adjacent to an oxygen atom, which is very electronegative and will lure electrons away that would otherwise surround the H atoms. These deshielded protons now experience the magnetic field to a greater degree, and their peak will be shifted downfield (to the left). In general, the closer a set of protons is to an electron-withdrawing group, the more deshielded they will be, and the farther left their peak will be found. Table 2 lists the chemical shifts associated with common functional groups on a ^{1}H NMR spectrum.

Functional group	Shift (ppm)
$-CH_3$	0.9
$-CH_2OH$	1.0-5.5
$-C{\equiv}CH$	2.0-3.0
$-CH = CH-$	4.5-6.0
Ar (aromatic ring)$-$H	6.0-8.4
$-CHO$	9.5
$-COOH$	10.5-12.0

Table 2. ^{1}H NMR chemical shifts

Finally, typically, the most confusing aspect of NMR is **splitting**. Until this point, we've explained ^{1}H NMR signals in a simplified way, implying that each signal is one clearly defined peak. In reality, each signal is affected by protons on atoms adjacent to the carbon to which the proton is attached. To predict splitting patterns, follow the n + 1 rule, which states that any peak will be split into a number of smaller peaks equal to the number of adjacent hydrogen atoms plus one. If a hydrogen atom is positioned on a terminal carbon adjacent to a carbon bound to one additional hydrogen atom, for example, the peak that represents the first hydrogen atom will be split into a doublet (1 adjacent hydrogen atom + 1 = 2). You can remember this rule by recognizing that a proton next to *zero* hydrogen atoms cannot yield a "zero peak." Instead, having no adjacent protons yields a singlet, as 0 + 1 = 1.

To elaborate, re-examine Figure 3. Here, the peak corresponding to the red hydrogen atoms is split into four smaller peaks (a quartet). We observe this because the red hydrogen atoms are positioned on a carbon adjacent to a carbon containing *three* neighboring protons in blue (3 + 1 = 4). Now consider the peak marked in green. These methyl protons represented by this peak are adjacent to the carbonyl carbon, which is not bound to any hydrogen atoms. As a result, the green peak is a singlet (0 + 1 = 1). Finally, the peak marked in blue is a triplet because it represents three protons that are *adjacent* to a carbon with two protons (2 + 1 = 3).

Let's try an example. How many peaks will appear on a ^{1}H NMR spectrum of ethanol? And how will each peak be split? First, we need to note that ethanol (CH_3CH_2OH) has three sets of equivalent protons. Thus, the ^{1}H NMR spectrum for ethanol should include three peaks. The hydroxyl hydrogen is not adjacent to any hydrogens, so it will be a singlet. The two protons on carbon 1 have three neighboring protons (three from –CH$_3$), so their peak will be a quartet. Finally, the three protons on carbon 2 will correspond to a triplet due to the two neighboring hydrogens.

Let's wrap up with a brief discussion of ^{13}C NMR spectroscopy, which is far less likely to appear on the MCAT. As this NMR type is tested less frequently than ^{1}H NMR, you must only know a few key pieces of information. Most carbon on Earth exists in the form of ^{12}C, but ^{13}C is used because only nuclei with an odd number of protons have nuclear spin.

If you were to encounter ^{13}C NMR on the MCAT, it would likely appear as a spin-decoupled spectrum in which all peaks exist as singlets. Be careful, though—just as equivalent protons corresponded to a single peak in ^{1}H NMR, equivalent *carbon* atoms appear as a single peak in ^{13}C NMR. Symmetrical compounds may have multiple sets of equivalent carbons that are mirror images of each other. The scale of a ^{13}C NMR spectrum is also larger than that of a ^{1}H spectrum, ranging from 0–200 ppm. As in ^{1}H NMR, the signals of deshielded carbon atoms are shifted downfield and vice versa.

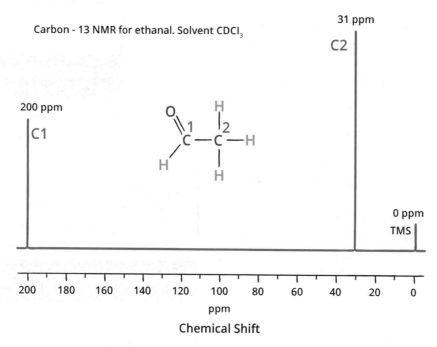

Figure 4. The ^{13}C NMR spectrum of ethanal

2. Ultraviolet-Visible Spectroscopy and Mass Spectrometry

IR and NMR spectroscopy are the highest-yield MCAT analytic techniques, but we must mention a few other techniques. To begin, **ultraviolet-visible (UV-Vis) spectroscopy** is a technique that analyzes the absorbance of visible or ultraviolet light by organic compounds. UV light is slightly higher in frequency than visible light, so UV rays from the sun can damage biological molecules. Since frequency and wavelength are inversely proportional, UV light also possesses a *shorter* wavelength than visible light, with a range of 10 nanometers (nm) to 400 nm (Recall from physics that the wavelength of visible light spans from 400 to 700 nm!).

On a UV-Vis spectrum, the absorbance, or the proportion of light absorbed by the sample, is plotted against the wavelength of this light. Conjugated compounds with alternating single and double bonds tend to readily absorb UV-Vis light due to the delocalization of π electrons. Beta-carotene, a biologically relevant example of such a compound, is shown in Figure 5.

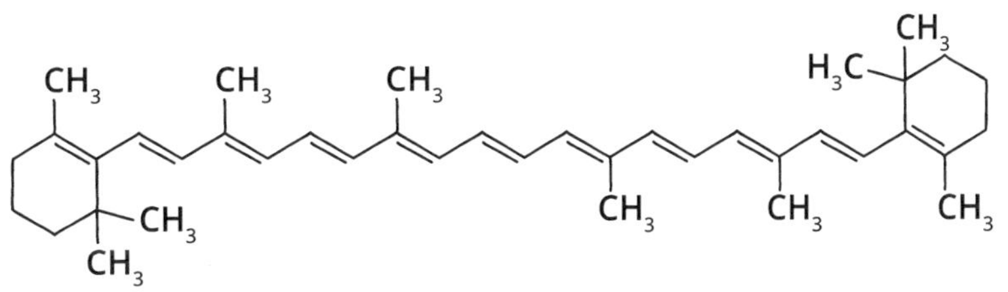

Figure 5. Beta-carotene, a conjugated compound

Lastly, let us wrap up our discussion of spectroscopic techniques with **mass spectrometry**, an incredibly useful method for identifying unknown organic compounds. In this technique, a sample is injected into a mass spectrometer, which exposes the molecules to a beam of electrons. These high-energy electrons cause the sample molecules to ionize or become charged. Removal of one electron from the parent molecule creates the M^+ cation, which has the same molecular weight as the uncharged parent molecule. Sample molecules also fragment into a variety of smaller charged species.

The mass and charge of the fragments are measured and plotted on a mass spectrum (Figure 6). The x-axis shows the mass-to-charge ratio (m/z) of the fragments, and the y-axis displays their relative abundance. The peak with the highest m/z value is usually the M^+ peak, which lets us know the molecular weight of the unknown molecule. The peak corresponding to the most abundant fragment is the base peak. The locations of these peaks give researchers information about the size and functional groups of a compound, though in-depth analysis of mass spectra is outside of the scope of the MCAT.

> **MCAT STRATEGY >>>**
>
> On the current MCAT, UV-Vis spectroscopy often appears in the context of identifying aromatic amino acids. Since these amino acid residues have conjugated side chains, they give a distinctive reading on a UV-Vis spectrum. Aromatic amino acids include phenylalanine, tyrosine, and tryptophan.

> **>> CONNECTIONS <<**
>
> Chapter 2 of Biochemistry

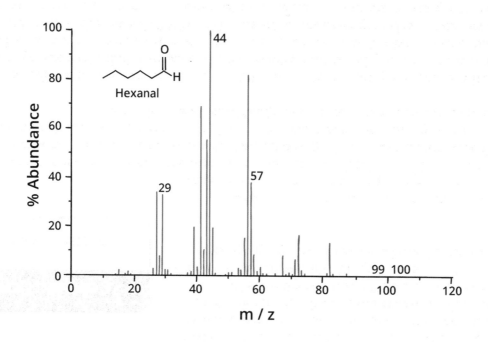

Figure 6. The mass spectrum of hexanal

3. Separations: Distillation

With your newfound knowledge of spectroscopy, you may now be able to identify some compounds based on their IR or NMR readings alone (and you certainly have sufficient information to ace MCAT questions)! However, this information would be next to useless if you were first presented with a mixture of organic compounds—your desired product along with side products, leftover reactants, and other contaminants. How can you isolate a single product? To do so, we use **separation techniques**.

To determine which technique is best for a given situation, first consider the phases of the compounds involved. For example, is the desired product a solid immersed in liquid? Is it a solid with solid impurities? Or is it a liquid in solution with other liquids? If the answer to this last question is "yes," you may be able to utilize **distillation**. Most distillation procedures aim to separate one liquid from another by utilizing the difference between the two liquids' boiling points. A distillation apparatus is shown in Figure 7.

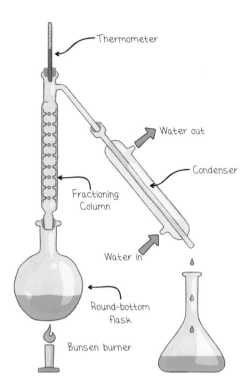

Thermometer

Water out

Condenser

Fractioning
Column

Water in

Round-bottom
flask

Bunsen burner

Figure 7. A distillation apparatus and setup

Let's deeply examine this figure. Imagine that you are separating two liquids, Liquid A and Liquid B. Liquid A has a boiling point of 80°C, while Liquid B has a boiling point of 125°C. Both liquids are initially held in the same round-bottom flask or the distilling flask. To begin the procedure, the flask is positioned above a heat source, typically a Bunsen burner. The top of the flask connects to a column, which leads to a downward-sloping glass condenser. The condenser is held within a glass casing through which cold water is pumped. As the round-bottom flask is heated, the liquid with the lower boiling point (here, Liquid A) will begin to vaporize, and its vapor will travel up the column. Some vapor will pass into the condenser; the adjacent cold water will then cause the vapor to condense into a liquid. Since the condenser slopes downward, the liquid travels down directly into an empty flask that is positioned below its opening. This vessel is aptly called the receiving flask. Over time, more of Liquid A will pass into the receiving flask, while the majority of Liquid B will remain in the liquid phase in the distilling flask.

> **CONNECTIONS**
>
> Chapter 5 of Chemistry

But how can we be certain that 100% of Liquid A will vaporize, re-condense, and enter the receiving flask before any of Liquid B begins to vaporize? After all, some liquid molecules are constantly escaping into the vapor phase, even at temperatures below the liquid's boiling point. Well, truthfully, we can't ensure that. In fact, distillation is an imperfect technique. For example, we may end up with 90% Liquid A and 10% Liquid B in the receiving flask, which is fairly impure. To obtain as close to a pure component as possible, repeated distillations are usually necessary.

Let's now discuss the "fractionating" column. While all distillation procedures include a vertical glass structure that connects the round-bottom distilling flask to the condenser, not all procedures include a fractionating column. This brings us to the distinction between simple and fractional distillation. **Simple distillation** is used when the liquids in question have very dissimilar boiling points and for the sake of the MCAT, they should be at least 25°C apart (In other words, their vapor pressures are very far apart at a given temperature). A simple distillation procedure does not include a fractionating column. Instead, the receiving flask is connected close to the opening of the condenser, resulting in an apparatus that is shorter in height. As the boiling points are so different, the compound with the lower boiling point will vaporize, rise the short distance, and enter the condenser before the majority of the other compound with a higher boiling point.

Fractional distillation, in contrast, is utilized when the compounds to be separated have boiling points separated by less than 25°C. In such cases, simple distillation is not sufficient; both compounds will vaporize and travel the short distance to the condenser, at least to some extent, and the contents of the receiving flask would thus contain significant proportions of both liquids. To prevent this, a long glass fractionating column—often filled with beads and insulated with foil—is placed between the distilling flask and the top of the condenser. Consider, for example, a distillation procedure involving acetone (BP = 56°C) and methanol (BP = 65°C). The distilling flask is heated, and a significant amount of acetone—along with some methanol—enters the vapor phase and rises through the column. Since the fractionating column is long and filled with packing materials that form available condensation sites, the compound with the higher boiling point (methanol) will tend to condense within the column and fall back down to the distilling flask. On the other hand, at least some of the lower-BP acetone molecules will make it to the top of the column and enter the condenser. While this procedure takes longer than simple distillation, it provides for better separation between the two liquids (In fact, the longer the fractionating column, the better the separation).

The third MCAT-relevant distillation technique is **vacuum distillation**. To understand this method, recall the definition of boiling point: boiling occurs at the temperature at which the vapor pressure of the liquid in question (P_{vap}) is equal to the atmospheric pressure of the surroundings (P_{atm}). Imagine that you are trying to separate two liquids with boiling points greater than 400°C. If their boiling points are very different, we might predict that simple distillation would be effective, while if they are similar, we may need to use fractional distillation. Regardless, however, it is not feasible to use a Bunsen burner to heat a liquid to a temperature of 400°C or more. When we cannot raise the temperature (which increases the vapor pressure), we must instead *decrease* the atmospheric pressure to meet the vapor pressure. This can be accomplished by attaching a vacuum to the distillation apparatus. Lowering the ambient pressure of the surroundings results in a decreased boiling point for all compounds involved, allowing us to then conduct a typical distillation procedure.

4. Separations: Extractions

From the information presented in this chapter so far, we now know that liquids with different boiling points may be separated using distillation. However, many liquid mixtures do not fit this criterion. Instead, the two (or more) liquid components may differ from each other with regard to *other* physical or chemical characteristics. One such trait is solubility in aqueous or organic media. On the MCAT, compounds with disparate solubility characteristics are most often separated using **liquid-liquid extraction**. To conduct an extraction, one must utilize a device known as a

separatory funnel (Figure 8). The funnel is hung vertically, with an opening at the top through which solutions may be poured and a stopcock at the bottom that can be opened to let liquid out.

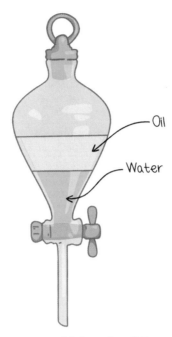

Figure 8. A separatory funnel containing two immiscible liquids: oil (lower density) and water (higher density)

Several variants of extraction procedures exist, but for the sake of the MCAT, understand that liquid-liquid extractions that take advantage of acid-base characteristics. Let's walk through an example. Imagine that you just finished an organic chemistry lab, and you now have a flask that contains acetic acid (CH_3COOH, a carboxylic acid) and aniline ($C_6H_5NH_2$, an amine) in the same solution, with a diethyl ether solvent. Diethyl ether ($CH_3CH_2OCH_2CH_3$) is relatively nonpolar. To separate the acetic acid from the aniline using extraction, you must first add an aqueous solvent, most often simply water; extractions require two immiscible liquid layers, and nonpolar organic solvents are not miscible with water. You first transfer your organic mixture to a separatory funnel, then add water, and this aqueous solvent settles in its own layer below the organic solution.

> **MCAT STRATEGY >>>**
>
> As you will learn in physics, a key fact about fluids is that less dense liquids or objects tend to float, while more dense objects or liquids sink. Diethyl ether has a density of approximately 713 kg/m³, while water has a density of 1000 kg/m³. (You do not need to memorize the density of diethyl ether, but be certain to know that of water.)

You now have a separatory funnel that contains an aqueous layer below an ether-based organic layer. However, how has this brought us any closer to separating acetic acid from aniline? Both are somewhat soluble in ether, so significant proportions of both compounds remain in the organic solvent. If we are to separate the two, we must move one compound into the aqueous layer and pour it off. We can accomplish this by taking advantage of the compounds' acid-base properties. On the MCAT, one key concept is that charged compounds are highly polar, much more so than their uncharged states. If we can make one of the two compounds charged, most of its molecules will move into the aqueous layer.

At this point, we have a choice: acetic acid is an acidic molecule, while aniline is basic. While it does not particularly matter, let's opt to move the acetic acid into the aqueous layer. To do so, we can add a strong base (for example,

NaOH) and shake the funnel. This will deprotonate the acetic acid, forming its conjugate base, CH_3COO^-. The negatively charged compound is now far more soluble in the polar aqueous layer than the organic ether layer, so it will move to the aqueous layer of the funnel. Now, we can open the stopcock to release the aqueous layer into a beaker waiting below the separatory apparatus. Like distillation, extraction usually must be conducted multiple times to ensure that the product mixtures are as pure as possible.

>> CONNECTIONS <<

Chapter 7 of Chemistry

Although our imaginary procedure is now complete, let us continue the same example to ensure that this technique is understood. What if we had chosen to move the aniline to the aqueous layer rather than the acetic acid? Predictably, just as we added a strong base to deprotonate the acetic acid and move it to the aqueous layer, we can add a strong *acid* to protonate the basic aniline molecules. As charged species (albeit positively rather than negatively charged), they will then transition to the aqueous layer, which can be poured off as we explained above.

Acetic acid is acidic, while aniline is basic, and this allows for easy separation. But could extraction be effective even if we needed to separate two acids?" Absolutely! Consider an imaginary solution of benzoic acid and phenol, again dissolved in a diethyl ether solvent. Moving this mixture to a separatory funnel and adding water will yield the two immiscible layers that we now expect to form. Both benzoic acid and phenol are somewhat acidic, with benzoic acid (a carboxylic acid) being significantly *more* acidic than phenol (an aromatic alcohol). To ensure that one of the compounds exits the organic phase, simply add a weak base. The weak base will be sufficiently basic to deprotonate the stronger benzoic acid, but it will leave the weakly acidic phenol molecules untouched. Benzoic acid, being deprotonated and thus negatively charged, will now move into the aqueous layer, where it can be poured from the funnel. Phenol, the weaker and thus less reactive acid, will largely remain in the original ether layer.

5. Separations: Chromatography

Our next separation technique is **chromatography**, which is a broad category that contains several different methods. Chromatography is often used to separate amino acids and proteins, and as such, it is described in great detail in your biochemistry book. In this chapter, we discuss chromatography techniques with a focus on their relation to chemistry.

>> CONNECTIONS <<

Chapter 5 of Biochemistry

Throughout this discussion, note the common features of these methods. In particular, chromatography involves two phases: a mobile phase, or moving fluid, and a stationary phase, or solid that does not move. A sample is passed through the apparatus, and its components travel at different rates depending on their affinities for the mobile and stationary phases. For each type of chromatography that is discussed, be certain to ask yourself what constitutes the mobile phase and what makes up the stationary phase.

Arguably the most often-discussed organic chemistry chromatography method is **thin-layer chromatography** or TLC. The stationary phase in a TLC procedure is a glass or plastic plate coated in adsorbent, most commonly polar silica gel (SiO_2). A chemical sample is dabbed onto the plate, which is then placed in a beaker containing a nonpolar solvent, such as hexane. Capillary action draws the solvent up the plate, bringing the components of the sample with it. As the mobile phase is nonpolar, nonpolar components are attracted to it and travel farther down the plate; in contrast, polar components have a higher affinity for the polar plate and thus do not travel as far. Figure 9 depicts a typical TLC plate after thin-layer chromatography of a mixture. Note that the plate must undergo subsequent visualization treatment if the compounds involved are colorless; otherwise, their corresponding spots would not be visible. Such treatment typically involves exposure to ultraviolet (UV) light or iodine.

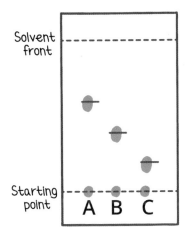

Figure 9. A TLC plate after chromatography. Assuming a nonpolar solvent and a polar plate, compound A must be the most nonpolar, followed by B, then C

Thin-layer chromatography allows us to make rough measurements of the relative polarities of compounds. The main such measurement is termed the retention factor or R_f. R_f is equal to the distance traveled by a compound down the plate from its starting position divided by the distance traveled by the solvent (often called the "solvent front"). For example, imagine that a TLC plate is 10 centimeters long. If the solvent traveled 8 cm while Compound C traveled 2 cm, the R_f of Compound C is (2 cm)/(8 cm) = 0.25. Assuming that the solvent is nonpolar, a higher R_f denotes a more nonpolar compound since traveling a large distance implies that the compound has a marked affinity for the nonpolar mobile phase.

Although thin-layer chromatography is an effective way to compare the polarities of compounds or detect impurities within a sample, it does not allow us to isolate any separated components for later use. To do this, we can instead utilize **column chromatography**, in which the stationary phase is a solid adsorbent packed within a vertical column and the mobile phase is a liquid solvent. Again, the many forms of column chromatography are described in detail in Chapter 5 of our biochemistry book since these techniques are most often tested in relation to protein analysis. First, **size-exclusion chromatography** is used to separate the components of a mixture by physical size. Its stationary phase consists of pore-studded gel beads; smaller molecules become trapped in the pores and elute through the column slowly, while large molecules pass through rapidly. Two additional forms of chromatography, both grouped under the heading of ion-exchange chromatography, center around electrostatic interactions. **Cation-exchange chromatography** is utilized to trap positively charged molecules within the column, and as such, it includes a negatively charged stationary phase. On the other hand, **anion-exchange chromatography** uses a positively charged stationary-phase rosin to trap negative molecules, or anions, within the column. Finally, the most specific form of column chromatography is **affinity chromatography**, in which ligands designed to bind to a compound of interest are attached to the beads that make up the column's stationary phase.

The final variations on chromatography that we discuss in this chapter are **gas-liquid chromatography** (also known as gas chromatography, or GC) and **high-performance liquid chromatography** (HPLC). Do you recall the beginning of this chapter, where we urged you to focus on the phases of matter involved in each separatory

> **MCAT STRATEGY >>>**
>
> We have described the most common form of TLC, in which the stationary phase (plate) is polar and the mobile phase is nonpolar. However, be certain to understand that the opposite scenario is possible. If a passage mentions a nonpolar stationary phase, then, you can assume that the mobile phase of the TLC procedure is polar.

technique? **Gas-liquid chromatography** is the only separatory technique in this chapter to include a gaseous mobile phase, often consisting of helium or nitrogen. The sample to be analyzed is also vaporized into a gaseous state, then passed through an apparatus consisting of a column coated in a thin layer of polymer or liquid (The polymer or liquid constitutes the stationary phase). The time taken for the sample to move through the apparatus is measured and used to estimate its affinities for the gaseous mobile and liquid/polymer stationary phases. A longer elution time implies a higher affinity for the stationary phase and vice versa. One final note on gas chromatography: for this method to work properly, the sample must be one which we can force into the gas phase fairly easily. A liquid that does not vaporize below 700°C, for example, would therefore be a poor choice of sample.

MCAT STRATEGY >>>

As always, when reading MCAT content, ask yourself, "Why?" Here, we might ask why helium or nitrogen are chosen for the carrier gases that make up the GC mobile phase. The answer relates to the inert nature of these gases, which prevents them from reacting with the sample in unwanted side processes.

Finally, **high-performance or high-pressure liquid chromatography (HPLC)** involves passing a liquid mobile phase through an adsorbent-packed column, just like many forms of chromatography that we discussed earlier. The distinction, however, is that HPLC takes place under high pressure, allowing the resolution of the sample's components to occur more rapidly. Note that "regular" HPLC shares the characteristics of TLC in that its stationary phase is polar while its mobile phase is nonpolar. Watch out, however; an alternative technique termed reverse-phase HPLC (RP-HPLC) also exists, and it includes a *nonpolar* stationary phase and a *polar* mobile phase.

	Normal phase	**Reverse phase**
Stationary phase	polar	non-polar
Mobile phase	non-polar	polar

Table 3. Normal and reverse phase chromatography

6. Other Separation Techniques

We have almost finished our discussion of the separation techniques used in MCAT organic chemistry. Only two methods remain, neither of which fit perfectly within a larger category. The first technique is recrystallization. Until now, we have placed our focus on the separations of liquid and gaseous samples. Often, however, an organic procedure will leave us with a solid product. This solid is likely to contain solid impurities. To purify the compound, we must remove them—but how? The answer lies in a foundational aspect of the solid structures formed by chemical compounds. When a typical solid precipitates out of solution, it forms a specific, ordered crystalline structure. If a solid can be made to precipitate multiple times, it will gradually increase in purity, as every crystallization will exclude additional impurities from the structure.

>> CONNECTIONS <<

Chapter 5 of Chemistry

The procedure of a simple **recrystallization** is as follows: The desired solid product is placed in a liquid solvent and heated, causing it to dissolve. The solvent-product mixture is cooled upon full dissolution, and the solid once again forms as a precipitate. This process is facilitated by scratching the side of the flask, which provides rough "seed" regions for crystals to begin to form. The recrystallization process may be repeated multiple times, with the solid becoming progressively higher in purity.

One key decision to make when planning a recrystallization procedure is the identity of the solvent to use. An ideal recrystallization solvent is one in which our desired product is highly soluble at high temperatures (if this were not the case, it wouldn't dissolve at all)! At the same time, however, our product should be relatively *in*soluble in this solvent under low-temperature conditions, or it will never precipitate back out of solution when the mixture is cooled.

Once we are satisfied with our solid product, we may need to isolate it from the liquid solvent in which it is held. This brings us to our final separation technique: filtration. This simple process is used to separate a solid product from unwanted fluids. To conduct a filtration process, set up a filter (often a single piece of filter paper) through which liquid, but not solid, can pass. Pour the liquid-solid mixture over this filter, and the desired solid will remain on the surface of the paper while the liquid will pass through to a flask below to be discarded.

7. Must-Knows

> Analytic techniques: identify features of a molecule or the molecule's identity.
  — Often render the sample unusable in the future.
  — Examples: IR, NMR, UV-Vis, mass spec.
> Separation techniques: convert a mixture into multiple separate, pure samples (to the extent to which this is possible):
  — Samples can then be analyzed or otherwise used later.
  — Examples: distillation, extraction, chromatography, recrystallization, filtration.
> Infrared (IR) spectroscopy:
  — Uses radiation with a frequency lower than that of visible light to vibrate bonds.
  — C=O → 1700 cm^{-1}, sharp; O-H → 3200-3600 cm^{-1}, broad.
> Nuclear magnetic resonance (NMR) spectroscopy:
  — Left side of spectrum = "downfield" = deshielded = close to e$^-$ withdrawing groups.
  — Right side of spectrum = "upfield" = shielded = far from e$^-$ withdrawing groups.
  — Area under peak corresponds to number of equivalent hydrogens.
  — Splitting (singlet, doublet . . .) is determined by number of hydrogens on adjacent atom.
> Ultraviolet-visible (UV-Vis) spectroscopy:
  — Useful to discern presence of conjugated/aromatic species.
> Mass spectrometry:
  — Helps determine molecular weight (m/z peak).
> Distillation: separates liquids based on boiling point (BP).
  — For BPs > 25° apart, use simple distillation.
  — For BPs < 25° apart, use fractional distillation.
  — For very high BPs, use vacuum distillation to lower atmospheric pressure (lower P → lower BPs).
> Extraction: separates liquids based on solubility/acid-base properties:
  — Requires immiscible aqueous and organic layers in a separatory funnel.
  — To send an acid into the aqueous layer, add base (deprotonate it).
  — To send a base into the aqueous layer, add acid (protonate it).
> Chromatography involves a mobile phase and a stationary phase with different properties.
  — TLC: stationary phase is polar (usually silica) while mobile phase is a nonpolar solvent.
    • R_f = (distance traveled by compound) / (distance traveled by solvent).
  — Size-exclusion, cation-exchange, anion-exchange, and affinity chromatography are all forms of column chromatography.
  — Gas chromatography (GC) vaporizes sample and passes through a column, then measures retention time.
  — HPLC = rapid method of column chromatography; polar stationary phase and nonpolar mobile phase for regular process; nonpolar stationary phase and polar mobile phase for reverse process (RP-HPLC).
> Other separation techniques: recrystallization and filtration.

End of Chapter Practice

The best MCAT practice is realistic, with a focus on identifying steps for further improvement. For those reasons, we recommend completing practice questions in an online setting that simulates the real MCAT interface, and taking advantage of advanced analytic features to help you determine how best to move forward in your MCAT study journey.

With that in mind, online end-of-chapter questions for Biology, Biochemistry, Chemistry + Organic Chemistry, Physics, and Psychology/Sociology are available through your Blueprint MCAT account.

As a further supplement, given the importance of active learning for effective studying, we also suggest that you consult the Must-Knows as a basis for creating a study sheet, in which you list out key terms and test your ability to briefly summarize them.

IMAGE ATTRIBUTIONS

Chapter 1: Atomic Structure and Periodic Trends

Figure 1: https://en.wikipedia.org/wiki/Helium#/media/File:Helium_atom_QM.svg

Chapter 7: Acid-base Chemistry

Figure 4: https://en.wikipedia.org/wiki/Phenolphthalein#/media/File:Phenolphthalein-at-pH-9.jpg

INDEX

103, 106, 109, 118-121, 138-147, 151-155, 161-169, 172-174, 179-188, 196-199, 202, 204, 206-208, 216-227

mole fraction 77, 79

N

Nernst equation 124
neutralization reactions 39, 54, 120
neutrons 1, 2, 3, 218
Newman projections 147
NMR spectroscopy 218, 220
noble gases 9, 12, 13
nonmetals 11, 12, 21
nonpolar covalent bonds 21, 118
normality 131
nucleophiles 174, 195, 209, 210
nucleophilic addition 176, 177, 195, 196, 200, 210, 212, 207-209
nucleophilic substitution 118, 120, 185, 186, 188, 196, 200, 201, 202, 208

O

octet rule 19, 20
open systems 56
orbital 6, 7, 8, 10, 20, 22, 29, 30, 100
orbital hybridization 29, 30
osmotic pressure 79, 80
oxidation 11, 39, 41, 89, 100, 108, 117-131, 141, 164, 165, 167, 168, 175
oxidation-reduction reactions 108
oxidation state 117-131, 165
oxidizing agents 122, 168, 174, 191

P

partial pressure 53, 77
percent composition 38
percent yield 45
periodic table 2, 3, 6, 9, 10, 12, 13, 21, 27, 28, 37, 39, 41, 43
periodic trends 2, 3, 6, 9, 10, 12, 13, 21, 27, 28, 37, 39, 41, 43, 119
phase changes 39, 40, 69, 70-74
phase diagrams 73, 74
phases 40, 69, 70, 71, 72, 74, 75, 222, 226, 227
phenols 144, 166, 167, 168, 189, 191
pH scale 103, 104
pKa 163, 181
Planck's constant 5
polar aprotic solvents 198
polar covalent bonds 21, 118

polar protic solvents 21, 198
polyatomic ions 4, 118
polyprotic acids 109
priority rules 151, 154
protecting groups 169
protons 1-4, 8, 12, 38, 102, 105, 109,112, 131, 163, 218-220

Q

quantum numbers 6

R

racemic mixture 154, 177, 197
Raoult's law 79
rate constant 87, 88, 92, 93
reaction balancing 42
reaction coordinate diagrams 89
reaction coordinates 91
reaction order 94
reaction quotient 51, 63, 81, 133
recrystallization 228, 229
redox reactions 39, 41, 117, 118, 120, 121, 122, 123, 127, 130, 131
redox titrations 117, 130, 131, 132
reducing agents 118, 122
reduction 165, 174, 175, 184, 206, 207
reduction potentials 117, 122, 123
replacement reactions 40
resonance 27, 28, 29, 137, 143, 144, 146, 166,167, 173, 174, 178, 181, 182, 188, 189, 191, 201, 205, 206, 207, 209, 215, 218
retro-aldol reaction 179, 180, 191, 208
reversibility 49
Robinson annulation 208, 209, 210
Rydberg formula 5

S

saponification 181
second-order reactions 92, 94
semimetals 11
single displacement 39, 40, 120
solids 50, 51, 53, 56, 60, 69, 70, 74, 78, 80, 82, 92, 102
solubility 69, 78, 80, 81, 82, 99, 224
solution(s) 21, 40, 56, 57, 69, 78-82, 88, 91, 99, 100, 102-110, 112, 120, 125-132, 147, 154, 211, 222, 225, 226, 229
specific heat capacity 56, 72, 73
specific rotation 153, 154

spontaneous 60-63, 89, 91, 123, 124, 127, 129, 130, 132, 133, 163, 206, 207
staggered conformations 147, 148
stereochemistry 137, 138, 145, 199
stereoisomers 147, 152, 154, 157
stoichiometry 32, 37, 41-45, 49, 50, 111, 184, 203, 204
strong acids 12, 81, 103-106
strong bases 103, 104
structural isomers 145, 146, 157
sublimation 71, 74
supersaturated solutions 78
synthesis reactions 39, 40

T

tautomerism 146, 147, 191, 204, 205, 211
tautomers 146, 189, 205
temperature 11, 12, 40, 51-57, 60, 62, 63, 65, 70-82, 87, 88, 91, 102, 105, 146, 223, 224, 229
theoretical yield 53
thermodynamic control 64, 65, 178, 179
thermodynamics 55, 56, 60, 64, 69, 132
thin-layer chromatography 226, 227
thioesters 190
thioethers 190
thiols 158, 190
titration curves 109-112
titration 108-111, 131, 132
transesterification 187, 191
transition complex 88
transition metals 9-11
triple point 73, 74

U

ultraviolet radiation 224
UV-vis spectroscopy 152, 220, 221, 230

V

valence electrons 2, 9, 10-13, 19, 20, 26-29, 119, 195
Van der Waals equation 77
vapor pressure 74, 79, 89, 224
vapor pressure reduction 79
voltaic cells 124, 128, 129, 132
VSEPR theory 19, 29, 30, 41

W